Interrogating Trauma

Throughout the past century, traumatic experiences have been re-enacted frequently by evolving media and art forms. Now there is a significant body of theory across academic disciplines focused on the representation of cataclysmic European and US historical events. However, less critical attention has been devoted to the representation of havoc outside the West, even though depictions of Third-World disasters saturate contemporary media and art around the globe.

This book considers traumatic histories internationally in a broad range of creative arts and visual media representations. Deploying diverse applications of the conventional theories of trauma, it examines the theoretical limitations at the same time as considering alternative methodologies. *Interrogating Trauma* is concerned with the examination of the concept of trauma, and how it is (often unproblematically) used to theorise the cultural representation of disaster and atrocity. It offers a theorisation of trauma, in order to reappraise the relationship between cultural representation and the socio-historical processes which are marked by violence, conflict and suffering.

This book was published as a special issue of *Continuum: Journal of Media and Cultural Studies*.

Mick Broderick is Associate Professor and Research Coordinator in the School of Media, Communications & Culture at Murdoch University, where he is Deputy Director of the National Academy of Screen & Sound (NASS). He has published editions of the reference work *Nuclear Movies* and, as editor, *Hibakusha Cinema*.

Antonio Traverso is Senior Lecturer in Film and Television studies in the School of Media, Culture and Creative Arts at Curtin University, Perth, Australia. He co-edited a special issue of *Social Identities*: "Living Through Terror: (Post)Conflict, (Post)Trauma and the South", and has produced several short films, including the award-winning *Tales from the South.*

Interrogating Trauma

Collective Suffering in Global Arts and Media

Edited by Mick Broderick and Antonio Traverso

Routledge
Taylor & Francis Group
LONDON AND NEW YORK

First published 2011 by Routledge
2 Park Square, Milton Park, Abingdon, Oxon, OX14 4RN

Simultaneously published in the USA and Canada
by Routledge
605 Third Avenue, New York, NY 10017

Routledge is an imprint of the Taylor & Francis Group, an informa business

First issued in paperback 2013

This book is a reproduction of *Continuum*, vol.24, issue 1. The Publisher requests to those authors who may be citing this book to state, also, the bibliographical details of the special issue on which the book was based

Typeset in Times New Roman by Value Chain, India

British Library Cataloguing in Publication Data
A catalogue record for this book is available from the British Library

ISBN13: 978-0-415-58278-0 (hbk)
ISBN13: 978-0-415-84532-8 (pbk)

CONTENTS

Notes on Contributors

Mick Broderick is Associate Professor and Research Coordinator in the School of Media, Communications & Culture at Murdoch University, where he is Deputy Director of the National Academy of Screen & Sound (NASS). His major publications include editions of the reference work *Nuclear Movies* (1988, 1991) and, as editor, *Hibakusha Cinema: Hiroshima, Nagasaki and the Nuclear Image in Japanese Film* (1996, 1999). In 2007 his experimental screen installation concerning the Rwandan genocide, *Exhale*, was exhibited at Revelation 10: the Perth International Film Festival. Broderick's curated exhibition of Cold War material culture artefacts, *Atomicalia*, was recently on show in Hiroshima during 2009.

Adam Brown teaches literature, history and communication studies at Deakin University and works in the testimonies department at the Jewish Holocaust Centre in Melbourne. He publishes critical and creative works, and has written a PhD on Holocaust representation, focusing on how moral judgements are revealed in portrayals of 'privileged' Jews in different media.

David Carlin is a writer, filmmaker and Senior Lecturer in the School of Media and Communication at RMIT University, Melbourne. David has recently published in *Overland, Text* and *Senses of Cinema*. His plays have been performed in Australia, Europe and South America, his documentary *Out of Our Minds* (2000) screened internationally, and in 1997 he directed the contemporary circus *Circus Oz's* New York and Australian seasons. His PhD (University of Melbourne, 2009) focused on issues of the representation of traumatic memory in narrative. His first book of creative non-fiction *Our Father Who Wasn't There* was published by Scribe in 2010.

Catherine Ann Collins received her PhD from the University of Minnesota in 1977. She is a Professor in the Department of Rhetoric and Media Studies at Willamette University and writes and teaches in the areas of visual rhetoric, the rhetoric of war, memory and memorials, and media framing. Recent publications are in *Media International Australia*, *Interdisciplinary Aspects of Climate Change*, and *International Dimensions of Mass Media Research*.

Felicity Collins teaches Cinema Studies in the School of Communication and Critical Enquiry, La Trobe University, Melbourne. She is the author of *Australian Cinema After Mabo* (with Therese Davis) and Chief Investigator of an Australia Research Council Discovery Project on Screen Comedy and the Nation (with Sue Turnbull and Susan Bye). Recent publications focus on allegorical truth and ethical violence in settler colonial cinema.

Vivien Green Fryd is Professor and Chair of History of Art at Vanderbilt University. She has published *Art and Empire: The Politics of Ethnicity in the U.S. Capitol, 1815-1860* and *Art and the Crisis of Marriage: Georgia O'Keeffe and Edward Hopper*, as well as numerous articles published in *American Art, Art Bulletin, Common-place, National Women's Studies Association Journal, Traumotology, Winterthur Portfolio*, among other journals. She was the Spence and Rebecca Webb Wilson Fellow at the Robert Penn Warren Center of the Humanities and director of its year-long seminar on Trauma Studies, 2008-2009. She is currently completing a book manuscript, *Reenacting and Performing Sexual Trauma in Second-Wave Feminist Art*.

Sophie Anne Oliver recently completed an interdisciplinary PhD at the University of London. Her doctoral research examined the possibility of an ethics of secondary witnessing, in particular in relation to embodiment and the cultural memory of atrocity. Awarded a Research Fellowship by the Alexander von Humboldt Foundation, she is currently working on a new project about the aesthetics of secondary witnessing and memorial culture in Berlin. She has published a number of articles in peer-reviewed journals, and is a contributor to various edited books on a range of themes including human rights, cultural theory and media representations of trauma.

Alexandra Opie is Assistant Professor of Art at Willamette University. She teaches video art, installation and photography. She received her Masters in Fine Arts in video art from the School of the Museum of Fine Arts, Boston, in 2000.

Iliana Pagán-Teitelbaum, from Puerto Rico, currently teaches courses on global citizenship and film at the University of Pennsylvania, USA. During a Mellon Postdoctoral Fellowship (2007–2009) she conducted research on violence in Caribbean literature and film, in the Department of Romance Languages at the University of Pennsylvania. Her PhD dissertation, entitled 'The disposable city: The hidden side of urban violence in narrative and film of two Latin American cities' (Harvard University, 2006), analyses how literary and filmic texts from Brazil and Peru represent violence, exclusion, and citizenship.

Suvendrini Perera (Curtin University, Australia) completed her BA at the University of Sri Lanka, Kelaniya, and her PhD at Columbia University, New York. She has published widely on topics relating to race, ethnicity, multiculturalism and refugees. Her latest book is *Australia and the Insular Imagination* (New York: Palgrave Macmillan, 2009).

Susannah Radstone teaches in the School of Humanities and Social Sciences at the University of East London. Recent publications include: *The Sexual Politics of Time: Confession, Nostalgia, Memory* (2007); (ed.) with Katharine Hodgkin, *Memory Cultures* (2005); and (ed.) with Katharine Hodgkin, *Memory, History, Nation* (2005). With Bill Schwarz, she has recently completed *Memory: Histories, Theories, Debates*, a large edited volume on approaches to memory research (Fordham University Press, 2010). She is currently completing a project on new approaches to trauma, to be published as *Getting over Trauma*.

Mark Straw is a PhD student in the Department of American and Canadian Studies at the University of Birmingham, UK. He has taught courses on film theory, North American cinema and national identity, and has published articles on contemporary American cinema and its relationship to US foreign policy.

Antonio Traverso teaches Screen Studies at Curtin University. Born in Chile, he has lived in Australia since 1987. Traverso has published essays on political cinema and written and directed short experimental videos. In 2008 Traverso was convenor (with

Mick Broderick) of the *Interrogating Trauma: Arts & Media Responses to Collective Suffering* International conference, Perth. In addition to the present collection, he has edited (with Mick Broderick) a special issue of the online journal *Intersections: Gender and Sexuality in Asia and the Pacific*, titled *Arts and Media Responses to the Traumatic Effects of War on Japan* (June, 2010), and a book anthology, *Trauma, Media, Art: New Perspectives* (Cambridge Scholars Press, 2010). Currently, Traverso is working on a monograph about post-dictatorship Chilean cinema and two edited collections on political documentary in Latin America.

Janet Walker is Professor of Film and Media Studies at the University of California, Santa Barbara, where she is also affiliated with Feminist Studies and the Environmental Media Initiative of the Carsey-Wolf Center for Film, Television and New Media. Her books as author or editor include *Feminism and Documentary* (with Diane Waldman); *Westerns: Films through History*; *Trauma Cinema: Documenting Incest and the Holocaust*; and most recently, *Documentary Testimonies: Global Archives of Suffering* (with Bhaskar Sarkar). Walker also directs an ongoing project, *Video Portraits of Survival*, to create expressive, testimony-based documentaries about local residents who are survivors and refugees of the Holocaust, and is working on a book about space, place, geography and documentary film.

Abstracts

Caché: Or what the past hides
SUSANNAH RADSTONE

Michael Haneke's film *Caché (Hidden)* (2005) has provoked a good deal of criticism and debate, much of it focusing on the question of the 'hidden' to which the film's title refers. Responses to the film have tended to focus on *Caché's* relations with colonial history as trauma, aligning the film's 'hidden' with the dissociated memory of France's 'dirty war' against Algeria. The psychoanalytic theory of Jean Laplanche offers the Humanities an approach to culture that diverges from the version of trauma theory drawn on by many of *Caché's* commentators. This essay takes up Laplanche's ideas in the context of a critique of trauma theory and aims to demonstrate their potential to shed light not only on *Caché* but also on culture's relations with temporality, violence, and the enigmatic.

Torturous dialogues: Geographies of trauma and spaces of exception
SUVENDRINI PERERA

How are suffering, damage and disaster produced and made visible across different sites, and how are they made to count, to matter? This essay considers certain philosophical, historical and geopolitical coordinates that locate trauma and disaster in the context of the Indian Ocean tsunami of 2004. Trauma in its various significations – the banal, the aesthetic, the philosophical, the medicalized, the political, the pathologized – is an essential form of currency in the torturous dialogues that make, define and delineate the contours of disaster, damage and suffering. These are constitutively geopoliticized, as they are racialized and gendered, processes. Trauma is a medium that enables dialogue and exchange; it is eminently transactable, mobile and adaptable in its circulation between the refugee camp and the disaster victims' camp; it ramifies, with uneven meanings and effects, across and between subjects, scenes, sites, practices and relations. This essay considers the geopolitics of the tsunami as a globalized trauma-event and asks how the biopolitics of trauma, as a set of institutionalized practices for managing and ordering the life and health of populations, plays out across the necropolitical terrain of global inequality and in relation to those it locates as bare life.

Moving testimonies and the geography of suffering: Perils and fantasies of belonging after Katrina
JANET WALKER

This essay explores the use of situated testimony in documentary films and videos about belonging, displacement, and return while calling for a 'spatial turn' in trauma studies. Through an analysis of selected works about Hurricane Katrina (Spike Lee's *When the Levees Broke*, Tia Lessin and Carl Deal's *Trouble the Water*, and the activist video *New Orleans for Sale!* by Brandan Odums, Nik Richard, and the group 2-cent), this paper extrapolates from Cathy Caruth's insights about psychoanalytic 'belatedness' and critical human geography's anti-essentializing conceptions of place to expose the concomitant materiality and unassimilability of traumatic space. The essay questions assumptions about home and right of return, ultimately advocating what architect Eyal Weizman has called a new mode of 'practising space' in the service of social justice.

After the apology: Reframing violence and suffering in First Australians, Australia, and Samson and Delilah
FELICITY COLLINS

This article explores the cinematic reframing of media images that normalize violence and suffering in remote Aboriginal communities. It proposes that, in the light of the 2007 Northern Territory Emergency Response and the 2008 apology to the Stolen Generations, the archival history series *First Australians*, the postmodern blockbuster Australia, and the arthouse drama *Samson and Delilah* contribute to an anti-colonial politics by creating cinematic spaces for affective and ethical response to issues of 'bare life' that tend to be exhausted, rather than worked through, in media temporality.

Confronting 'choiceless choices' in Holocaust videotestimonies: Judgement, 'privileged' Jews, and the role of the interviewer
ADAM BROWN

'Privileged' Jews include those prisoners in the camps and ghettos who held positions which gave them access to material and other benefits. Subject to extreme levels of coercion, these victims were compelled to act in ways that have been judged as both self-serving and harmful to fellow inmates. Such situations, which exemplify what influential theorist Lawrence Langer terms 'choiceless choices', are the chief concern of Primo Levi's paradigmatic essay on the 'grey zone'. In light of these key conceptualizations of the ethical dilemmas of Holocaust victims, the paper analyses the representation of 'privileged' Jews in several videotestimonies recorded at the Jewish Holocaust Museum and Research Centre (JHMRC) in Melbourne, Australia. It will be shown that judgements of victims in extremis cause considerable problems for attempts to testify to the complex situations and experiences of 'privileged' Jews. The role of the interviewer is a crucial factor in this, particularly when interviewers are themselves Holocaust survivors. The paper reveals that while it might be argued that moral evaluations of 'privileged' Jews should be suspended, judgements are often imposed on Holocaust testimonies in various ways and have a significant impact on their content.

The guilt zone: Trauma, masochism and the ethics of spectatorship in Brian De Palma's *Redacted* (2007)
MARK STRAW

The main question of this paper is the fraught psychological realm of the combat veteran or soldier in the Brian De Palma film *Redacted*. This will explore how a traumatic male subjectivity is constructed and is rendered explicitly in the staging and dramatization of the film. It will also explore how this trauma impacts on the communities inscribed in the film and the implied community of the films' spectators. This paper will therefore deal with the issue of how war is memorialized, processed and critiqued through deploying traumatized male subjectivity in cinema. I will deal with this question by referring to a now well-established critical discourse of 'trauma cinema', influenced especially by

E. Ann Kaplan and Ban Wang, Janet Walker, and Thomas Elsaesser, and also to Deleuze's model of masochism. I intend to argue that (as mentioned previously) masochistic male subjectivity is deployed in films in which the central male protagonist is ostensibly traumatized. I also argue that, given the recent 'turn to ethics' in film studies, this masochistic subjectivity has important implications for the spectatorship of catastrophe and suffering. *Redacted*, in particular, seems to be aware of its ethical position through its reflexivity and forced collision with genuine images of death. The value of this is to show how spectators are sited in relationship to film images of death and suffering and to point out the ethical complexities of 'consuming trauma'. It is also of use in that the position of masochistic spectatorship offers a route out of the binding power relations which inflict inaction and passivity on consumers of contemporary visual culture.

When places have agency: Roadside shrines as traumascapes
CATHERINE ANN COLLINS AND ALEXANDRA OPIE

This essay focuses on roadside shrines as places where time seems to replay itself and the experiences of loss are continuously re-experienced – what Foucault would term heterochronias where the evocation of the initial trauma leaves the past open in the present, constraining individual agency while giving agency to place. The located memorials are also symbolic spaces when adorned with ceremonial, domestic, and personal artefacts that sacralize them. These traumascapes help the pilgrim negotiate the chaotic and traumatic event of the past and hold out the possibility of a bearable future.

Trauma, bodies, and performance art: Towards an embodied ethics of seeing
SOPHIE ANNE OLIVER

The question of how to be an ethical witness to the suffering of distant others is one that has long been a preoccupation of trauma studies scholars. This paper addresses the problem of (un)ethical spectatorship of the traumatized body by engaging with the theory and practice of contemporary performance art. Rejecting the fantasy of the ideal moral witness, the author turns to models of embodied spectatorship suggested by performance-body art to propose ways of seeing that acknowledge and accept the necessary ambivalence of the distant spectatorship of suffering, while at the same time promoting a sense of 'response-ability' and self-reflection.

Poetic witnessing in the archive: The database narrative of *Life after Wartime*
DAVID CARLIN

In this paper I analyse the textual strategies employed in Ross Gibson and Kate Richards's interactive database narrative project *Life after Wartime* (2002), which I argue generates a form of narrative that embodies a 'poetics of haunting'. Shifting juxtapositions of image and text, archive and fiction within Life after Wartime serve to foreground the ambiguities within testimony and to set in motion the connections we make with the past. I explore whether Life after Wartime may be productively viewed as a distinctive new media model of a 'trauma text', one eschewing notions of narrative or therapeutic closure, in which complex interconnections between memory, history and fantasy are played out.

Bearing witness to the trauma of slavery in Kara Walker's videos: Testimony, Eight Possible Beginnings, and I was transported
VIVIEN GREEN FRYD

This essay shows that Kara Walker creates in her film and video work a repetitive traumatic site that surrounds, involves, and challenges the viewer to witness, acknowledge, and remember the individual and transgenerational trauma of slavery and contemporary racism in the United States, contributing to cultural remembrance and forcing the viewer to bear witness to her topsy-turvy world. Walker represents the 'intergenerational transmission of trauma' as postmemory, which is defined as the relationship of previous generations to powerful, often traumatic, experiences that preceded their births but that were nevertheless transmitted to them so deeply as to seem to constitute memories in their own right, though they can never be fully understood nor re-created. In doing so, she creates art that functions as a ritualized site for a kind of witnessing that becomes visible in her films and videos, a medium that by its own nature performs the act of bearing witness. The paper goes on to show that in her film and video work Walker disrupts conventional US histories and embodies formally and textually trauma's capacity to disrupt, thereby re-enacting or performing the phenomenological structure of trauma. Rather than suggest an opening or release of trauma's repetitive cycles, Walker embodies the hopeless and helpless repetition of trauma among individuals and generations who lack the healing potential often implied in the act of testimony. The viewer is, therefore, unable to imagine trauma as residing solely in the past but rather witnesses it as relentlessly and continuously invading the present in the form of post-traumatic slave syndrome (PTSS), thus failing to enable recovery, healing, or closure.

Depiction or erasure? Violence and trauma in contemporary Peruvian film
ILIANA PAGÁN-TEITELBAUM

Most of the 70,000 people who died or disappeared during the 1980–2000 civil war in Peru were Indigenous Quechua speakers. It is still proscribed to talk about the violent conflict in this Latin American country on the Pacific, where the high levels of poverty that may have triggered the war continue to affect 40% of the population. In this paper, I discuss the effort of three Peruvian films to respond to the trauma of misery, racism, forced migration, and dirty war experienced by both civilians and soldiers. I analyse how the films *Gregorio* (Grupo Chaski, 1984), *The Lion's Den* (Francisco Lombardi, 1988), and *Days of Santiago* (Josué Méndez, 2004) depict or erase the persons and bodies of the Andean individuals who have suffered violence.

Dictatorship memories: Working through trauma in Chilean post-dictatorship documentary
ANTONIO TRAVERSO

This essay discusses the representation of traumatic memory in Chilean post-dictatorship documentary. It argues that Chilean political memory documentaries of the post-dictatorship period, beyond their necessary depiction of the traumas and suffering of victims and survivors, consistently reveal productive attributes of life under dictatorship, such as the people's creative capacities of agency, resilience and imagination. In order to illustrate this proposition the essay offers an encompassing critical review of post-dictatorship documentaries directed by Chileans both in Chile and abroad between 1990 and 2007, focusing in particular on the films' representation of strategies of working through that counterbalance the acting out of suffering and damage that is characteristic of trauma cinema.

Acknowledgements

This collection of essays stems from an interdisciplinary conference, screen programme and art exhibition held in Perth, Australia in December 2008, entitled ‘Interrogating Trauma: Arts & Media Responses to Collective Suffering’ (wwwmcc.murdoch.edu.au/trauma). The conference and associated media and arts activities sought to provide a space of critical reflection about the potentials and limitations of various modes of creative and theoretical engagement with histories and experiences of mass suffering. International and local keynote speakers, panel chairs and presenters were invited to consider cross-disciplinary methodologies, orthodoxies and openings in order to articulate creative strategies for imagining the beyond of trauma through the arts and the media.

We would like to thank our sponsors, the various departments and organizations linked to Murdoch University and Curtin University, which have generously provided financial and in-kind support to make the conference and this publication possible. From Murdoch: the School of Media Communication and Culture; the Faculty of Creative Technology and Media; the National Academy of Screen and Sound; the Kulbardi Aboriginal Centre; and the Institute for Sustainable Societies Education and Politics. From Curtin: the Centre for Advanced Studies in Australia, Asia and the Pacific; the Faculty of Humanities; the School of Media, Culture and Creative Arts; the Centre for Aboriginal Studies; and the Sustainability Policy Institute. Thanks are also due to our conference co-convenor Dr Miyume Tanji (Curtin), our plenary debate chair Dr Roseanne Kennedy (ANU), conference administrators Silvia Rosenstreich (Murdoch) and Girish Lala (Murdoch), and website coordinator Mark Busani (Murdoch). We would also like to recognize the efforts of conference assistants and session chairs at Murdoch and Curtin Universities, the work of the art and media exhibition coordinators, and the support of the Film and Television Institute, the Round House, and Kidogo Art Gallery in Fremantle. Our gratitude goes also to all the performers, visual artists and filmmakers who contributed with their works to the exhibitions and screenings accompanying the conference, and in particular to visual artists Vicky Smith (England) and Thomas Delohery (Ireland), who respectively provided the images for the conference programme and this publication’s front cover. The conference and the present collection would not have been possible without the stimulating contributions from the authors assembled here, and many others whose works will appear in future publications. Our sincere thanks to the editors of *Continuum: Journal of Media & Cultural Studies* and to all our external peer reviewers. Finally, special thanks go to our Publications Coordinator Dr Christina Houen (Curtin) for her diligence, patience and professional editorial assistance.

M.B. and A.T.

Interrogating trauma: Towards a critical trauma studies

Antonio Traverso[a] and Mick Broderick[b]

[a]*School of Media, Culture and Creative Arts, Curtin University, Perth, Australia;* [b]*School of Media, Communication and Culture, Murdoch University, Perth, Australia*

In a French arthouse film an Algerian man draws out a large kitchen knife and cuts his own throat. In a short Sri Lankan art video the goddess of destruction, Kali, and a woman soldier surface from the ocean and walk towards a small seaside village. Shaky images of a video documentary bear witness to the muddied streets and flooded buildings of a poor, black neighbourhood of the Southern United States. In a low-budget Australian film written and directed by an Indigenous filmmaker two homeless, petrol-sniffing Aboriginal youths walk aimlessly on the streets of an outback town. We encounter the modern world and its history via depictions of catastrophe, atrocity, suffering and death. During the past 100 years or so, traumatic historical events and experiences have been re-imagined and re-enacted for us to witness over and over by constantly evolving media and art forms. Perhaps due to the ubiquity and multiplication of such images and narratives in modern and post-modern culture, questions about the impulse to behold and depict both the suffering of others and of the self, as well as more general questions about the ontological status of the representation of trauma, have increasingly been raised within intersecting, inter-disciplinary fields of study over the past two decades.

However, while these ongoing debates have produced a body of theoretical and testimonial literature of vast dimensions, their focus has been markedly restricted by an interest in the narrative and visual traces of cataclysmic European and US historical events, such as the Holocaust, the Vietnam War, 9/11 and the post-9/11 *war on terror*. In contrast, substantially less theorization has been devoted, by and large, to the representation of suffering as a result of political conflict outside the West, even though depictions of Third World disasters saturate contemporary media and art around the globe.[1] In addition, when critical attention has been given to the latter, largely the same conventional theory of trauma developed in Holocaust and trauma studies, namely a theory of subjective dissociation initially derived from Freudian psychoanalysis, has been used, with only limited attempts to develop alternative conceptualizations applicable to localized, culturally specific representations of suffering.[2]

Consequently, this collection joins a critical trend in twenty-first-century traumastudies to redress the balance (Blocker 2009; Douglas, Whitlock, and Stumm 2008; Guerinand Hallas 2007; Ball 2007; Winter 2006; Bennett 2005; Hodgkin and Radstone 2005; Tumarkin 2005; Kaplan 2005; Kaplan and Wang 2004; Collins and Davis 2004;

Bennett and Kennedy 2003; Douglass and Vogler 2003; Huyssen 2003; Eyerman 2001; Weibel and Kaltenbeck 2000; Robben and Suárez-Orozco 2000). Firstly, the collection focuses on media and artistic representations of political conflict and disaster in a diversity of regions around the world. Secondly, it seeks to interrogate the methodological limits of the dominant theory of trauma as a way of critically engaging with diverse expressions and depictions of political conflict and the representation of the personal and social suffering the latter produces.

It is important to clarify at the onset that the phrase 'interrogating trauma' in this collection's title implies neither a sociological nor historical analysis of specific events and experiences of trauma, nor the intent to relativize the past and continuing suffering of human groups around the world as a direct effect of political conflict and violence. Rather, the essays in this collection indirectly consider traumatic histories and experiences by focusing more specifically on a broad range of representations of political conflict and suffering realized through creative arts and visual media. In this sense, the interrogation of trauma alluded to in our title refers more precisely to the examination of the *concept* of trauma used – often unproblematically – to theorize the cultural representation of human suffering and atrocity.

Furthermore, this collection's 'interrogation' of the significance of the dominant theory of trauma for artistic and media representation does not involve a blind rejection of this theory. On the contrary, most of the contributions assembled here engage in varying degrees with a wide range of uses and applications of the theory of trauma. At the same time, each essay examines the potential limitations of this theory's use, while considering alternative conceptual and methodological possibilities. The effect of this, we hope, is a critical opening – rather than abandonment or rejection – of the conventional theory of trauma, as a means to facilitate the critical reappraisal of the relationship between cultural representations and their referent in socio-historical processes marked by violence, conflict and suffering.

Trauma, memory and culture

Trauma has progressively become a key notion in discussions that interrogate the links between social history, subjective experience, and cultural representation. Several decades ago, humanities scholars became interested in the outcomes of research about traumatic memory conducted within the confines of psychology and psychiatry, with many concepts developed in the mental health sciences being translated into the study of history, society, and culture. Since then, a constantly evolving, multidisciplinary field known as *trauma studies* has grown to great proportions. A broad look at the field of trauma studies shows that while the application of the notion of trauma to the analysis of history, culture and politics is widespread, the methodological distinction between this term's original psychological denotation and its analogical use in relation to the socio-cultural realm is often ambiguous if not altogether obscure. This is particularly so in debates concerning the representation of trauma in media such as photography and film. In this regard, Robert Rosenstone observes that '[u]nlike the word, the filmic image cannot abstract and generalize. The screen must show specific images … not the working class but a specific British family grappling with the problems of depression, unemployment, war, and recovery' (1995, 8). However, in their specificity, images also possess the capacity to generate abstract meaning and, in fact, more often than not the visual and narrative rendition of the pain of individual characters is interpreted as a synecdoche for the suffering of a people, culture or nation.

Trauma studies has developed in close partnership with memory studies, a field that has also increased its size and influence exponentially in the last couple of decades. Reflecting a broader cultural interest – an obsession some may say – in memory as a phenomenon at once neuronal, psychological, cultural, and socio-political, the academic study of memory has seen scholars from diverse disciplines attempt to understand a subject that constantly challenges the traditional disciplinary boundaries on which academic research is based. Indeed, the past two decades have seen the emergence of hundreds of new publications about memory, not only books and articles but journals and editorial series, as well as seminars, conferences, and both undergraduate and graduate courses. All of them seem to be articulated by a common central focus on the multiple ways in which memory comes to be expressed and known and, more broadly, on how the personal and cultural worlds come to be constituted through memory. A quick look at the contents of many memory studies publications immediately shows that the discussion of trauma, both in its psychological and cultural forms, is a recurrent sub-topic.[3] Conversely, the same can be said for trauma publications, courses and projects where memory normally features as a key category.[4] Thus, this interpenetration of trauma studies and memory studies makes the boundaries of these two fields difficult to draw, and it is, in fact, virtually impossible to separate them out; their underlying difference being more of emphasis than any intrinsic specificity to be delineated from a historical, thematic or methodological perspective.

The fact that trauma studies and memory studies constantly intersect each other is possibly due to an inherent affinity between their subjects: although not all memory is traumatic, trauma generally is described as a kind of memory (from this view, trauma studies would have to be postulated as a department of memory studies). Even though some clinical definitions of trauma stress the traumatic event or experience, as opposed to its aftermath, that is, its belated manifestation, most approaches appear to agree in understanding trauma as a kind of memory. At the same time, most also concur that this is an exceptional form of memory; not a memory formed through symbols and narratives but one closer to the nature of an injury, a fact that is further supported by the Greek etymology of the term *trauma*, which means *wound*. Thus, essentially understood as a form of damage, traumatic memory is often described as a wound: a painful mark of the past that haunts and overwhelms the present. Significantly, it is the analogical physicality of the traces left by the past in traumatic memory – a violent latency of the past in which memory is imagined as a wounded body – that complicates attempts to understand trauma in terms of cultural representation. This is so because trauma's inherent nature would be to neutralize the habitual processes of symbolization and narrativization through which personal, family and cultural memories and identities are woven.[5]

Initially coined in physical medical science, this notion of a past, latent wound was then analogically transposed to case studies of psychiatric patients, notably in the late nineteenth century.[6] In this way, trauma became a key concept in clinical psychology, particularly in Freudian psychoanalysis, as it analogically described a psychological injury produced by the experience of an external event that damaged the individual's sense of self, and continued to produce belated negative effects that manifested themselves in the form of involuntary symptoms, for example, as disturbing nightmares and flashbacks. This way of understanding psychological trauma in terms of dissociation (between the subject and its present, conscious experience), due to the pervasive, involuntary irruption of disturbing, incomprehensible memories, thus became hegemonic in psychological discourses of trauma, and greatly contributed to the dominant conception of trauma in a socio-cultural sense.

The adoption and adaptation of the notion of trauma into debates about history and culture between contemporary Western thinkers in the humanities took place at significant moments during the twentieth century, often as a response to the morbid spectacle of war. According to Matthew Sharpe, since 'the last century as a whole was arguably a century of traumas ... [a] sense of trauma, unsurprisingly, pervades much of twentieth century European thought' (2007, 1).[7] An early and notable case is the reflection on the paradigm-shifting impact of modernity on human life found in the writings of Walter Benjamin. According to Anca Pusca, the German philosopher was not only one of the first to consider the underlying significance of modern trauma, but his assessment of *shock*, which is for him the basis of trauma, constitutes a *revealing* alternative to Freud's negative perspective on it (2007, 346).[8] Nevertheless, the comparatively lesser attention given in the field of trauma studies to philosophical theories on angst, shock and death may perhaps be explained by the greater historical influence that Holocaust studies have so far had on trauma scholars.

The continuing historical and philosophical reflection initiated in the aftermath of the Second World War has seen the field of Holocaust studies reach extraordinary proportions. In fact, in the course of this development, other distinct fields have surfaced from within the depths of the former, for example, the comparative field of genocide studies. Similarly, it is possible to affirm that the emergence of trauma studies occurred when scholars engaging critically with the concept of trauma within Holocaust studies began to apply trauma-related debates – initially elaborated in unique reference to the Holocaust – to other catastrophic historical experiences.[9] Since that development, the 1990s debates about how historical and political events, in particular catastrophic ones, connect with trauma and memory, both at the subjective and cultural levels, have increased in quantity, intensity, and complexity. Thus, the specific study of cultural trauma appears today as a critical, self-reflexive and vastly inter-disciplinary field. Still, what humanities scholars in disciplines that range from history, anthropology and social science to philosophy, cultural studies and media studies have in common is a vested interest in the problems that traumatic memory and its cultural and political expression pose to critical theory at the level of individuals, communities, nations and global networks. The broad range of contributions to this collection is a sign of this expanding diversity.

Cultures of political memory and the limits of the trauma framework

As stated above, this collection's specific focus is the way in which trauma is – or fails to be – represented, for example, in direct-witness video testimonies, or in photography and narrative film. This is in fact one of the most debated topics in trauma studies, and as such it has triggered a series of productive intersections between trauma studies and other fields, such as studies of literature, visual culture and film. In this context, it is not surprising that the Holocaust, which has been given rapt attention in historical and philosophical works as the key event of twentieth-century history, arguably continues to be the most depicted in literature, art, and screen culture. By the same token, analyses of visual, narrative, poetic and even musical engagements with the Holocaust are by far the most commonly found examples in the critical literature. According to Guerin and Hallas (2007), the emphasis given to the Holocaust in twentieth-century trauma scholarship may be the reason behind the fact that until relatively recently 'scholars have paid more attention to the written and spoken word as the most appropriate communicative forms for bearing witness to and remembering the suffering of the traumatised subject' (7).[10] However, it is significant that the sub-field of inquiry into trauma's representation in visual culture has arguably begun to displace the traditional attention given to written testimonials and reflections. In this sense, the forms most commonly debated in the field of visual culture studies are sites such as memorials and museums,[11] photography,[12] modern and contemporary arts,[13] the mass media[14] and cinema. Perhaps cinema (film and video included) is the visual form that most often, most vividly and through the most diverse range of approaches has represented and explored the myriad ways in which trauma manifests in subjective experience and culture. Thus, the critical literature on films about the trauma of the Holocaust and, more generally, the Second World War, Vietnam and other European and US wars is, in the first place, copious.[15] However, no less profuse is the developing literature that opens up the inquiry to include cinematic representations of traumatic histories and experiences elsewhere.[16]

In the midst of such abundance of scholarship, it is hardly surprising that the trauma framework is sometimes presented as an all-inclusive master paradigm, a grand model that would fit and fulfil all cases. Needless to say, such an approach is limited. The cultural articulation of the human response to political oppression, abuse, and atrocity (as in colonialism, war, concentration camps, torture, terrorism, and genocide) or other overwhelming experiences, such as intra-family violence (particularly, rape and child abuse) and environmental catastrophes (tsunamis, floods, earthquakes and fires)[17] is not the exclusive territory of trauma studies. It is, as well, routinely approached from alternative disciplinary perspectives: political science, ethics, historical studies, and anthropology, to name just a few. These diverse approaches to what is basically the same matter of study, that is, the cultural representation of human life as troubled by devastation and mayhem, do not necessarily emphasize trauma and suffering, but often focus rather on experiences of survival, resilience, struggle, and recovery. As Andreas Huyssen points out, the preferential focus given to trauma 'confine[s] our understanding of memory, marking it too exclusively in terms of pain, suffering, and loss [denying] human agency and [locking] us into compulsive repetition' (2003, 8). Thus, to reduce all representation of memories and experiences marked by conflict, violence and atrocity to trauma is problematic, as it emphasizes a victim position and potentially fails to give due attention to the expression of agency.

Whereas trauma discourses and cultures often constitute the way in which individuals and communities work through their histories and memories of conflict, catastrophe and suffering, at the same time, these histories and memories are often engaged from active positions of political agency. This may involve the articulation of legal discourses that emphasize the establishment of truth and delivery of social and institutional justice, or ethical discourses that stress ideas such as witnessing, recognition, apology, reconciliation, reconstruction and compensation. In this context, cultural representation naturally makes use of all its discursive possibilities, from trauma and healing to truth and justice. Several of the authors in this collection stress cultural processes and expressions that actively work through trauma over those that endlessly insist on acting it out (see, for example, the essays by Felicity Collins and Antonio Traverso).[18]

Towards a critical trauma methodology

The development of a critical methodology for the study of cultural trauma involves the recognition of the fact that the theory of trauma is not a single, homogeneous entity but that, on the contrary, an array of perspectives has been developed within diverse disciplinary traditions. Critical mappings of the field, which disallow the possibility of collapsing diverse concepts of trauma into a single, undifferentiated one, have been undertaken efficiently by many in the field (see, especially, Radstone 2007; Leys 2000).

A précis of the main theoretical and methodological approaches often identified in the vast literature on trauma in the humanities would include the following: concepts of trauma developed in psychoanalysis and, more broadly, psychology;[19] applications of post-structuralist and deconstructive concepts and methods to psychoanalytic and neurological models of trauma;[20] philosophical reflections on historical trauma;[21] psychoanalytic and philosophical concepts of trauma reworked through the discipline of history;[22] and the application of a sociological framework to the understanding of cultural trauma, as a distinct category from psychological trauma.[23] While the differences among these various approaches can be substantial, as pointed out above, often the concept of trauma used in a context of cultural inquiry remains largely undefined. Despite some specific exceptions, uses of the expressions 'cultural trauma' and 'collective trauma' are generally no more than problematic analogical extensions of medical and psychological trauma concepts. In a relatively recent article, Susannah Radstone, one of the contributors to this collection, critiques the widespread use of a vocabulary developed to describe subjective memory to refer to social and cultural phenomena (2005). The effect of this reifying use of language, Radstone argues, is that it renders as literal 'what might better be regarded as a series of compelling metaphors – the "traumatisation" of a nation, for instance, or the "healing" of a culture' (137). At the same time, she stresses, it problematically diverts 'attention away from the processes of articulation through which past happenings and the meanings and affects associated with them are discursively produced, transmitted and mediated' (137). In a similar vein, Jay Winter warns against the 'loose usage of the term "collective memory" [as it has been] framed to mean virtually anything at all – in every corner of the arts and the humanities' (2006, 4). Thus, the unproblematic use of metaphors of memory and trauma in a cultural context invariably results in the avoidance of the task of elaboration of a more adequate definition of cultural trauma. What does it mean to say that a society or community is traumatized?

Perhaps the most deliberate effort to elaborate a definition of cultural trauma that unambiguously differentiates it from psychological trauma is the sociological model articulated by Jeffrey Alexander and his collaborators (2004). Their constructivist proposition is that, against lay naturalistic understandings of trauma (which, according to Alexander, pervade scholarly accounts, especially psychoanalytically inflected ones), cultural trauma is not the naturally occurring response of a community or society to cataclysmic events. Rather, a culture of trauma is activated by symbolic and imaginative work and, therefore, is separate from the event that may have caused it. In this way, they argue, cultural trauma can be studied in terms of its material and symbolic manifestations in social processes and structures, while remaining separate from the vicissitudes of the traumatic symptoms and experiences of individual sufferers. However, if trauma in its socio-cultural dimension is to be generalized to such an extent as to broadly denote a culture of memorialization whose content refers to specific politicized histories and experiences of human suffering – which nevertheless always involve resilience and struggle as well as trauma – then the use of the term *trauma* to refer to this culture seems arbitrary. There are, in fact, other established sociological and anthropological models, such as *social suffering*, *conflict*, *violence* and *genocide studies*, which consider the social and cultural responses of communities to catastrophic events, while avoiding the psychologizing connotations implied by concepts of trauma.[24] Thus, a radical sociologizing and de-psychologizing of cultural trauma is not without its own complications.[25]

In addressing the methodological problem of analogical articulations between concepts of psychological and cultural trauma, Dominick LaCapra radically suggests that psychoanalysis could be a discourse that has more affinity with the social and cultural realm than with the level of the individual psyche (LaCapra 1994, 173–4). Similarly, Joshua Hirsch, who considers LaCapra's suggestion, attends to this problem through the category 'discourse of trauma', which

> as one encounters it in conversation, in reading, in film – gives one a language with which to begin to represent the failure of representation that one has experienced [...] It is in the discourse of trauma that we can move from the notion of individual responses to traumatizing events toward the notion of collective responses. (2004, 18)

The present collection, therefore, is animated by a concern with conceptual and methodological issues underlying the critical understanding of historical experiences of conflict and suffering and their remembrance in various forms of collectively, that is, discursively, produced representations.

At a time when important voices in the field (Radstone forthcoming; Bennett 2005; Huyssen 2003)[26] are revealing a movement away from the persistent attention given to traumatic memory in historical and cultural studies at least since the late 1980s, more than ever there is an urgent need to reassess the study of the cultural engagement with historical suffering caused by political conflict, in terms of new inter-disciplinary and inter-cultural methodological perspectives. Thus, this collection seeks to contribute to this movement *beyond* trauma –not in the ethically and politically unsustainable sense of turning away from ahumanistic concern with social suffering and social justice but in the sense of opening up the scope of interpretation mostfamiliar to traumastudies.The contributions to this collection aim at doing just this, by expanding the discussion regarding artistic and media representations of the suffering of peopleina diversity of political contextsinSouth and North America,Southern Asia, Australia and Europe. At the same time, each of the essays that follow takes in its own specific way amore or less pronounced critical, theoretical and methodological distancefrom the conventional trauma theory, while remainingfaithful to the ethicaland politicalconcerns of acriticaltrauma studies.

This 'Interrogating Trauma' collection also shows the resolve of scholars in various areas of the study of culture to reinvigorate the interest in trauma representation by revalorizing the use of established disciplinary methodologies of analysis, as well as traditional fruitful collaborations between dissimilar disciplines, such as screen studies, history and anthropology. It also highlights two of the most important critical considerations to be kept in mind when engaging with trauma from within the humanities. Firstly, the perception that trauma studies – or the turn to trauma of many humanities fields primarily concerned with cultural expression – would have allowed a critical (non-naive) return to the real after the detour taken by post-structuralist and post-modern theory. However, implicit in the collection is a call for caution that warns of the risks involved in this perception, in the sense that this *return* could be just another illusion created by the same metaphysical essentialism that post-structuralism sought to dethrone in the first place. The second consideration alludes to the fact that with its pervasive medical connotations, most probably due to its entrenched origin in the physical and psychological health sciences, the expression *trauma* continuously tends to psychologize, and therefore, potentially, depoliticize the discussion and analysis of socio-historical phenomena and their representation.

The collection's first four contributions are those of the scholars who delivered the keynotes at the 'Interrogating Trauma' conference in Perth in 2008. In the first essay, '*Caché*: Or What the Past Hides', Susannah Radstone produces a detailed analysis of Michael Haneke's *Caché (Hidden)* (2005) – a film that through a mysterious narrative and an unfathomable subversion of formal levels addresses the trauma of colonial history, in particular 'the dissociated memory of France's 'dirty war' against Algeria'. Radstone uses her discussion of Haneke's film as an occasion to invite the humanities to consider Jean Laplanche's psychoanalytic theory of the *enigmatic signifier* as a productive alternative to dissociative trauma theory in the understanding of the relationship between subjective and cultural memory. Radstone's piece is followed by an essay by Suvendrini Perera, 'Torturous Dialogues: Geographies of Trauma and Spaces of Exception', which considers historical, ideological, and geopolitical elements that contribute to the necro-political and bio-political ordering of suffering and damage – whereby trauma becomes a transactable currency – in the context of maritime disasters, in particular the Indian Ocean tsunami of 2004. Janet Walker's essay, 'Moving Testimonies and the Geography of Suffering: Perils and Fantasies of Belonging after Katrina', continues the exploration of the underlying political structures of human suffering in the context of so-called natural disasters by focusing on the use of testimonial documentary film and video to come to terms with trauma and devastation in the aftermath of Hurricane Katrina in 2005. Felicity Collins's essay, 'After the Apology: Re-framing Violence and Suffering in *First Australians*, *Australia*, and *Samson and Delilah*', complements Radstone's and Walker's focus on cinematic media, as well as the critical attention that Perera gives to discursive construction, by considering media images of remote Aboriginal communities that normalize violence and the suffering of people positioned as 'bare life'. Conversely, Collins argues for the potential of three recent Australian cinematic texts to work through the traumatic past.

Adam Brown's 'Confronting "Choiceless Choices" in Holocaust Videotestimonies: Judgement, "Privileged" Jews, and the Role of the Interviewer' explores the ethical and political dilemmas involved in the production of Holocaust video testimonies in cases where the survivor interviewees were prisoners who held positions involving benefits that common prisoners did not have. In considering these dilemmas, Brown engages ethical concepts from Holocaust studies, such as Lawrence Langer's 'choiceless choices' and Primo Levi's 'grey zone'. Moving the attention away from testimonial video and towards commercial cinema, Mark Straw's 'The Guilt Zone: Trauma, Masochism and the Ethics of Spectatorship in Brian De Palma's *Redacted* (2007)' provides an analysis of this controversial Iraq War veteran film. Straw discusses the screen construction of a traumatized/masochistic male subjectivity by combining trauma cinema studies (Kaplan and Wang 2004; Walker 2005; Elsaesser 1996) with Gilles Deleuze's creative theoretical reworking of the concept of masochism. In 'When Places Have Agency: Roadside Shrines as Traumascapes' co-authors Catherine Collins and Alexandra Opie depart from cinematic culture to consider one form of what Maria Tumarkin (2005) has denominated *traumascapes*. Invoking Foucault's concept of *heterochronia* for the purposes of trauma studies, Collins and Opie reflect on the urban cultural phenomenon of roadside shrines that proliferate on back roads of the United States. The reflection on the embodied performance of traumatic memory, as well as a concern with the ethics of spectatorship of the suffering of others, is continued in Sophie Oliver's essay, 'Trauma, Bodies, and Performance Art: Towards an Embodied Ethics of Seeing', where she discusses ways in which performance art embraces a model of embodied, self-reflective and ethical spectatorship. David Carlin's contribution, 'Poetic Witnessing in the Archive: The Database Narrative of *Life after Wartime*', considers the ethics of witnessing by returning to the analysis of screen arts – this time neither documentary video nor narrative cinema, but an Australian interactive database narrative project, which, as Carlin proposes, can be seen as a new model of *trauma text*, one which avoids either narrative or therapeutic closure.

The final group of essays returns to cinematic culture. Vivien Fryd's 'Bearing Witness to the Trauma of Slavery in Kara Walker's videos: *Testimony*, *Eight Possible Beginnings*, and *I was transported*' discusses three cinematic works by the controversial African-American artist Kara Walker. Fryd claims that through these works the artist forces her viewers to witness the transgenerational trauma of slavery and racism in the United States by embodying trauma's disruptive potential. In 'Depiction or Erasure? Violence and Trauma in Contemporary Peruvian Film', Iliana Pagán-Teitelbaum discusses three narrative films made in this impoverished South American country. These films depict the traumatized bodies of Indigenous people, thus exploring 'the trauma of misery, racism, forced migration, and dirty war'. The final essay, 'Dictatorship Memories: Working through Trauma in Chilean Post-dictatorship Documentary' by Antonio Traverso, considers Chilean documentary cinema made in the period after the military dictatorship. Traverso claims that these documentaries, whose recurrent theme is the memory of that traumatic past, work through Chile's historical trauma by revealing 'productive attributes of life under dictatorship, such as the people's agency, resilience and capacity to imagine the future'.

In summary, this collection contributes to the broader project of a critical trauma studies by emphasizing – and also constituting – a set of aims and principles which include thematic and cross-cultural epistemologies that deepen the discussion about the relationship between individual memory/trauma and collective or cultural memory/-trauma. It engages with the potential of established methodologies in fields such as screen studies while embracing multi- and inter-disciplinarity, in recognition that there is not one but numerous theories and concepts of trauma. These collected writings cultivate methodological openings to alternative ways of approaching trauma representation, besides the conventional psychoanalytic theory of subjective dissociation. Examples of such openings, illustrated by the writings assembled here, include: Laplanchian psychoanalysis; contemporary performance theory; philosophical theorizations (for instance, concepts of the sublime, Benjamin's reflection on shock, Foucault's notion of heterochronia, Deleuze's theory of masochism, and Agamben's theory of biopolitics); Klein's critique of disaster capitalism; critical human geography; and the sociology and anthropology of social suffering, violence, conflict and resilience. As such, this collection is testament to the diversity and richness of the field, and to the ongoing desire for the continued analysis and application of theory to the representation of trauma and social suffering around the globe.

Notes

1. By 'the West' and 'the Third World' we mean not only the geographical enclaves of hegemonic, wealthy Western nations, such as Australia, Canada, Europe and the United States, in opposition to the poor nations of Africa, Asia, the Middle East, Latin America, and Oceania, but also the differing socio-cultural spaces that exist within national geographical boundaries, such as post-colonial Indigenous groups and disenfranchised racial and diasporic groups living in Western countries.
2. The concept of trauma based on a model of subjective dissociation – by virtue of which the traumatized subject's sense of self is violently estranged from its relation with present experience by the constant, unannounced irruption into conscious experience of the traces of a painful past – has been developed, firstly, in psychoanalysis and other psychological approaches in relation to the war phenomenon of *shell shock* and, more recently, as the basis of the clinical definition of post-traumatic stress disorder (PTSD).
3. See Radstone and Hodgkin (2005), Radstone (2000), and the journals *History & Memory*, *Memory Studies* and *Screening the Past* (www.latrobe.edu.au/screeningthepast/).
4. See Walker (2005) and Leys (2000).

5. The conventional theory of cultural trauma as a 'crisis of representation' is conveyed by Cathy Caruth, one of its best-known exponents (see Caruth 1995, 1996), for a lucid explanation of Caruth's theory, see chapter 8 in Leys (2000).
6. See Kaplan (2005), Kaplan and Wang (2004), Hirsch (2004), and Leys (2000).
7. Sharpe makes reference to the trauma or angst-inflected thought of some of the most iconic European thinkers of the twentieth century besides Freud, including Heidegger, Levinas, Adorno, Benjamin, Lacan, Lyotard, Jameson, Žižek, and Derrida (2007, 1–2)
8. Also see Pusca (forthcoming 2010); and for two recent cases of engagement with Benjamin's theories in the context of cultural trauma studies, see Kaplan (2005) and Collins and Davis (2004).
9. On the origin of trauma studies: 'Trauma studies originated in the context of research about the Holocaust' (Kaplan 2005, 1); on the origin of genocide studies: 'early [genocide] literature drew upon more than a decade of intensive research on the Jewish Holocaust' (Jones 2006, 14).
10. A recent double special issue of the journal *Life Writing* is devoted entirely to *trauma* as the theme of a 'vigorous and widespread turn to the practice and theory of life writing (a term that covers biography, autobiography and variants and mutations of both)'; see Douglas, Whitlock, and Stumm (2008, 1).
11. See Winter (1995), Young (1993) and Samuel (1994).
12. See Butler (2009), Khun and McAllister (2006), Sontag (1977, 2003) and Zelizer (1998).
13. See Trezise and Wake (2009), Saltzman and Rosenberg (2006) and Bennett (2005).
14. See Randell and Redmond (2008) and Michalski and Gow (2007).
15. See Winter (2006), Torner (2005), Hirsch (2004), Hornstein and Jacobowitz (2003), Vice (2003), Walker (2005), Zelizer (1998, 2001), Sturken (1997), Elsaesser (1996), Caruth (1995), Reimer and Reimer (1992), Avisar (1988) and Insdorf ([1983] 1989).
16. Kaplan (2005), Lowenstein (2005), Kaplan and Wang (2004), Collins and Davis (2004), Douglass and Vogler (2003), Stacey (2003), Radstone (2000, 2001) and Rosenstone (1995).
17. The contributions by Perera and Walker to this collection, which respectively discuss the Indian Ocean tsunami of 2004 and Hurricane Katrina in the United States in 2005, make it clear that the separation between 'natural' and 'human-induced' disasters is a problematic one because the inner structure of human suffering is invariably political. See also Giblett (2009) and Pearson (2008).
18. This emphasis on working through trauma texts and strategies is noticeable in the work of many established trauma scholars, among whom one of the most influential is Dominick LaCapra (1997, 2001).
19. See Kaplan (2005) and Walker (2005), among many others.
20. See Caruth (1995, 1996) and Felman and Laub (1992).
21. See Sharpe et al. (2007); this is an edited collection of essays originally presented at the Australian Society for Continental Philosophy conference, Deakin University, 2006; also see Collins and Davis (2004), where the authors use 'Benjamin's theories of history, modernity and shock' (8) in their discussion of what they call 'post-*Mabo* cinema', that is, recent Australian films that engage with the history of race relations in this country.
22. See the extensive work of LaCapra (1994, 1998, 2001) on trauma and history.
23. Best illustrated by the work of Jeffrey Alexander, Neil Smelser and others at the Centre for Advanced Studies in the Behavioural Sciences at Yale University; see Alexander et al. (2004) and Eyerman (2001).
24. See Das (2007), Jones (2006), Wilkinson (2004), Hinton (2002), Das et al. (2000), Das et al. (2001), Kleinman, Das, and Lock (1997) and Fein (1993).
25. Alexander et al. seem to discard important aspects – for example, that the analogy between psychological trauma and cultural trauma is not a fortuitous one. On the contrary, it is because there are actual traumatized individuals – generally survivors and direct witnesses – within those communities where a trauma culture purportedly develops, that this culture represents and often resembles the traumatic symptoms of sufferers. Additionally, the argument of a complete separation between the cultural elaborations produced in response to a catastrophic event and the event itself contains crucial political implications, as it may provide theoretical tools to genocide and atrocity deniers.
26. As indicated by Radstone in her biographical note, 'she is currently completing a project on new approaches to trauma, to be published as *Getting over Trauma*'; Bennett toys with the idea of trauma culture's passing out of fashion within the art world (2005, 149); and Huyssen suggests that the privileged attention hitherto given to trauma has resulted in 'a thick discursive network' that stresses 'repression, spectres, and a present repetitively haunted by the past' (2003, 8).

References

Alexander, Jeffrey, et al. 2004. *Cultural trauma and collective identity*. Berkeley: University of California Press.

Avisar, Ilan. 1988. *Screening the Holocaust: Cinema's images of the unimaginable*. Bloomington and Indianapolis: Indiana University Press.

Ball, Karyn. 2007. *Traumatizing theory: The cultural politics of affect in and beyond psychoanalysis*. New York: Other Press.

Bennett, Jill. 2005. *Empathic vision: Affect, trauma, and contemporary art*. Stanford: Stanford University Press.

Bennett, Jill, and Rosanne Kennedy. 2003. *World memory: Personal trajectories in global time*. Basingstoke and New York: Palgrave Macmillan.

Blocker, Jane. 2009. *Seeing witness: Visuality and the ethics of testimony*. Minneapolis: University of Minnesota Press.

Butler, Judith. 2009. *Frames of war: When is life grievable?* London: Verso.

Caruth, Cathy, ed. 1995. *Trauma: Explorations in memory*. Baltimore and London: Johns Hopkins University Press.

———. 1996. *Unclaimed experience: Trauma, narrative, experience*. Baltimore and London: Johns Hopkins University Press.

Collins, Felicity, and Therese Davis. 2004. *Australian cinema after Mabo*. Cambridge: Cambridge University Press.

Das, Veena. 2007. *Life and words: Violence and the descent into the ordinary*. Berkeley and London: University of California Press.

Das, Veena, et al., eds. 2000. *Violence and subjectivity*. Berkeley and London: University of California Press.

———, eds. 2001. *Remaking a world: Violence, social suffering, and recovery*. Berkeley and London: University of California Press.

Douglas, Kate, Gillian Whitlock, and Bettina Stumm, eds. 2008. Trauma in the 21st Century. Special issue, *Life Writing* 5, nos 1/2.

Douglass, Ana, and Thomas A. Vogler. 2003. *Witness and memory: The discourse of trauma*. London and New York: Routledge.

Elsaesser, Thomas. 1996. Subject positions, speaking positions: From *Holocaust, Our Hitler*, and *Heimat* to *Shoa* and *Schindler's List*. In *The persistence of history: Cinema, television and the modern event*, ed. Vivian Sobchack, 145–83. London and New York: Routledge.

Eyerman, Ron. 2001. *Cultural trauma: Slavery and the formation of African American identity*. Cambridge: Cambridge University Press.

Fein, Helen. 1993. *Genocide: A sociological perspective*. London: Sage.

Felman, Shoshana, and Dori Laub. 1992. *Testimony: Crises of witnessing in literature, psychoanalysis, and history*. London and New York: Routledge.

Giblett, Rod. 2009. *Landscapes of culture and nature*. Hampshire and New York: Palgrave Macmillan.

Guerin, Frances, and Roger Hallas, eds. 2007. *The image and the witness: Trauma, memory and visual culture*. London and New York: Wallflower Press.

Hinton, Alexander, ed. 2002. *Annihilating difference: The anthropology of genocide*. Berkeley and London: University of California Press.

Hirsch, Joshua. 2004. *After image: Film, trauma and the Holocaust*. Philadelphia: Temple University Press.

Hodgkin, Katharine, and Susannah Radstone, eds. 2005. *Contested pasts: The politics of memory*. London and New York: Routledge.

Hornstein, Shelley, and Florence Jacobowitz, eds. 2003. *Image and remembrance: Representation and the Holocaust*. Bloomington and Indianapolis: Indiana University Press.

Huyssen, Andreas. 2003. *Present pasts: Urban palimpsests and the politics of memory*. Stanford: Stanford University Press.

Insdorf, Annette. 1989/1983. *Indelible shadows: Film and the Holocaust.* 2nd ed. Cambridge: Cambridge University Press.
Jones, Adam. 2006. *Genocide: A comprehensive introduction.* London and New York: Routledge.
Kaplan, E. Ann. 2005. *Trauma culture: The politics of terror and loss in media and literature.* New Brunswick, NJ: Rutgers University Press.
Kaplan, E. Ann, and Ban Wang, eds. 2004. *Trauma and cinema: Cross-cultural explorations.* Hong Kong: Hong Kong University Press.
Khun, Annette, and Kirsten E. McAllister, eds. 2006. *Locating memory: Photographic acts.* New York: Berghahn Books.
Kleinman, Arthur, Veena Das, and Margaret Lock, eds. 1997. *Social suffering.* Berkeley and London: University of California Press.
LaCapra, Dominick. 1994. *Representing the Holocaust: History, theory, trauma.* Ithaca, NY: Cornell University Press.
———. 1997. Lanzmann's *Shoah*: 'Here there is no why'. *Critical Inquiry* 23, no. 2: 231–69.
———. 1998. *History and memory after Auschwitz.* Ithaca, NY: Cornell University Press.
———. 2001. *Writing history, writing trauma.* Baltimore and London: Johns Hopkins University Press.
Leys, Ruth. 2000. *Trauma: A genealogy.* Chicago: University of Chicago Press.
Lowenstein, Adam. 2005. *Shocking representation: Historical trauma, national cinema, and the modern horror film.* New York: Columbia University Press.
Michalski, Milena and James Gow. 2007. *War, image and legitimacy: Viewing contemporary conflict.* London and New York: Routledge.
Pearson, Chris. 2008. *Scarred landscapes: War and nature in Vichy France.* Hampshire and New York: Palgrave Macmillan.
Pusca, Anca. 2007. Shock, therapy, and postcommunist transitions. *Alternatives* 32: 341–60.
———. Forthcoming 2010. *Walter Benjamin and the aesthetics of change.* London and New York: Palgrave Macmillan.
Radstone, Susannah, ed. 2000. *Memory and methodology.* Oxford and New York: Berg.
———, ed. 2001. Trauma and screen studies: Opening the debate. *Screen* 42, no. 2: 188–216.
———. 2005. Reconceiving binaries: The limits of memory. *History Workshop Journal* 59: 134–50.
———. 2007. Trauma theory: Contexts, politics, ethics. *Paragraph* 30, no. 1: 9–29.
Radstone, Susannah. Forthcoming. Getting over trauma.
Radstone, Susannah, and Katharine Hodgkin, eds. 2005. *Memory cultures: Memory, subjectivity and recognition.* New Brunswick, NJ: Transaction.
Randell, Karen, and Sean Redmond, eds. 2008. *The war body on screen.* New York and London: Continuum.
Reimer, Robert, and Carol Reimer. 1992. *Nazi-retro film: How German narrative cinema remembers the past.* New York: Twayne; Toronto: Maxwell Macmillan.
Robben, Antonius, and Marcelo Suárez-Orozco. 2000. *Cultures under siege: Collective violence and trauma.* Cambridge: Cambridge University Press.
Rosenstone, Robert A., ed. 1995. *Revisioning history: Film and the construction of a new past.* Princeton: Princeton University Press.
Saltzman, Lisa, and Eric Rosenberg, eds. 2006. *Trauma and visuality in modernity.* Hanover and London: University Press of New England.
Samuel, Raphael. 1994. *Theatres of memory.* Vol. 1*: Past and present in contemporary culture.* London and New York: Verso.
Sharpe, Matthew. 2007. Why 'trauma' now? In *Trauma, history, philosophy*, ed. Matthew Sharpe et al., 1–7. Newcastle: Cambridge Scholars.
Sharpe, Matthew, et al., eds. 2007. *Trauma, history, philosophy.* Newcastle: Cambridge Scholars.
Sontag, Susan. 1977. *On photography.* New York: Farrar, Straus, Giroux.
———. 2003. *Regarding the pain of others.* New York: Farrar, Straus, Giroux.
Stacey, Jackie, ed. 2003. The trauma debate II. *Screen* 44, no. 2: 200–28.

Sturken, Marita. 1997. *Tangled memories: The Vietnam War, the AIDS epidemic, and the politics of remembering*. Berkeley and London: University of California Press.
Torner, Carles. 2005. *Shoa: cavar con la mirada*. Barcelona: Editorial Gedisa.
Trezise, Bryoni, and Caroline Wake, eds. 2009. After effects: Performing the ends of memory. Special issue, *Performance Paradigm* 5, no. 1.
Tumarkin, Maria. 2005. *Traumascapes: The power and fate of places transformed by tragedy*. Carlton: Melbourne University Publishing.
Vice, Sue, ed. 2003. *Representing the Holocaust*. London and Portland: Vallentine Mitchell.
Walker, Janet. 2005. *Trauma cinema: Documenting incest and the Holocaust*. Berkeley: University of California Press.
Weibel, Peter, and Franz Kaltenbeck, eds. 2000. *Trauma und erinnerung/Trauma and memory: Cross-cultural perspectives*. Vienna: Passagen.
Wilkinson, Iain. 2004. *Suffering: A sociological introduction*. Cambridge and Malden, MA: Polity.
Winter, Jay. 1995. *Sites of memory, sites of mourning: The Great War in European cultural history*. Cambridge: Cambridge University Press.
———. 2006. *Remembering war: The Great War between memory and history in the twentieth century*. New Haven and London: Yale University Press.
Young, James E. 1993. *The texture of memory: Holocaust memorials and meaning*. New Haven and London: Yale University Press.
Zelizer, Barbie. 1998. *Remembering to forget: Holocaust memory through the camera's eye*. Chicago and London: University of Chicago Press.
———, ed. 2001. *Visual culture and the Holocaust*. New Brunswick, NJ: Rutgers University Press.

Caché: Or what the past hides

Susannah Radstone

School of Humanities and Social Sciences, University of East London, London, UK

Michael Haneke's film *Caché* (*Hidden*) (2005) has provoked a good deal of criticism and debate, much of it focusing on the question of the 'hidden' to which the film's title refers. Responses to the film have tended to focus on *Caché*'s relations with colonial history as trauma, aligning the film's 'hidden' with the dissociated memory of France's 'dirty war' against Algeria. The psychoanalytic theory of Jean Laplanche offers the Humanities an approach to culture that diverges from the version of trauma theory drawn on by many of *Caché*'s commentators. This essay takes up Laplanche's ideas in the context of a critique of trauma theory and aims to demonstrate their potential to shed light not only on *Caché* but also on culture's relations with temporality, violence, and the enigmatic.

> But, in the enigmatic signifier, there is not only an explicit message, but also an implicit message, and the child cannot but understand that there is something hidden in it ... (Laplanche, in Fletcher and Stanton 1992, 22)

> The key question that confronts Haneke's film is the following: what, exactly, is caché? (Khanna 2007, 237)

What might it mean to speak of the 'hidden'? If Michael Haneke's provocative and much commented upon film *Caché* (*Hidden*) (2005) invites speculation on this theme, much of the film's criticism has responded by naming, locating, identifying the 'hidden' to which *Caché* is understood to refer. But *can* the 'hidden' be named? Can it be found? Can it be located? And if so, in what sense? These are questions that, if we descend from the abstract to the more concrete, can be seen to bear forcefully on those debates about history, memory and representation that have been inflecting humanities research for some time. Particularly in the field of trauma theory,[1] the quest to find traces of lost and hidden past experiences – lost and hidden, on this account, because too terrible to be directly recalled – has animated much recent research. In film, literary and media studies, as well as in branches of history, sociology and elsewhere, research has been transformed into acts of bearing (secondary) witness to testimonies that only the dialogics of reading or spectating can begin to interpret (Felman and Laub 1992; Caruth 1992, 1995). This critical turn has radically altered understandings of what texts *and* criticism can and ought to do. At stake in these interpretative projects is a model of temporality in which past traumatic experiences are considered to belatedly make their presence felt, an epistemology that holds that past experiences of trauma can, if only with difficulty and to a degree, pass from the unknowable to the knowable, from the inchoate to the specifiable, and from the hidden to the light, and an ethics that deems it a critical duty to bear witness to the sufferings of the past. But, as I've already begun to ask, does 'the hidden' bear belated witness to the traumatic past? Can it be located, named, interpreted? And is the quest to bear witness and to speak of the hidden, understood in these terms, either realizable by, or a duty of, criticism?

Caché is a film that makes great play of what is, and remains hidden – to its characters, to its camera and to its spectators. This formal and thematic motif extends from *Caché*'s much commented upon opening credits sequence – a long shot of a house, seen (but by whom?) from across a Parisian street, to its closing frames – another long shot, again from across the street, of children on the steps outside their school, from which 'crucial plot information was apparently hidden within the background activity of the image' (Cousins 2007, 223). The film, in the apposite words of Libby Saxton, 'turns on a series of attempts to uncover the identity and motives of a *hidden* presence who observes, films and even, in a certain sense, directs the action from beyond the frame' (2007, 7; emphasis added). But if this presence, and more besides, remains hidden beyond the temporal and spatial frames of *Caché*'s closing shots, the comparatively precipitate revelation of other story information only contributes to the film's inscrutability. *Caché* is not a film that can adequately be summed up, then, nor does the provocation of its final shot bring its story to an end. This radical openness, though it stretches beyond the film's formal ending, can be foreclosed *or* redeemed, however, by a criticism of 'the hidden'. This essay explores how criticism might acknowledge what *remains* hidden in *Caché* and seeks to demonstrate why such a critical turn might matter.

Trauma and the hidden

Haneke's much awarded film *Caché* is not a work that lends itself to easy generic categorization or summary. That, indeed, is the point, in a sense, of what I want to go on to say. Part art movie, part thriller, *Caché* concerns itself with a couple, Georges (Daniel Auteuil) and Anne (Juliet Binoche) who, as the DVD jacket has it,

> live the perfect life of comfort and security in modern day Paris. They have a teenage son and Georges hosts a popular literary review TV programme while Anne works in publishing. One day, they start receiving packages on their doorstep that contain video surveillance footage shot secretly from their street, accompanied by disturbing drawings. (Dendy/Madman 2005)

As *Caché* unfolds, it begins to seem that these tapes – although authorially 'unmarked' and altogether lacking definitive signs of their origin or meaning – may be linked with Georges's temporary adoptive step-brother Majid, whose apartment appears in one of the deposited tapes and who Georges eventually visits and aggressively confronts. Majid, the child of Algerian parents murdered in the Paris massacre of protestors demonstrating for Algerian independence in October 1961,[2] was, so Georges reveals, taken in by Georges's parents after the massacre, but was subsequently expelled to an orphanage on the basis of Georges's fabricated accusations. It was he, Georges discloses, who turned his parents against Majid by persuading him to kill one of the family's chickens and by falsely claiming that Majid was coughing up blood – a sign of tuberculosis. Georges ultimately confesses something of this guilty past to his wife Anne, before going once more to Majid's apartment at his request, whereupon Majid, after insisting that the tapes were not his work, slits his own throat with a knife, sinking to the floor before a motionless Georges, who, after heading to the cinema,[3] returns home to what appears to be an increasingly disintegrating life.

Much of the literature on *Caché* returns to the theme of France's war with Algeria. But *Caché* was made and released in the year of the 'banlieu riots', that uprising of protests against racism and unemployment that shook Paris, and then France, in 2005 and in which at least two North African youths lost their lives. It's not hard to propose that, with its closed-in camerawork, its aesthetic and narrative concerns with surveillance, its claustrophobic interiority, its defended, or even barricaded domestic *mise-en-scène*, and its scenes of explosive conflict between Georges and a North African cyclist, *Caché* 'describes' those tensions – critically perhaps – from the point of view of the privileged and anxious white middle class.

The linearity of *Caché*'s narrative is punctuated by what appear to be temporally unplaceable and ambiguously motivated short sequences and shots of a boy, sometimes with bleeding face – and by shots of strange, childish drawings of a bloodied face and a bleeding chicken that accompany some of the videotapes. These shots and sequences, which later become placeable as still ambiguously motivated flashbacks relating to Majid and the killing of the chicken, have led critics to take *Caché* as a trauma film[4] belonging to the history of a French and Algerian cinema 'punctuated' by the trauma of the Algerian war (Austin 2007, 529). Martine Beugnet has proposed, for instance, that those critics who have 'account[ed] for the effect of the disincarnated presence ... that the film's apparatus creates, merely in terms of the sadistic inclination of a demiurgic filmmaker intent on manipulating his audience' (Beugnet 2007, 228) disregard the trauma embedded in the film.

Though the theme of the hidden – inflected, as it has become, by the paradigm of trauma theory – permeates *Caché*'s voluminous criticism, a range of political and theoretical imperatives have informed commentators' responses to the question of what it is that is hidden in, or by, the film. Focusing on audience conversations prompted by the film, Mark Cousins diverges from the majority in suggesting that the film's concern with colonial guilt hides its provocation – for middle-class privileged audiences at least – of more abstract and philosophical anxieties about the apparent meaning of its narrative and the trustworthiness of its narration. Far more commonly, and in line with trauma theory's focus upon victims, perpetrators and the injunction to remember the wounds of the past, *Caché*'s 'hidden' is read in relation to the trauma of violence perpetrated upon the colonized and the guilt that now ought rightfully to be acknowledged by the colonial power. Paul Gilroy expresses a minority view when he argues that *Caché*'s apparent censure of colonialism hides its 'horrible accommodation' (Gilroy 2007, 233) by means of an equation of colonial atrocities with the childish acts of a six-year-old (235). More frequently, critics have read *Caché*'s concealed cameras, its ambiguous points of view, its embedded videos and, for some, its complex imbrication with childhood, as strategies through which the hidden traumas of colonial violence begin, after what is commonly agreed to have been 'a long-lasting silence' (Beugnet 2007, 227), to make their presence felt or, relatedly, to make visible and to confront spectators with colonialism's amnesic modes of disavowal (Beugnet 2007; Saxton 2007).

For Martine Beugnet, it is the video images themselves that inscribe trauma into the body of the film (2007, 228). This is a trauma hidden by the apparent comfort of Georges and Anne's comfortable-looking house, itself 'partly hidden behind a thick privet hedge' (227), and, like the set for Georges's TV review programme, 'cloaked' by walls of books. Recorded by 'a mysterious, hidden observer ... an enigmatic presence' (229), the video image 'does not so much "puncture" through this cloak, but rather weaves itself into it, and reveals it for what it is' (230) – a screen hiding the traumas of colonial perpetration and victimhood.

If, for Beugnet, it is video itself that becomes, in Haneke's vision, 'the obstinate witness to the everyday denial of intolerable realities and memories' (Beugnet 2007, 228) and the transmitter, by means of its enigmatic recording presence, of the hidden, or even purposively forgotten agony of the oppressed (231), for others it is the link between the video footage –

or, in one case, the drawings – (Austin 2007) and a child's eye view that lifts the cloak. On this account, *Caché*'s 'other' emerges, not as the victim of colonial violence but as 'the Child, who remains the ultimate locus of knowledge and judgement' (Mecchia 2007, 132). This 'child-director', is not, as has also been suggested, Haneke as 'concealed sadistic child playing with images' (Rehm, qtd in Beugnet 2007, 231). The child-director acts, rather, as the bearer of 'the implacable gaze of a relentless and scandalously innocent onlooker, this time hidden behind the mechanical eye of the camera' (Mecchia 2007, 132), and serves as what Mecchia, following Rancière, terms a 'restorer of appearances'. Under the watchful gaze of a child-witness who hides within all of us (140), *Caché*'s child-director reveals, on Mecchia's account, truths of colonial guilt – truths that might otherwise remain concealed by the 'adult world of prejudice and deception' (131, abstract).

If, for Mecchia, Beugnet's observing yet enigmatic presence becomes the much less enigmatic child-director, the hidden truth that both find revealed by the video camera's look is that of traumatic colonial violence and guilt – a guilt and violence indissociably linked with the after-effects of France's dirty war and, in particular, the October massacres. On these accounts, this is a 'hidden' that can, if only with difficulty, come to be located, named, known.

Other readings of Haneke's work and of *Caché* place greater stress on the viewing positions opened up by his particular manipulations of the camera, the image and the look. Lebeau's recent essay on Haneke directs our attention to that formative relay of looks exchanged between mother and child. Following the psychoanalytic theory of D.W. Winnicott, Lebeau proposes that within this process of exchange the reflected image of both mother and child may be too present *or* too absent, creating a deadness in place of life (2009). Lebeau's suggestion that Haneke's work attempts to acknowledge and address a pathology within contemporary regimes of looking which might be equated with a foundational and primary pathology of the visual, sustains an association between Haneke's work, childhood and looking while embedding this within a psychoanalytic frame. But, even though Lebeau alludes to Haneke's concerns with violence – 'violence', she suggests, 'is never far from Haneke's screen' (Lebeau 2009, 42) – in this universalist approach to the psychoanalytics of the visual, relations *between* historical violence, visual culture and the negation of 'coming to life' (37) remain obscure.

Focused, too, on the spectatorial relations opened up by *Caché*, and upon the 'enigmatic look [that] is at once the origin and the blind spot of the narrative', Libby Saxton's (2007) discussion of the film moves on to contemplate the enigma posed more generally by *Caché*'s play on what remains hidden in off-screen space, suggesting that it 'emerges as the site of a historical trauma' (9). Yet as Saxton goes on to point out, off-screen space remains a 'repository of latent meaning', provoking the film's spectators to acknowledge their blind spots (15). But can off-screen space be resolved as a site of historical trauma, while remaining replete with latent meaning? Can that which continues to remain hidden be specified in this way? And is that 'hidden' to which *Caché*'s commentators and trauma theory have addressed themselves best understood as the trace of a traumatic past? The writings of the French psychoanalyst Jean Laplanche can help us to explore these questions.

Enigmatic signification and the hidden

Laplanche's psychoanalytic theory has not been drawn on as extensively as it might have been by trauma theorists. Yet his work offers the opportunity to reconfigure trauma theory's understandings of temporality, history, culture and, in particular, the role of the critic. Laplanche's radical re-thinking of Freudian psychoanalysis overturns previous understandings of the constitution of the unconscious, of trauma, and of the transmissions that constitute culture *and* the earliest and most formative of infantile experiences. These insights provide us with new ways of understanding what might be meant by 'the hidden' in culture, in the unconscious and, not least, in *Caché*.

For Laplanche, the unconscious is constituted from the residues of attempts to translate enigmatic signifiers embedded within messages addressed to us by the other.[5] The Laplanchian other refers not to Lacan's abstractly formulated 'Other' but to that actual other, primarily the earliest caretaker, with whom the infant shares its foundational experiences and from whom the infant receives its first communications. If we think of the example given by Laplanche of a child feeding at the breast, a dimension of this experience screened by earlier psychoanalytic understandings, but stressed by Laplanche, is the formative nature for the child of its experiences of the sexuality and desire of the breast-feeding mother or nurse. Aspects of this scenario and this experience remain enigmatic both for the child *and* for the mother, argues Laplanche. As Fletcher explains:

> [t]he messages directed towards the infant are enigmatic, not just because the infant has no access to a code to determine their meaning, or because they outstrip its capacities for understanding, but because, compromised by the unconscious wishes of the other, they are opaque to the adult as well. (Fletcher 1999, 12)

Laplanche's description of the process through which the child becomes caught up with these enigmatic messages as a seduction (Laplanche 1989; Fletcher 1999; Fletcher and Stanton 1992) signals the absolute relevance of his writings for trauma theory. Purposively conversing with and revising both the Freud of recovered memory *and* the Freud of the seduction fantasy, Laplanche's 'seduction' refers neither to the child's actual sexual abuse by a parental figure, nor to the child's repressed sexual fantasies concerning the parent but to the infant's entanglement with those enigmatic messages to which it is passively exposed and that it struggles to translate. That these translations will *always* remain partial and incomplete is a premise of the seduction theory that begins to converse with and unsettle trauma theory. Laplanche introduces us to a world of interminable translation – interminable because, as Fletcher explains, 'the child's attempt to substitute a signifier or signifying sequence of its own, for the enigmatic signifier or message of the other, always leaves something untranslated; ... the *à traduire*, the yet-to-be-translated' (Fletcher 1999, 16). The Laplanchian unconscious is formed neither from the traces of inadmissible sexual fantasies nor from the imprint of unacknowledgeable encounters with actual adult seducers; it is constituted neither from fantasy nor from dissociated reality but from what remains untranslatable in the enigmatic messages it receives from the other. For Laplanche, the ego is formed in this process of translating these earliest messages (Caruth 2001, 36). Later traumas (where Laplanche uses the term) come to be experienced from the perspective of these enigmatic messages. But this is *not* to say that the meanings given to traumas are derived simply from the past. Laplanche's concept of 'afterwardsness' (Fletcher 1999, esp. 261ff.; Fletcher and Stanton 1992, 217–27; Caruth 2001) describes a process of translation that brings forwards *and* refers back to the earliest residues of translation, continuously attempting to re-translate the untranslated in revised terms.

At a stroke, Laplanchian seduction theory – Laplanche frequently substitutes the term seduction, where an interlocutor has referred to trauma[6] – destabilizes trauma theory's sometimes problematic[7] understandings of temporality and experience. If trauma theory posits a traumatic temporality of belatedness or latency, suggesting that trauma holds the present captive to a dissociated or unrepresentable past, seduction theory posits, rather, a temporality of afterwardsness – a synthesis of deferred action with 'after-the-event' understanding (Caruth 2001, 11–23) prompted by those enigmatic messages from the other, and by 'what is radically not known, both at the beginning, and later' (Caruth 2001, 18). On the question of traumatic experience, seduction theory moves us some way from trauma theory's emphasis either on the actuality or on the experienced actuality of traumatic events. 'Why do I speak of translation and not of interpretation?' Laplanche asks, before responding that '[i]nterpretation may mean that you interpret some factual situation. Translation means that there is no factual situation that can be translated. If something is translated, that's already a message' (Caruth 2001, 108). That this understanding extends even to those experiences that are regarded, by trauma theory, as overwhelming and unrepresentable traumas is confirmed when Laplanche, responding to Caruth's direct questions about how he conceives of traumatic events, takes up the example of the recent Mexican earthquake, commenting:

> I mean that, ultimately, a trauma like that may be – and this is very strange – in consonance with something like a message. After all, even an earthquake could be taken in as a message. Not just something that is factual, but something that means something to you. (Caruth 2001, 51)

Emphasizing, as he does, the formative impact of those first messages from the other, the temporality of the translations and re-translations that, for Laplanche, constitute the essence of psychical life, confound our binaries of past or future orientation. 'I see the translation drive', Laplanche explains,

> as the root of the temporalisation of the human being, and I consider its driving force to lie not in the translator but in the internal, non-temporal, simultaneous disequilibrium of the enigmatic message, which supplies the force of a 'to be translated'. (Fletcher 1999, 190)

Laplanche's theory of enigmatic signification radically revises psychoanalytic understandings of temporality by eschewing both a radical determinism of the present by the past and the radical relativism of hermeneutics' construction of the past by the present. With its emphasis on even the 'primary moment ... as a proto-understanding' (Fletcher 2003, 7), and on the equivalence of traumas to enigmatic messages, Laplanchian theory opens the door to a new approach to 'the hidden', understood not as the trace of a past traumatic event or experience but as the *à traduire*, the signifier of an otherness that remains opaque both to the sender of the enigmatic message as well as to its addressee. This 'hidden' resists localization either to a past of primary seduction, or to those present agitations of re-translation (even this formulation risks too temporally linear a representation of the interweaving of deferred action and retrospection constitutive of Laplanchian translation). It is a 'hidden' that resists, also, as we've seen, the interpretative strategies of classical psychoanalysis. What, then, can Laplanchian seduction theory contribute to our understanding of *Caché*'s 'hidden'?

As several critics have noted, *Caché* was one of those films that 'gets you talking, and keeps you talking for days afterwards' (Cousins 2007, 223; see also Ezra and Sillars 2007a, 211; Gilroy 2007, 233). The film's plotting and narration provoke the spectator to countless acts of revision, as it prompts, in subsequent scenes or shots, 're-translations' of the story the film has previously seemed to tell. Take the opening and much discussed credits sequence, for instance. A long shot, objective motionless camerawork framing an urban scene – a house, faint sounds of street life match diegetic sound with space, through certain sounds – a door closing? – seem to belong to an interior, rather than an exterior shot. A cyclist crosses the camera's field – a woman leaves the house. To all intents and purposes an establishment shot introducing the spectator to the film's fictional world – not 'classical', for the shot is of markedly and discomfortingly longer duration than might be expected, and the sound a little too ambiguous – perhaps an 'art film', we might think. And on the sound track: '*Alors*? [Well?]', asks a male voice, to be responded to in the irritated tone of a female interlocutor with '*rien* [nothing]'. Then – 'where was it?' and the response – 'in a plastic bag on the porch'. And a cut to the same house at night – a man coming out and looking around, a woman emerging behind him – before back to the house in daylight. But then, in mid-frame, the familiar distorting lines across the screen of a fast-forwarded video-tape disrupt our understanding, prompting us to re-translate what we had been lulled into assuming was the opening up, by an apparent establishment sequence, of the diegetic space of an illusory 'real world' that we now re-translate as the screening of a video.

Secrets, intromission and the hidden

'I hate this word "applied"', exclaims Laplanche (Fletcher and Stanton 1992, 34):

> applied means you find all the information somewhere and you just apply it like you apply something to skin ... psychoanalysis 'outside the walls', or outside the cure, should have the ambition to have findings of its own: that is, to find other methods, for, as I have said, the main method you don't have, because you don't have a person to give you free associations. But you have many other ways: for instance, trying to define the effect of the work ... This is not just applied, because after all you have to invent. (Laplanche, in Fletcher and Stanton 1992, 34–5)

Thus Laplanche challenges and assists cultural theory. But he goes further still, overturning our previous understandings of the relations that psychoanalysis constructs between individual psychical life and culture. In place of an approach that 'applies' to culture a psychoanalysis rooted in clinical work with individuals, Laplanche proposes that culture might best be conceived of *itself* in the terms of enigmatic signification. 'One of the major dimensions of the cultural domain', suggests Laplanche, is

> this provocation by the enigma of the other. The cultural message, the artistic 'creation' is situated beyond a purely pragmatic aim ... It is in its depths, provoked by the 'nameless public', 'scattered into the future', who will receive (or not) this message in a bottle. (Fletcher 1999, 111)

Speaking of the relation between clinical and cultural analysis, Laplanche goes further, suggesting that clinical analysis may be, in a sense, secondary to the analysis of culture:

> We wish to transpose the model of clinical transference onto what lies beyond it ... but maybe transference is already, 'in itself', outside the clinic. If one accepts that the fundamental dimension of transference is the relation to the enigma of the other, perhaps the principal site of transference, 'ordinary' transference, before, beyond, or after analysis, would be the multiple relation to the cultural, to creation, or, more precisely, to the cultural message. (Fletcher 1999, 222)

If culture in its entirety is constituted by Laplanchian theory as a field of enigmatic signification, then I want to propose, provisionally, that *Caché* might be regarded both as a film *about* and as a film *of* enigmatic signification.[8] If we say that the process of enigmatic signification, translation and re-translation is figured by the characters' responses to the intrusions and provocations of those video-tapes and drawings, then we can say that *Caché* is literally 'about', or a metanarrative of, Laplanchian seduction theory. If we wanted to substantiate this claim further, we could point to Georges's job as a TV literary review chat show host and Anne's as a literary editor – there is a surfeit of evidence to support a reading of *Caché* as a film about the attempt to translate and re-translate enigmatic signifiers. But if we focus on the enigmas surrounding the subjectivity or objectivity of the video-camera and the film's final shot's apparent suggestion of a friendship between

Majid's son and Georges's and Anne's son, another perspective emerges. The foregrounding of those aspects of the film that have provoked spectators into that endless talking 'for days afterwards', as commented upon by Cousins and others, produces a differently nuanced account of *Caché*. From this perspective, *Caché* emerges as a film that is both 'of' as well as 'about' enigmatic signification – a film that literalizes, perhaps, the agitating properties of the enigmatic signifier, initiating the spectatorial quest for that which the enigmatic signifier 'hides'.

But I said that I'd only provisionally propose that we read *Caché* as a film that is both 'of' and 'about' enigmatic signification. Now – true to the spirit of Laplanche, and provoked by all that my initial proposal leaves untranslated, I find I must re-visit the enigma that *Caché* poses for me.

If culture *is* a field of enigmatic signification – its messages addressed to a 'nameless future public' – what does it mean to find oneself drawn to discuss a particular film *in the very terms* of enigmatic signification – what does it mean to read *Caché* as enigmatography? I've said that there is almost a *surfeit* of evidence to support this reading but there is also much that remains to be seen. Attention to those elements that remain redundant to a reading of *Caché* as 'simple' enigmatography may help us to remain *alive* to what *remains* hidden in *Caché*.

In the opening sequence, this redundancy extends through a range of filmic elements. At the level of *mise-en-scène*, it includes the scene's bleached-out tonality and colour, Georges's and Anne's dowdy appearance and baggy, ill-fitting clothes and Georges's slumped posture. In the field of performance, elements that fall outside my previous reading include the staccato and inexpressive delivery of dialogue, together with a sense of conversation 'going nowhere', of stalling, and of the frequent recurrence of 'unresponsive responses' such as '*alors*?' or '*quoi*?', accompanied by shrugs of irritated, impatient incomprehension. Overall, the impression this scene – and much of the rest of the film – conveys, is one of interruption, stagnation, immobility, stalling. Though we might read all of this in terms of *Caché*'s evocation of an anxious middle class, claustrophobically barricaded within a postmodern, postcolonial world of inescapable surveillance, surfaces, screens, and, one might add, affectlessness, what is most striking is the contrast evident between the endless conversations prompted by the film and its evocation of deadlock, impasse, blockage – of a certain deadness. A surfeit of evidence first drew me to associate *Caché* with enigmatic signification. But perhaps that surfeit was itself symptomatic – perhaps it is only when a machine goes wrong that it draws itself to our attention.

Included in Laplanche's account of psychical life as the translation and re-translation of enigmatic 'signifiers' is a discussion of the more pathological variant of these processes:

> Implantation [of enigmatic signifiers] is a process which is common, everyday, normal or neurotic. Beside it, as its pathological variant, a place must be given to intromission. While implantation allows the individual to take things up actively, at once translating and repressing, one must try to conceive of a process which blocks this, short-circuits differentiation of the agencies in the process of their formation, and puts into the interior an element resistant to all metabolisation. (Fletcher 1999, 136)

Laplanche's account appears to describe a process affecting the very formation of the psyche – a process that must therefore be taken to occur in early infancy, rather than one that can be located within culture, conceived of as acting upon, or acting 'like' an already 'formed' psyche. Yet *Caché*'s 'arrested' dialogue, with its blockages, its '*alors*?' and its '*riens*', its multiply static qualities of camera and of bodies, its colourlessness, its lack of 'life', make me wonder about the film's – and culture's – relations with intromission rather than, or better, as well as, with translation.

Can intromission, understood in Laplanche's terms, be associated with the cultural? Or is the concept's use to be restricted only to processes occurring in early childhood? As we've seen, at points, Laplanche's account of the psyche/culture relation seems to overturn the psychoanalytic view of culture as a *secondary* field within which the primary processes of infancy are repeated, revised, or worked through. Laplanche announces, for instance, that

> [t]he biological individual, the living human, is saturated from head to foot by the invasion of the cultural, which is by definition intrusive, stimulating and sexual. How has analysis been able to lose sight of this truth, which was ready to emerge alongside the theory of seduction? (Fletcher 1999, 225)

As we have also seen, Laplanche has advised the cultural critic, particularly where the effects of a text are in question, that 'you have to invent' (Fletcher and Stanton 1992, 35). Taking courage from Laplanche's own counsel, I will step further, allowing my intuitive sense of *Caché*'s intromissive qualities – of *mise-en-scène*, of performance, and more – to lead me to my own response to the enigma of *Caché*'s 'hidden'. For, if we allow that something akin to intromission *may* bear upon culture,[9] then Laplanche can help us to see that what is 'hidden' in *Caché* – or, perhaps better put, the absence around which *Caché* pivots – is that of 'the hidden' itself.

In his sharply argued dismissal of *Caché*, Paul Gilroy has reminded us that: '[s]ince Fanon, we have known that colonialism brings out the worst in everyone it touches' (Gilroy 2007, 235). For Gilroy, *Caché* fails because 'it offers precious little beyond that simple insight' (235). Contrasting *Caché*'s aestheticism, and even its colonialist collusion (234), with an imagined cinema that might do better justice to the dead and to the complexity of postcolonial politics, Gilroy comments that:

> When the Majids of this world are allowed to develop into deeper, rounded characters endowed with all the psychological gravity and complexity that is taken for granted in ciphers like Georges, we will know that substantive progress has been made towards breaking the white, bourgeois monopoly on dramatizing the stresses of lived experience in this modernity. (234)

As we can see, though Gilroy acknowledges the 'horrible shallowness of the adult Georges' (235), Gilroy's hostility (233) towards *Caché* is provoked by the film's silence concerning Majid's motivations, its depthless view of his character, its refusal to grant him an inner life. What would it mean – what would it do to our understanding of *Caché* – to re-read Gilroy's critique in Laplanchian terms? As we have seen, for Laplanche, coming to life is constituted through the attempt to translate enigmatic signifiers – signifiers that come to us bearing the hidden and untranslatable traces of the otherness *of* the other. In place of 'deepness' and 'roundedness', the Laplanchian lexicon would refer, rather, to a 'hollow[ness] in the object' (Scarfone 2003, 76). Referring to the mother, and speaking for the infant, Scarfone explains that what seduces

> ... is that *other thing* which emanates from her, but which *isn't her and which troubles me.* The source object of my drives, the object of my desires, is what is beyond my mother; it is what makes my mother hollow, which makes her other, which gives her a complexity, a thickness, or a depth; which makes her psychically *real.* This is a reality posed from the beginning in its *negativity.* (72; final emphasis added)

As we have observed, Guy Austin's analysis of *Caché* linked the child drawings with the belated emergence of Georges's trauma and guilt, before concluding that 'what remains almost entirely unspoken ... is the trauma suffered by Majid' (Austin 2007, 534). When I first read Austin's conclusion, I knew that it simply didn't come anywhere close to my own sense of the film but I knew I needed to return to Majid and my sense of there being something that I had yet to understand about the *uncompromising* aspect of that suicide scene.

Discussing with a friend my *own* stalling around *Caché*'s relations with enigmatic signification and intromission and my sense of this being linked with colonial and postcolonial violence – the dirty war, the banlieu riots – as well as with Majid and that *terrible* suicide scene, enacted before either Georges or the spectator can in any way prepare themselves for it, my friend said 'that's it – Majid's suicide – it's *in your face*'. And that is 'it' – the violence of France's colonial past, re-translated in continuingly violent times with its unmetabolized kernal not 'just' borne, here, by the body of the 'other', Majid, but violently and desperately enacted in Georges's and in the spectator's face. But what does it mean for something to be 'in your face' and how might this be linked with *Caché*'s 'hidden'?

Critics of *Caché* have associated the violence of France's Algerian war and, in particular, the October massacre, with a 'hidden' (Ezra and Sillars 2007b, 215) or 'public' (Khanna 2007, 240) '*secret*': the tapes, argue Ezra and Sillars,

> appear to show little more than the unexceptional surface of their everyday lives, yet they serve to unlock a *secret from the past*, a *hidden story* of colonial suffering – and in doing so expose the structures of oppression and complicity on which their lives are built. (215; emphasis added)

In this way, criticism points to the state's disavowal of the brutality by means of which colonialist dominance is maintained. In an elaboration of Laplanche's concept of intromission, Dominique Scarfone explores how Laplanchian psychoanalysis might approach the idea of the secret. In the primary scene, enigmatic signification involves the sending by the adult to the child of a message described by Scarfone as 'compromised'.[10] An important feature of this process is that 'the adult of the compromised message must also be the adult who allows a compromise-formation ... "translat[ing] for the infant", while transmitting to the child that which is destined to remain enigmatic' (Scarfone 2003, 73). It is through this process that the reality-testing to which Scarfone refers – 'a reality posed from the beginning in its *negativity*' (72) comes into play. In contrast to this process, Scarfone describes a scenario where 'there are things about which the future psychotic is not allowed to exercise his autonomous thinking'. But, continues Scarfone, 'for this prohibition to be effective, the forbidden things cannot be identified' (74). This process, associated by Scarfone with that of intromission and with the transmission of signifiers that are 'enigmatic certainly, but *without compromise*' (73), is constituted through the violence not of the message but of its sender (74). If implantation produces, in the receiver, the capacity to metabolize 'the hidden', and, in so doing, to touch upon the 'negative reality' of the otherness of the other – a reality that can be sensed but not translated – in intromission, by contrast, '[A] *void* is ... created in the subject's thinking, soon filled in by delusional thoughts' (73–4).

Scarfone's account of the delusions and paranoia resulting from the violence of intromission brings us back to *Caché*. Describing the effects of violent intromission in terms that could constitute an account of the film's aesthetics, its themes and its central couple, Scarfone states that:

> [p]aranoid hypervigilance seems to me to translate this state of affairs. The feeling of transparency in relation to others, the delusion of observation ... maybe as a direct expression of the non-differentiation of the psychical agencies ... or else as a projection of its own permanent observation of the movements of the always menacing other. (75)

With that latter possibility, Scarfone opens the door, I suggest, to a reading of culture – and of *Caché* – in the terms of intromission. But what is the *difference* between a colonialist 'public secret' and colonialist intromission? This is a difference that hinges on the question of violence and 'the hidden'. If the colonial 'public secret' can be specified, as we have repeatedly seen, in the terms of a guilty violence associated with the hidden traumas of its perpetrators and its victims, intromission's violence is of a very different order, for what its message without compromise forecloses – what it hides – is what is hidden within and by the enigmatic message: 'the reality of the other as other' (Scarfone 2003, 76), both to themselves and to 'us'.

Caché fails, Gilroy tells us, because it offers little beyond the insight that 'colonialism brings out the worst in everyone it touches' (235), but colonialism's effects *upon* others are hardly uniform or equal. This is a reality that we can take from the message *without compromise* of Majid's dreadful suicide – a suicide that constitutes, on the terms I have been proposing, a tragic but powerful response to colonialist intromission's effects on the colonized. But perhaps the film goes further, offering the spectator something more than this disturbing vision. With its paradoxical evocation of all that cannot be felt or known, *Caché* transmits to us a sense of what happens when the hidden *is* hidden, but also the beginnings of a glimpse *of* a hidden, the absence of which has, one might say, animated the film; a hidden destined *never* to be known. Perhaps this is what we begin to talk about, but also fail to see, when we seek out, as so many have done, what it is that *Caché* 'hides': we, *Caché*'s spectators, are provoked not by a hidden that can be known, located, specified, but by the glimmer of an *à traduire*, an intimation that *could* animate a different future.

Acknowledgements

With heartfelt thanks to Amal Treacher for sharing with me her profoundly helpful insights about *Caché* at critical moment in the writing of this paper. I am also very grateful to Magdalena Zolko for drawing my attention to Laplanche's explicit use of the term 'hidden' and to John Fletcher for his encouragement and for pointing me in very useful directions. The research drawn on in this article was made possible by an award from the Arts and Humanities Research Council (UK)'s Research Leave Scheme, for which I am very grateful.

Notes

1. For a longer discussions of trauma theory, see Radstone (2007) and Hodgkin and Radstone (2003). For a thoughtful and provocative recent essay collection on theories of trauma, see Ball (2007).
2. On 17 October 1961 a peaceful demonstration by supporters of Algeria's National Liberation Front (FLN) was violently put down by the police. Many of the protestors were murdered, and their bodies flung into the Seine. Jim House and Neil MacMaster's recent book *Paris 1961* (2006) explores the memorial legacy of this atrocity and Libby Saxton's essay on *Caché* (2007) also engages with the film's relations with this event.
3. A scene that has been associated by one commentator with Haneke's acknowledgement of cinema's inevitable limitations as a 'process of thought' (Beugnet 2007, 231).
4. For useful discussions of trauma cinema see Kaplan and Wang 2004 and Walker 2005.
5. For a clear introduction to Laplanche's writings on enigmatic signification, see Fletcher (1992, 1999).
6. This is particularly noticeable in his interview with Cathy Caruth (2001) in which Laplanche often responds to Caruth's questions about trauma by elaborating his theory of seduction.
7. Elsewhere I have written at greater length on the question of trauma theory's blind spots and problematic aspects, see particularly Radstone (2001, 2007).

8. Here we need to distinguish this approach from film theory's routine designation of the questions that propel narrative forwards, provoking spectatorial curiosity or suspense as 'the enigma'. Here, we are dealing with an enigma that provokes but cannot be defined – or analysed – in these terms, an enigma that may extend to the ontology of the image.
9. I am aware that this proposition requires a fuller elaboration than space permits. A longer version of this essay will appear in my forthcoming book, *Getting over Trauma.*
10. Scarfone refers to several linked meanings of the term compromised: the message is a compromise between two parties, as well as being compromised by the unconscious of the adult (Scarfone 2003, 73).

References

Austin, Guy. 2007. Drawing trauma: Visual testimony in *Caché* and *J'ai 8 ans*. *Screen* 48, no. 4: 529–36.

Ball, Karyn. 2007. *Traumatizing theory: The cultural politics of affect in and beyond psychoanalysis.* New York: Other Press.

Beugnet, Martine. 2007. Blind spot. *Screen* 48, no. 2: 227–31.

Caruth, Cathy. 1992. *Unclaimed experience: Trauma, narrative and history.* Baltimore: Johns Hopkins University Press.

———, ed. 1995. *Trauma: Explorations in memory.* Baltimore: Johns Hopkins University Press.

———. 2001. An interview with Jean Laplanche. *Postmodern Culture* 11, no. 2. http://pmc.iath.virginia.edu/text-only/issue.101/11.2caruth.txt. 1-142 (numbers refer to numbered points rather than pages).

Cousins, Mark. 2007. After the end: Word of mouth and *Caché*. *Screen* 48, no. 2: 223–6.

Dendy Films/Madman Films. 2005. *Hidden*. Australia. DVD jacket notes.

Ezra, Elizabeth, and Jane Sillars. 2007a. Introduction to *Caché* dossier. *Screen* 48, no. 2: 211–3.

———. 2007b. *Hidden* in plain sight: Bringing terror home. *Screen* 48, no. 2: 215–21.

Felman, Shoshana, and Dori Laub. 1992. *Testimony: Crises of witnessing in literature, psychoanalysis and history.* New York: Routledge.

Fletcher, John. 1992. The letter to the unconscious: The enigmatic signifier in the work of Jean Laplanche. In Fletcher and Stanton 1992, 93–120.

———. 1999. Introduction: Psychoanalysis and the question of the Other. In *Jean Laplanche: Essays on otherness*, ed. John Fletcher, 1–52. Warwick studies in European philosophy. London and New York: Routledge.

———. 2003. Recent developments in the general theory of primal seduction. *New Formations* 48 (Winter): 5–25.

Fletcher, John, and Martin Stanton, eds. 1992. *Jean Laplanche: Seduction, translation and the drives.* Trans. Martin Stanton. London: Psychoanalytic Forum, Institute of Contemporary Arts.

Gilroy, Paul. 2007. Shooting crabs in a barrel. *Screen* 48, no. 2: 233–5.

Hancke, Michael. 2005. Dendy Films/Madman Films, Australia. Notes from inside DVD jacket.

Hodgkin, Katharine, and Susannah Radstone. 2003. Introduction to 'Remembering suffering: Trauma and history'. In *Contested pasts: The politics of memory*, ed. Katharine Hodgkin and Susannah Radstone, 97–103. London and New York: Routledge. Re-published as *The politics of memory: Contested pasts* (New Brunswick: Transaction, 2005).

House, Jim, and Neil MacMaster. 2006. *Paris 1961: Algerians, state terror and memory.* Oxford and New York: Oxford University Press.

Kaplan, E. Ann. 2005. *Trauma culture: The politics of terror and loss in media and literature.* New Brunswick, NJ: Rutgers University Press.

Kaplan, E. Ann, and Ban Wang, eds. 2004. *Trauma and cinema: Cross-cultural explorations*. Hong Kong: Hong Kong University Press.
Khanna, Ranjana. 2007. From Rue Morgue to Rue des Iris. *Screen* 48, no. 2: 237–44.
Laplanche, Jean. 1989. *New foundations for psychoanalysis*. Trans. David Macey. Cambridge: Basil Blackwell.
Lebeau, Vicky. 2009. The arts of looking: D.W. Winnicott and Michael Haneke. *Screen* 50, no. 1: 35–44.
Mecchia, Giuseppina. 2007. The children are still watching us: *Caché*/Hidden in the folds of time. *Studies in French Cinema* 7, no. 2: 131–41.
Radstone, Susannah. 2001. Social bonds and psychical order: Testimonies. *Cultural Values* 5, no. 1: 59–78. Re-printed in Ball 2007, 101–26.
———. 2007. Trauma theory: Contexts, politics, ethics. *Paragraph* 30, no. 1: 9–29.
Saxton, Libby. 2007. Secrets and revelations: Off-screen space in Michael Haneke's *Caché 2005*. *Studies in French Cinema* 7, no. 1: 5–17.
Scarfone, Dominique. 2003. 'It was *not* my mother': From seduction to negation. In Jean Laplanche and the theory of seduction, ed. John Fletcher. *New Formations* 48 (Winter): 69–76.
Walker, Janet. 2005. *Trauma cinema*. Berkeley and Los Angeles: University of California Press.

Torturous dialogues: Geographies of trauma and spaces of exception

Suvendrini Perera

Department of Communication & Cultural Studies, Curtin University, Perth, Australia

How are suffering, damage and disaster produced and made visible across different sites, and how are they made to *count,* to matter? This essay considers certain philosophical, historical and geopolitical coordinates that locate trauma and disaster in the context of the Indian Ocean tsunami of 2004. Trauma in its various significations – the banal, the aesthetic, the philosophical, the medicalized, the political, the pathologized – is an essential form of currency in the torturous dialogues that make, define and delineate the contours of disaster, damage and suffering. These are constitutively *geopoliticized*, as they are racialized and gendered, processes. Trauma is a medium that enables dialogue and exchange; it is eminently transactable, mobile and adaptable in its circulation between the refugee camp and the disaster victims' camp; it ramifies, with uneven meanings and effects, across and between subjects, scenes, sites, practices and relations. This essay considers the geopolitics of the tsunami as a globalized trauma-event and asks how the biopolitics of trauma, as a set of institutionalized practices for managing and ordering the life and health of populations, plays out across the necropolitical terrain of global inequality and in relation to those it locates as bare life.

People are in a hurry to pack their things
And to be shifted to another camp
May be the third or fourth one
Within a month

Trauma and counseling are
The talk of the town

S. Jeysankar, 'Talk of the Town Or City of Batticaloa'

This discussion of the meanings, politics and resonances of the Indian Ocean tsunami of 2004 takes its title from Alain Corbin's analysis of the aesthetic and affective topicality of the shipwreck in eighteenth-century Europe. Corbin's *The Lure of the Sea* traces the emergence of 'a type of pleasure' in the ocean and the ways in which the 'unconscious desires and obsolete emotions' of European publics came to be performed on the 'coastal stage' from the mid-eighteenth century (1994, 282). Although the period of Corbin's study is coextensive with the heyday of maritime expansion, his is a resolutely Eurocentric production. Its attention is turned on the shores of England, France and Italy, despite the tacit acknowledgement that Turner's sea paintings or the shipwreck fictions of the *Tempest* or *Robinson Crusoe* all refer to an oceanic realm that is thoroughly imbricated with the imperial and the global. Corbin's identification of the complex emotions inspired by the spectacle of the shipwreck and the 'dense network of practices' that situate it, however, extends further than the limits of his text. It reveals the emergence of a form of affectivity and of what he calls a 'dramaturgy of feelings', a repertoire of responses associated with conditions of spectatorship on the 'coastal stage' (234–6).

'Towards the middle of the eighteenth century', according to Corbin, 'the shipwreck became the second most evocative figure of catastrophe, after the earthquake, and sensitive souls were moved by any mention of it' (234). Corbin's reference to the earthquake as the *primary* figure of catastrophe is an unspoken reminder of the Lisbon earthquake and tsunami of 1755, a formative event for European modernity to which I will return. The emotional responses to the Lisbon earthquake/tsunami are gathered into what Corbin calls the 'rhetoric of pity' associated with the shipwreck (234), one that developed out of the form of spectatorship that characterized this period. Many shipwrecks occurred within sight of land, from where 'the spectators could ... watch the tragedy unfold from the shore and hear the cries and prayers of the survivors' (234). Yet the watching crowds

> did not consider the shore as merely a place from which to view the sublime anger of the elements; they also experienced it as a vast stage surrounded by the headlands, with the infinite expanse of water as a backdrop. Contemplating nature's excesses created the dramaturgy of feelings. There gestures of farewell, nostalgic posturing ... and especially the horror of the shipwreck could be easily staged. (236)

In the theatre of coastal catastrophe spectators too became actors, performing a repertoire of emotions, through words, cries and gestures, so that '[b]etween those who were perishing and those who were watching, torturous dialogues could sometimes develop' (235). Corbin's description of the shore as a theatre from which the 'sublime anger of the elements may be viewed' merges the aesthetic sublime of Burke with the Kantian understanding of the sublime as a moment in which the viewing subject achieves a transcendence over the awe and terror of nature.

In this essay I suggest that there are a number of ways in which the 2004 tsunami restages Corbin's torturous dialogues in a contemporary global arena, dialogues that are echoed, amplified and refracted by the technologies that enable direct and indirect spectatorship. Characterized by conditions of desperate asymmetry and elemental disparity, these torturous exchanges are marked by interruption, distortion and mutual unintelligibility between shore and sea, between here and there; between those who perish in the disaster and those who, in acting as spectators and witnesses, also achieve a form of mastery over it. In these tortuous dialogues, the tsunami as sublime spectacle is both linked to and distinguished from other scenes and associations that are enabled, magnified and resignified by new exchanges on the coastal stage.

In effect what Corbin brings into focus in the spectacle of the shipwreck is one of the constituent aspects of Western modernity: the turning of the world into picture and representation. Even in the context of the most 'ungovernable' of disasters (such as the storm or the tsunami) nature is rendered into a picture that at once domesticates nature by *enframing* it and, simultaneously, guarantees, through this process of enframing, the position of the spectator who watches the drama unfold from the safety of the shore or, as discussed below, as the magisterial viewer of a 'wall of screens' (Natali 2006, 100–1). The Heideggerian concept of enframing is a term that not only signifies the 'construction of a type of framework through which something is transmuted into an object of knowledge and thereby made intelligible, but ... a term which underscores the process by which something is summoned, ordered, objectified and made "calculable in advance"' (Perera and Pugliese 1998, 84, quoting Heidegger 2007, 21).

In an eloquent essay written shortly after the 2004 tsunami, Asma Abbas makes a critical point that is often lost in moments of emergency and crisis where the pressures to feel, respond and act can be overwhelming:

> How a disaster is ascertained, named, defined and assessed involves historically sanctioned processes of representation and translation ... The question of suffering – how to experience it, accost it, and respond to it – has repeatedly proven that the concepts and categories of dominant philosophical, religious, political, economic, hence ethical, discourses are not passive mediators between our intellect and the world, but actively construct the way we sense it in the first place ... Asking the question of how we sense and attend, and how our senses, access, and attention are themselves sculpted, may disarm us by forcing us to acknowledge our complicity in making, defining, and producing suffering, damage, and disasters in the way we do. (Abbas 2005)

Processes of conceptualization, representation and translation are central to the question of suffering: 'how to experience it, accost it, and respond to it'. How are suffering, damage and disaster produced and made visible across different sites, and how are they made to *count*, to matter? Trauma in its various significations – the banal, the aesthetic, the philosophical, the medicalized, the political, the pathologized – is an essential form of currency in the torturous dialogues that make, define and delineate the contours of disaster, damage and suffering. These are constitutively *geopoliticized*, as they are racialized and gendered, processes of exchange. In Sivagnanam Jeysankar's poem above, trauma is the 'talk of the town' between the aid organizations, volunteers and media agencies – whether from Colombo or the global North – that flood the shattered east coast city of Batticaloa, like a 'second tsunami', and its inhabitants, the subjects of trauma, shunted endlessly between the camps they lived in last month or last year as refugees of the war and the new camps for tsunami survivors (Jeysankar 2005).

Trauma is a medium that enables dialogue and exchange; it is eminently transactable, mobile and adaptable in its circulation between the refugee camp and the disaster victims' camp; it ramifies, with uneven meanings and effects, across and between subjects, scenes, sites, practices and relations. What are the geopolitics of the tsunami as a globalized trauma-event? Or, more precisely, how does the biopolitics of trauma, as a set of institutionalized practices for managing and ordering the life and health of populations, play out across the necropolitical terrain of global inequality and in relation to those it locates as bare life? Trauma is a discourse of multiple significations and I do not mean to deny in posing this question that the naming and identification of trauma is of unquestionable importance for many who have suffered its effects, including those affected by the tsunami. What I pursue here are certain philosophical, historical, geopolitical coordinates that locate trauma, disaster and the tortuous dialogues across the various geographies and geoimaginaries in which the tsunami is located – elemental imaginaries of land and sea; geographies of distance and proximity, danger and disaster, aid and capital; of exception and bare life, terror and the sublime. The final section of the essay turns to how these torturous dialogues of trauma and geography, disaster and geopolitics, play out in Australian responses to its surrounding region. The discussion is grounded in responses to the tsunami in and around the town of Batticaloa in eastern Sri Lanka, a place that I have returned to at different stages of my life since childhood, and where I spent some weeks a short while after the tsunami. I begin, then, with some stories of this place, Batticaloa.

'On the border of some human rights violation'

In a tiny, hastily rebuilt restaurant, across from a beach piled high with rubble, in a landscape scattered with ruins of smashed buildings and the remains of coconut trees blighted by salt water, a group of male Muslim community leaders from Kalmunai, many of whom had lost close family and belongings in this, one of the worst affected small towns around Batticaloa, insisted on treating me to a banquet. It was in the middle of Ramazan, and none of them could eat a morsel, or even take a sip of water. But plates piled high with vegetable buriyani, chicken, eggs and mint sambol were placed before me. To forestall the embarrassment that they knew I would experience in eating alone, my hosts had invited another Jaffna Tamil woman, a Hindu not bound by the fast, to sit and eat with me. As I ate, with relish for the care my hosts had shown for me, they talked to me about the events of the last weeks and months. Listening to their stories I remembered a reflection made by another researcher about how recounting the experience of the 1978 cyclone in Batticaloa had enabled survivors to articulate other, unspeakable experiences of war and violence (Lawrence 2003). One terror shading into another, war and tsunami soon became interwoven in our talk.

Batticaloa in 2005 is a raw and fevered place. The dust of wrecked buildings and new construction mingles with fumes from four wheel drives bearing NGO logos and army vehicles transporting troops to and from the 'uncleared areas' (the territory of the Liberation Tamil Tigers of Tamil Eelam [LTTE]). Sharing the broken road with tanks and signs warning of unexploded mines along the way are tourist coaches. A source mentions that in the more scenic areas of the east in these post-tsunami months, 'Buses with tourists drive along the coasts handing out aid (anything from shoes to toys to toiletries)' (Dieltiens 2005). Between 2002 and 2007 the 25-year war was in a state of official truce.[1] In 2005, in the months after the tsunami, travel between the east and the capital city, Colombo, is easier than in previous years, but the marks of war are everywhere evident in scarred and limping bodies, the gouged out buildings and ever-present barricades and checkpoints. The war in the east is not only the official war between the LTTE and the Sinhala majoritarian state; there is also the war on the people by the LTTE with forced conscriptions of children and the infliction of other forms of terror on dissidents; there is the regional war in which a leader from the east, Karuna, heads a breakaway faction at war with the LTTE. And a bitter recent history of massacre and counter-massacre has split Tamil and Muslim communities here apart despite hundreds of years of sharing a language and a way of life rooted in a unique topography of interlinked coastal villages.

After the chain of massacres, after the rapes in temples and at well sides after the taking of children for the war, after the burning paddy fields, after the days of bodies set aflame at junctions and of hooded informers at the crossroads, Batticaloa is a city of no-go zones and partitions. There is now a local Tamil administration and a Muslim administration, a Tamil Hospital and a Muslim Hospital, a Tamil University and a Muslim University. There is fear on the streets every day. Mysterious killings and abductions happen all over town in ones and twos in these days of the truce.

The tsunami brought scores of new NGOs to this divided and damaged place. Aid money poured in with them. There is intense competition for their largesse, although many of the tsunami refugees are still in makeshift tents with earth floors that turn to sticky mud when it rains. There are bright new boats on the banks of the lagoon, though they will never sail on it – in their haste the donors failed to check that the hulls were the right sort for these waters. Any vacant building that survived the war and the tsunami now houses an NGO. Anyone in Batticaloa who speaks even minimal English is a 'consultant' to an international NGO. Perhaps this second tsunami has the town in the grip of what Tim Anderson describes as 'aid-trauma', a 'distinct social process [that] begins in a heavily aid-administered country' (Anderson 2008, 9).

The conversations at lunch dwell on how the spirit of the town has changed since the first days of the tsunami: then drowned bodies, identified by distinguishing marks such as the earrings worn by Tamil women, were returned intact to the appropriate villages. Sinhala soldiers risked, and sometimes lost, their lives trying to save Muslim and Tamil children from the waves; households who were themselves going hungry found food for those made destitute. Now, with the return of the state apparatus and the swarming NGOs, divisions between Muslim, Tamil and Sinhala are becoming even more deeply entrenched. People talk about the militarization of the Muslims, and the prospect of not one but two separatist movements, Muslim and Tamil, in this small place. They remind me many times that in Iraq and elsewhere it is Muslims who do the suicide bombing.

My hosts that day did not engage in NGO-bashing, a common-enough activity in Lanka, and one with deep roots in nativist, chauvinist and fundamentalist discourses. Reluctance to tap into these destructive rhetorics restrains many critics of NGO culture. But a young Lankan-American volunteer, Nimmi Gowrinathan, puts into words in her blog the questions that many hesitated to pose in the first months after the tsunami:

> Walking through rows of tents what is striking is not the living conditions which seem to lie on the border of some human rights violation. Rather, it is the similarity between these camps and those that existed last February, and the February before ... Large sums of money flow freely into post-tsunami Sri Lanka. These same funds which are the life blood of relief, reconstruction, and rehabilitation efforts are accessed to sustain arms build ups, military development, and continued violence. The Sri Lankan government may have been war weary in early 2002 when it conceded to a bilateral ceasefire, but it was also bankrupt ... It had neither the funds to continue the armed combat, nor to reconstruct damaged areas and serve their constituencies ... [Today] inflated state bank accounts with minimal regulations have permanently altered the incentive structure for the government to engage in and remain committed to a peaceful solution. (Gowrinathan 2005)

The resumption of the war in 2007, renewed aggression on all sides, a new campaign of bombs in Batticaloa and elsewhere: what is the relationship between the resurgent war and the millions of humanitarian dollars that flowed in with the second tsunami? The effects of humanitarian aid and NGO intervention cannot be isolated from the processes of war. At a deeper level, in more complex ways, the one reinforces the other. As Patricia Lawrence suggested a couple of years before the tsunami, in Batticaloa the 'language of order' employed alike by 'the military apparatus, in the peace process and in some discourses of international non-governmental organizations' all collude in the 'production of killable bodies' (Lawrence 2003, 3). I read Lawrence's comment as a reference to the underlying structure of the camp as a space where the right to save and the right to kill may be exercised alternately or in tandem, as operations of sovereign power over forms of bare life. Refugees who are first identified as oppressed and/or traumatized increasingly constitute contemporary forms of bare life (Agamben 1998; Malkki 1995). In recent years the naming of bodies as oppressed and/or traumatized has authorized and accompanied paired practices of violence and benevolence, as in the war on terror in Afghanistan (Perera 2002; Grewal 2003). Here I consider how the discursive formation of disaster, sometimes in conjunction with that of trauma, contributes to the production of bare life, and explore how the right to save and the right to kill are interrelated modalities through which sovereign power operates over bare life (Žižek 2002).

Disaster, bare life and the sublime

The Lisbon earthquake of 1755, and the tsunami and fire that immediately followed it, caused the death of about a quarter of a million people, prompting unprecedented outpourings of grief, terror, shock and empathy throughout Europe. The Lisbon earthquake was a formative event for Enlightenment philosophy, religion, politics and aesthetics, instigating a number of debates about fundamental questions of good and evil, the nature of the universe and the existence of god; of belief in providence and the possibility of progress. These debates involved some of the major thinkers of the age, including Voltaire, Rousseau and Kant (Nieman 2002; Ray 2004). In *Candide* (subtitled *The Optimist*) published only four years later, in 1759, Voltaire famously satirized belief in providence through the figure of Dr Pangloss, a disciple of Pope and Leibniz, who reiterates the unshakable conviction that all is for the best in the best of all possible worlds, even as he and Candide are shipwrecked off the coast of Lisbon, caught up in the earthquake and witness its trail of death and destruction.

The era of modernity that was inaugurated by the Lisbon earthquake/tsunami, Susan Nieman argues, found its terminus at Auschwitz; for Nieman these two events signify the poles of natural and moral evil in European intellectual history. Nieman argues that the Enlightenment responded to the crisis of belief caused by the Lisbon earthquake by establishing a fundamental distinction between two 'intellectual constellations': between the suffering caused by inexplicable natural disasters – 'acts of god' – and those produced by human actions (Nieman 2002, 2–3). This categorization paved the way for a critical differentiation between the deplorable but unpreventable suffering of 'innocent victims' and that of other subjects. Through this fundamental distinction that 'tells us which suffering was political and which was not', Abbas caustically points out, 'the Enlightenment's responses to Lisbon have left us a legacy of co-opting human suffering by imposing limits on which suffering and which parts of life matter, and on their admission into political discourse' (2005). Articulated in this distinction is a categorical split between 'nature' and the 'political' that effectively erases both their discursively constructed status and their geopolitical imbrications and effects. Such a distinction paves the way also for another founding differentiation that will prove critical in the ensuing era: between those who are the subjects of their own suffering, and those who simply suffer.

Mapped in Agambenian terms, these economies of suffering layer on to zones of bare life as that which lies outside the realm of the political: those deaths for which no one is to be held accountable; indeed, the deaths which do not *count*. This distinction between unpreventable suffering, whether decreed by a providential plan or as a consequence of the inevitable advance of progress, knowledge and civilization, provided the preconditions for the massive death tolls of native populations that would accompany the expansion of the Enlightenment into the dark places of the earth. In Achille Mbembe's terms, these are necropolitical 'location[s] par excellence where the controls and guarantees of judicial order can be suspended – the zone where the violence of the state of exception is deemed to operate in the service of "civilization"' (2003, 24). Here, violence and death are naturalized through an economy of the unavoidable-though-regrettable: the price dark regions must pay for their entry into the grand arena of the historical. The burden of the economy of the 'unavoidable-though-regrettable' brings into focus the Hegelian providential dialectic that justifies colonial expansion as the bringing of civilization even as it rationalizes the violence and death inflicted on native populations.

As a moment of shock followed by recuperation, the Lisbon earthquake leaves its traces simultaneously on the philosophico-aesthetic discourse of the sublime. Kant's *Critique of*

Judgment, Gene Ray argues, is haunted by the Lisbon earthquake, about which Kant as a young man had produced a series of scientific articles. Returning Kant's later writing to the context of the earthquake 'brings back into view a repressed textual burden in Kant's *Critique of Judgment*: the need to silence pessimism' (2004, 10–11). Ray comments on a key passage in the 'Analytic of the Sublime' that depicts the 'tremor' of the imagination before nature's abyss until it is recalled and recovered by reason: 'Kant needed to domesticate those eruptions of the sublime, of which the Lisbon earthquake was exemplary in his own century, in order to neutralize the threat they posed to a myth of progress grounded in natural law and a purported human nature' (11).

The sublime, as a form of overcoming or elevating the power of reason over nature, is another enabling trope of European expansionism. As Joseph Pugliese reveals in a powerful reading that situates this same passage in the context of Kant's other writings, the 'power of reason' that ensures a recovery of the imagination on the very brink of nature's abyss is a racialized attribute, one only available to the European mind. It serves to mark the 'sublime experience as something exclusive to the Western subject' (Pugliese 1999, 27). The sublime, as an effect produced by a complex exercise of imagination and reason achievable only by the Western subject, underwrites the Western advance through the awe-inducing and terrifying theatre of the natural world that it alone is biologically, mentally and materially equipped to confront and master. In the context of this terrifying theatre of sublime trauma as representational and affective spectacle, the Western subject is positioned as both spectator and actor, a benevolent interventionist (as colonizer, missionary, aid organization, or volunteer). In 'White panic or Mad Max and the sublime', Meaghan Morris describes the 'plot of the sublime' with reference to Australian history as

> a scenario in which a dynamic self, normalized white and male, is overwhelmingly threatened by a fearsome power of alterity; freezes in astonishment ... then bounces back with renewed strength and vigor by making sense of the threatening power, while appropriating it some of its force. (1998, 242)

As Kant makes clear, it is this raced ability to make sense of and to appropriate the terrifying alterity of nature that is the essence of the sublime.

The intellectual constellation of natural terror, non-political or unavoidable suffering and the raced category of the sublime inaugurated by the Lisbon earthquake/tsunami meshes with the mapping of colonial geographies as dangerous and inimical. Gregory Bankoff describes how in the production of disasters: 'tropicality', 'development' and 'vulnerability' form part of 'the same essentialising and generalising cultural discourse: one that denigrates large regions of the world as dangerous – disease-ridden, poverty-stricken and disaster-prone; one that depicts the inhabitants of these regions as inferior – untutored, incapable, victims; and that ... reposes in Western medicine, investment and preventive systems the expertise required to remedy these ills' (2002, 29). Yet, Bankoff argues,

> the disproportionate incidence of disasters in the non-Western world is not simply a question of geography. It is also a matter of demographic difference, exacerbated in more recent centuries by the unequal terms of international trade, that renders the inhabitants of less developed countries more likely to die from hazard ... No single term has yet emerged that defines the areas where disasters are more commonplace: the media often sensationalises a certain region as a 'belt of pain' or a 'rim of fire' or a 'typhoon alley', while scientific literature makes reference to zones of 'seismic or volcanic activity' ... or to meteorological conditions such as the El Niño ... Whatever the term, however, there is an implicit understanding that the place in question is somewhere else ... and denotes a land and climate that have been endowed with dangerous and life-threatening qualities. (24)

This somewhere else – 'belt of pain', 'typhoon alley' – is discursively and representationally rendered as *somewhere else* by the very enframing technologies of theatre, screen and spectacle discussed above. Technologies of enframing, and of rendering trauma and disaster into a theatre of the sublime, symbolically mark the line between the 'us' and 'them' that Bankoff underscores. As the responses to Hurricane Katrina in the United States demonstrated, these references to a *somewhere else* map racialized geographies on to spatial demarcations of 'East' and 'West'. Dangerous geographies are geographies of otherness and difference. The enframing technologies that produced geographies of danger simultaneously generate and sustain the illusion between a wild, undomesticated and disease-ridden nature, the locus of bare life, 'out there', in contradistinction to a civilized, scientifically superior and sanitary space that is the privileged home of the West. The sea itself figures among the most dangerous of these othered geographies because of elemental imaginaries of the ocean as a wild and ungovernable space distinct from land, one that is associated in Christian symbology with sin and error (as in the biblical flood).

The bare life located in dangerous geographies, lacking the ability to 'sublimate' their environment, are condemned to an eternal victimhood from which only superior powers of reason, and all the scientific, medical and material power that entails, can attempt to rescue them. At work here, then, are all the familiar violently unequal power relations of colonial power that, on the one hand enable, sustain and reproduce the possibility for strategic providential interventions, rescue missions, and acts of benevolence, while on the other demarcating disposable lives situated within necropolitical domains; marked with the unredeemable imprimatur of bare life. These lives can be either killed with impunity or be abandoned to innumerable forms of letting die.

The bare life that inhabit dangerous geographies, represented as incapable of mastering or overcoming their own environment ('nature'), consequently lack both self-sovereignty and subjecthood. This is the conceptual product of Hegelian dialectics in which, as Mbembe explains in 'Necropolitics', questions of 'becoming subject', sovereignty and death all interlink:

> In transforming nature, the human being creates a world; but in the process, he or she also is exposed to his or her own negativity. Within the Hegelian paradigm, human death is essentially voluntary. It is the result of risks consciously assumed by the subject. According to Hegel, in these risks, the 'animal' that constitutes the human subject's natural being is defeated. (2003, 14)

In geographies of danger – the Third World, the global South, the arc of instability – 'nature' is precisely that which can be neither negated nor transformed ('sublimated') through work and struggle. The inhabitant of the global South, marked by this 'failure', is she or he who consequently cannot overcome their 'animal' status in order to become human/subject and be 'cast into the incessant movement of history' (Mbembe 2003, 14). Their deaths, as in the world of non-human animals, cannot be 'essentially voluntary'; rather, they die the animal death of the creature caught in unmasterable relations of nature.

Within the Hegelian paradigm, mastery and control over the 'biological field … presupposes the distribution of human species into groups, the subdivision of the population into subgroups, and the establishment of a biological caesura between the ones and the others. This is what Foucault labels with the … term racism' (Mbembe 2003, 17). As Mbembe outlines with uncompromising clarity, what such a biological caesura enables is the division of the world into the domain of European juridical order (*Jus publicum Europaeum*) and the domain of unmastered nature and the uncivilized. In this context, the

Jus publicum rapidly assumed 'the form of a distinction between, on the one hand, those parts of the globe available for colonial appropriation and, on the other, Europe itself (where the *Jus publicum* was to hold sway)' (23–4). The centrality of this distinction, in enabling and legitimating the exercise of colonial violence, is brought into sharp focus by Mbembe when he concludes that it is 'crucial in terms of assessing the efficacy of the colony as a terror formation' (24). Mbembe in effect maps out here complex relations of colonial power that intersect along the seemingly unrelated lines of natural disaster, colonial war and terror. In the analysis of Naomi Klein, as I discuss below, these relations are elaborated in the form of a 'shock and awe' model of capitalism.

Terror, trauma and the disasterscape

Naomi Klein's *The Shock Doctrine*, an epic attempt to map the global operations of what she terms 'disaster capitalism', takes its two opening epigraphs from the Old Testament description of Noah's flood and from a now infamous text of military strategy, Harlan Ullman and James Wade's *Shock and Awe: Achieving Rapid Dominance*. Ullman and Wade describe shock and awe as 'actions that create fears, dangers, and destruction that are incomprehensible to the people at large ... or the leadership', specifying that 'Nature in the form of tornadoes, hurricanes, earthquakes, floods, uncontrolled fires, famine, and disease can engender Shock and Awe' (1996, 110). Appropriating and redirecting the terror of nature, Harlan and Ullman advocate 'shock and awe' as a military strategy aimed at achieving 'rapid dominance' over an enemy through the technology of 'brilliance' (1996, xxix). As a strategy designed to produce terror based on spectacular displays of techno-dominance, Shock and Awe is clearly premised on, and mobilizes, the effects of sublime terror as described above.

Ullman and Wade's text, Malini Johar Schueller writes, 'identifies the psychosexual and social coordinates of US imperialism' from Hiroshima and Nagasaki to the present (2007, 169). In *The Shock Doctrine* Klein more precisely maps these coordinates, drawing clear lines of connection between post-Katrina New Orleans and Baghdad in 2002, between Pinochet's Chile and the personal histories of those subjected to CIA-funded experiments of brainwashing and shock treatment. A chapter of Klein's text is devoted to her visit to the fishing village of Arugam Bay, just outside Batticaloa, where she documents the resistance of local communities to the government's proposal to establish a 'buffer zone' that would clear them from the beach while making room for tourist developments designed to transform the region into a 'South Asian Riviera' (Klein 2007, 388).

Klein's central thesis is that disaster capitalism moves into scattered scenes of natural wreckage, war and trauma to flatten or level pre-existing structures and modes of being. For Klein, the 'fundamentalist model of capitalism' represented by Chicago school economics has 'always needed disaster to advance' (2007, 9). The 'disaster capitalism complex' operates through a systematic and/or opportunist reliance on the effects of shock and awe – that is, terror – to reduce either entire populations or isolated subjects to submission. In the state of 'psychological shock or paralysis' induced by a 'traumatic or sub-traumatic experience which explodes, as it were, the world that is familiar to the subject as well as his image of himself in that world', disaster capitalism finds its moment:

> That is how the shock doctrine works: the original disaster – the coup, the terrorist attack, the market meltdown, the war, the tsunami, the hurricane – puts the entire population into a state of collective shock. The falling bombs, the bursts of terror, the pounding winds serve to soften whole societies much as the blaring music and blows in the torture cells soften up prisoners.

> Like the terrorized prisoner who gives up the names of comrades ... shocked societies often give up the things they would otherwise fiercely protect. (Klein 2007, 16–17)

Klein's linkage of a series of disparate landscapes of trauma through the concept of the 'disaster capitalism complex' and the systematic collaboration between governments and global corporations that trade in the business of disaster is utterly compelling. Her analysis deliberately ignores the distinctive emotional and affective responses that are associated with different forms of disaster, and the ways in which these in turn shape the modes in which 'reconstruction' is couched – that is, those responses that usually operate to mask the structural links between disasterscapes. These differing emotional and affective responses pivot on that fundamental, yet untenable, distinction between 'nature' and the 'political' that, as outlined above, Mbembe maps in his theorization of the relations between biopolitics and necropolitics. Situated in this Mbembian context, the populations of the global South who undergo the violence of earthquakes or tsunamis emerge as the 'innocent' traumatized victims of the forces of 'nature' – that wild and undomesticated 'nature' they have failed to master and control. Their trauma is one that is both affectively acknowledged *and*, as Klein makes clear, opportunistically exploited for economic and political reasons. The 'political' trauma of victims of war, in contradistinction to the trauma of the 'innocent' victims of 'natural' disasters, evokes an entirely other response: this politically marked trauma is rarely acknowledged or witnessed, aside from anonymous mass body counts; rather, this is a trauma that is framed by the 'acceptability of putting to death' (Mbembe 2003, 17).

Yet the distinctions between the biopolitical imperative to save and the necropolitical imperative to make or let die are also deeply enmeshed with each other. The Australian columnist Greg Sheridan could write immediately after the tsunami: 'This crisis will re-engage the US with Southeast Asia on a broader front than just the war on terrorism. That is a very good thing' (2005). Sheridan's description of the tsunami as a 'very good thing' for US (and by extension Australian) military power in the region offers a revealing insight into the economy of bare life as that which may be disposed of, acceptably put to death, *regardless* of innocence or guilt, in the service of the sovereign.

Sheridan's remark also reveals the underside of humanitarian aid as an act that cannot be isolated from both biopolitical and necropolitical imperatives. In Batticaloa after the tsunami, the principle that provided the overt rationale for humanitarian aid – that of distributing non-political assistance to innocent victims – in effect proved unworkable. Aid workers on the ground soon discovered the impossibility of operating in an uncontaminated environment. Rather, the humanitarian efforts of NGOs frequently entailed, in the telling words used by one of them, the obligation of 'dining with devils' (Korf 2006). Similarly, Gowrinathan, the volunteer cited above, soon lost any illusion 'that the corrupt world of politics exists in a vacuum detached from pure humanitarian work' (2005). Rather, she found that 'despite attempts to stave off impure intrusions, the war politics of Sri Lanka pervade every action and interaction' while at the same time 'international actors find their arms tied by U.S. imposed directives and stereotypes'. The most confronting effect of this discovery for Gowrinathan was that the realization that 'surviving rural children ... have been left to overcome far greater obstacles than a 30-foot wave' (2005).

For the local inhabitants, such as my hosts in the devastated village of Kalmunai, the realization that the obstacles posed by a 30-foot wave are compounded by and interwoven with other forms of destruction and exploitation is one intimately known and lived every day. Klein's interviews with the fishing communities of Arugam Bay indicate that they, too, comprehended very well the collusive forces of national 'development', transnational capital and colonial histories brought to bear on their immediate scene of natural disaster:

> Open land. In colonial times, it was a quasi-legal doctrine – *terra nullius*. If the land was declared empty or 'wasted', it could be seized and its people eliminated without remorse. In those countries where the tsunami hit, the idea of open land is weighted with this ugly historical resonance, evoking stolen wealth and violent attempts to civilize the natives. Nijam, a fisherman I met on the beach at Arugam Bay, saw no real difference. 'The government thinks our nets and our fish are ugly and messy, that's why they want us off the beach. In order to satisfy the foreigners, they are treating their own people as if they are uncivilized'. Rubble, it seemed, was the new *terra nullius*. (2007, 402)

The term *terra nullius* links the project of disaster capitalism to a history all too familiar to Australians, returning us to another landscape of exception where necropower operates through the fig leaf of legality provided by the doctrine of *terra nullius* (Osuri 2008, 6). At the same time, the image of *terra nullius* as empty, uncultivated land, a spectacle that produces an instant of ontological terror in the colonizing imagination before it is sublimated into action, is a reminder, via Morris's description above, of how the 'plot of the sublime' works in contemporary Australia (1998, 242). Morris further specifies that

> the sublime in ... Australia has had *practical* force as a story elaborated for a particular form of settler colonialism as it extended across the continent, Aboriginal land – and as immigrants from Europe began to think of themselves as 'close' to the vastness of 'Asia'. (242–3)

The 'vastness of Asia', reduced to rubble and waste as a new *terra nullius*, thus confronts Australians with an image of the sublime that is also the restaging of a scene from their colonizing past. As in the *Mad Max* trilogy, this return, mediated by another representational history of Western cinema, is a scene of an unacknowledged 'traumatic sublime' (Natali 2006).

The wash-up

On New Year's Day 2005 Bill Leak's cartoon in the *Australian* was a sardonic offering representing a buried hand emerging from a beach. Against a backdrop of wreckage and broken bodies swirling among the waves, the emaciated brown hand holds up a sign emblazoned with the words 'Happy New Year 2005' and an image of a glowing Harbour Bridge illuminated by Sydney's 'best in the world' fireworks display. The image returns me to Corbin's coastal stage and the tortuous dialogues between shore and sea. In Leak's cartoon, the buried hand, as a universalized symbol of trauma, intersects with the local geographies that allude to the relations of proximity and distance, rhetorical and geographical, between Australia and Asia, and to the illusion of Australia as an island fortress in the Indian Ocean.

At the localized level, the appearance of dead bodies and severed limbs in the shadow of the Harbour Bridge both disorients and reorients. It brings home a scene from a beach elsewhere, scenes where scores of Australians died in the tsunami, as it also recalls the shadow presences of other bodies, such as the drowned of SIEV X, in our waters (Perera 2006). Leak's image reorients its viewers to the geographies that connect them to other coastlines. The tsunami's effects, after all, were felt in the currents off Rottnest Island, not too distant from the location of the 'Interrogating Trauma' conference. Yet the Harbour Bridge and fireworks simultaneously underscore the vast distances of alterity that separate them from us, and that provoke us into displays of conspicuous compassion leading to an insistence on Australia's own distinctive national goodness, decency and superiority (Perera 2005). The 'vastness of Asia', so far and yet so near, so abject as a disaster zone and yet so fearsome in its alterity, is an image that produces anew, re-presents, the awe and terror that it historically induces in the Australian settler imagination; it reminds us of the workings of the 'plot of the sublime' and the 'phobic narratives' with which Australia as a white island in a dangerous geography confronts the proximity of 'Asia'.

In her essay on the imperial imaginary of the 'traumatic sublime' Natali deploys the image of 'a wall of screens in which each video frames an image of somewhere in the world' to suggest the simultaneity of contexts that mediatize global representations of war and disaster:

> Our screen-made memory is full of traumatic 'landscapes with figures' ... satellite images of landscapes, war, territorial scars and scenes of ethnic violence, each of which is erased but quickly returns. The visible earth on our screens is produced by a panoptical 'magisterial gaze' and disseminated on an infinite number of walls filled with screens. (2006, 100–1)

In Natali's analysis, such rapid conflations and seamless transitions between traumatic images of fantasy and live events subsume them within the realm of the spectacle, locating them precisely as *aesthetic effects*, and serving to obscure their materiality and their political causes and consequences. These images merge with the sense of awe and terror induced by the spectacle of US power to become projections of its unacknowledged underside. Such images of carnage and ruin shadow the colonizing imagination as portents of its own destruction; intimations of the end of empire, the unspeakable fears and phobias of dominance. As a number of commentators pointed out, the destruction of the World Trade Center in the 9/11 terror attacks had been already prefigured in dozens of Hollywood disaster spectaculars and in the scenarios of science fiction (Žižek 2002). In Morris's discussion, the *Mad Max* trilogy serves as an Australian version of this type of traumatic sublime where the histories of colonization are restaged in the form of fantastic fictions in which 'we replay our genocidal past as our apocalyptic future' (Morris 1998, 247).

Absorbed into the imaginary of the traumatic sublime, scenes of disaster play out as no more than a seriality of spectacles, enframed within the wall of screens of empire's self-reflections. Their persistent restaging of the hidden fears and phobias of empire, precisely because they remain unacknowledged, cannot be confronted or transformed. Within this panoptical view the fundamental inequalities and the entangled relations that produce the distinction between natural and political terror, while at the same time mystifying the processes of that production and reproduction, remain largely out of the frame.

'Making sublimity material'

Disasters such as the tsunami may inspire horror, grief and outpourings of sympathy, but this very 'garrulousness', to use Abbas's term, is produced by a range of enframing and objectifying technologies that enable us 'to remain silent about the inequality and the multiple ways of dying inflicted upon us by society and civilisation' (2005, 1). One way, then, to articulate the hidden inequalities inscribed in necropolitical ways of letting die and making die is to contest the distinction between political and non-political forms of suffering; or, as Abbas puts it, to acknowledge the political and material forces that underlie seemingly non-political, unavoidable or aestheticized forms of suffering, and to examine the epistemological and representational histories that define our categories of suffering and disaster. Reopening the discursive and intellectual histories that distinguish natural from political disasters would enable us to understand the processes that depoliticize the former, and work instead to make their sublimity material (Abbas 2005, 6).

Still for all, the intellectual constellations that organize the distinction between natural and political, sublime and social, remain deeply entrenched even in discourses that are sceptical about the role of aid and compassion:

> The race for aid and souls is supposedly on between Al Qaeda and USAID. Aid then is meant to construct a warning system for this terrorism as much as it is meant to construct one for the movement of the sea. Another front has opened up in the war on terror, once again fusing humanitarian aid with imperial ambitions, casting aid as the spread of freedom. Will our warning systems ever capture the magical realism of disaster? Will the Harvard political scientist know when to sound the alarm? Will we know which ocean to wiretap? (Roy 2005, 58)

Even as Ananya Roy's essay on the tsunami eloquently critiques the appropriation of humanitarian action into the agenda of militarism, and argues for a closer examination of the political motives that underlie aid initiatives, her words reinforce a divide between natural and political, casting the ocean as a realm untouched by politics, war, or science. The image of 'wiretapping the ocean' is rhetorically powerful, suggesting the futility and the hubris of attempting to control and direct the realm of nature. Yet for all its powerful rhetorical effect, the image redirects attention away from the ways in which the ocean is *already* traversed by political, military, scientific, and legal forces, as it also distracts us from identifying the fundamental political, environmental, and human security failures that channelled the destructive natural power of the tsunami against the most vulnerable populations of the region.

Roy's phrase the 'magical realism of disaster' is more evocative, however, suggesting the surplus or inexpressible excess that attaches to the deepest experiences, that which cannot be rendered in the prosaic terms of reportage or official inquiry. 'Magical realism' is also a term that refers to the surpassing or unmaking of normative classifications and one that exposes the inadequacy of taken-for-granted categories to register predicaments of heightened exigency or extremity. So in Batticaloa, a few months after the tsunami, war and tsunami were not regarded as distinct events but often became interwoven in conversation, shading one form of terror into another.

This is not to suggest that the inhabitants of Batticaloa are somehow insulated from the hegemonic and *naturalized* distinctions that demarcate political and natural disaster, but that these distinctions cannot be sustained at the level of their everyday lives or in the emotional and intellectual ways in which they process and make sense of experiences of extremity and terror. In her (pre-tsunami) research in Batticaloa Patricia Lawrence recounts that its residents often conflated their long experiences of war with memories of a severe cyclone that lashed their villages in 1978. Narrating the experience of the cyclone enabled survivors to articulate other, unspeakable experiences of violence in a climate of fear and intimidation so memories and sensations of one became fused into the other:

> As on many mornings, we could hear the Sri Lankan Air Force bombing Paduvankarai and the Thantahmalai jungle, and there was irritable disagreement among the gathering about whether we were hearing thunder or bombing, even though we could feel the vibrations of the impacts through the straw mats on the sand. (Similarly ... people sometimes saw black smoke on the horizon as cloud formations.) (Lawrence 2000, 188)

Piraliyam, a short film by the Lankan activist and poet sumathy, captures precisely this interpenetration of war and tsunami in its opening sequence as the goddess Kali emerges from the ocean to walk slowly towards a small village on the beach in Batticaloa. Her face is inscrutable. Her blood-red sari billows around her bare feet. Shadowing her is the figure of another woman of death, a uniformed soldier armed with a machine gun. On the white sand, the marks of her heavy boots overlie the footprints made by the goddess of destruction as the two advance steadily on the village.

Such accounts suggest the possibilities of producing images and histories that narrate experiences of the tsunami other-wise – a step towards understanding the biopolitical, necropolitical and economic relations of power in which war and natural disaster are both embroiled, and that are part of their torturous dialogue.

Acknowledgements

The research for this article was conducted with the aid of a Discovery Grant from the Australian Research Council between 2005–2008.

Note

1. In April 2009 the war in Lanka came to an end with the defeat of LTTE forces by the Sri Lankan military. I have, however, decided not to update this essay, originally written in late 2008 when the prospect of any such end to the fighting seemed remote. Although the incidents I discuss here occurred during 2005/2006, a period of official truce, the dominant mood was not one of anticipation of the end of war, but rather of foreboding.

References

Abbas, Asma. 2005. Damages Inc.: Making the sublime matter, *Politics and Culture* 2. http://aspen.conncoll.edu/politicsandculture/page.cfm?key=377

Agamben, Giorgio. 1998. *Homo sacer: Sovereign power and bare life*. Trans. Daniel Heller-Roazen. Stanford: Stanford University Press.

Anderson, Tim. 2008. *The limits of RAMSI*. Sydney: Aidwatch.

Bankoff, Gregory. 2002. Rendering the world unsafe: 'Vulnerability' as Western discourse. *Disasters* 25, no. 1: 19–35.

Corbin, Alain. 1994. *The lure of the sea: The discovery of the seaside in the Western world 1750–1840*. Trans. Jocelyn Phelps. London: Penguin.

Dieltiens, Ivy. 2005. 6 months in post-tsunami Sri Lanka. http://www.hpathy.com/papersnew/Dieltiens-tsunami-srilanka.asp

Gowrinathan, Nimmi. 2005. Refugee babies: The lasting effects of tsunami aid in Sri Lanka. http://www.international.ucla.edu/asia/article.asp?parentid=21403

Grewal, Inderpal. 2003. Transnational America: Race, gender and citizenship after 9/11. *Social Identities* 9, no. 4: 535–61.

Heidegger, Martin. 1977. *The question concerning technology and other essays*. Trans. William Lovitt. New York: Harper Torchbooks.

Jeysankar, Sivagnanam. 2005. Talk of the town or city of Batticaloa. http://womenscoalition batticaloa.blogspot.com/2005/01/talk-of-town-or-city-of-batticaloa-by.html

Klein, Naomi. 2007. *The shock doctrine*. Camberwell, Vic: Allen Lane.

Korf, Benedikt. 2006. Dining with devils? Ethnographic enquiries into the conflict–development nexus in Sri Lanka. *Oxford Development Studies* 34, no. 1: 47–64.

Lawrence, Patricia. 2000. Violence, suffering, Amman: The work of oracles in Sri Lanka's eastern war zone. In *Violence and subjectivity*, ed. Veena Das, Arthur Kleinman, Mamphela Ramphele, and Patricia Reynolds, 171–204. Berkeley: University of California Press.

———. 2003. *The ocean of stories: Children's imagination, creativity and reconciliation in Sri Lanka*. Colombo: International Centre for Ethnic Studies.

Malkki, Lisa. 1995. Refugees and exile: From 'refugee studies' to the national order of things. *Annual Review of Anthropology* 24: 495–523.

Mbembe, Achille. 2003. Necropolitics. Trans. L. Meintjes. *Public Culture* 15, no. 1: 11–40.

Morris, Meaghan. 1998. White panic or Mad Max and the sublime. In *Trajectories: Inter-Asia cultural studies*, ed. Kuan-Hsing Chen, 239–62. London: Routledge.

Natali, Maurizia. 2006. The course of empire: Sublime landscapes in the American cinema. In *Landscape and film*, ed. Martin Lefebvre, 91–123. New York: Routledge.

Nieman, Susan. 2002. *Evil in modern thought*. Princeton: Princeton University Press.

Osuri, Goldie. 2008. War in the language of peace and an Australian geo/politics of white possession. *ACRAWSA e-journal* 4, no. 1. http://www.acrawsa.org.au/journal/acrawsa%205-5.pdf

Perera, Suvendrini. 2002. What is a Camp...? *Borderlands e-journal* 1, no. 1. http://www.borderlands.net.au/vol1no1_2002/perera_camp.html

———. 2005. The good neighbour: Conspicuous compassion and the politics of proximity. *Borderlands e-journal* 3, no. 3. http://www.borderlands.net.au/vol3no3_2004/perera_good.htm

———. 2006. They give evidence. Bodies, borders and the disappeared. *Social Identities* 12, no. 6: 637–56.

Perera, Suvendrini, and Joseph Pugliese. 1998. Parks, mines and tidy towns: 'Post'colonialism, enviro-panopticism and the politics of heritage in Australia. *Journal of Postcolonial Studies* 1, no. 1: 69–100.

Pugliese, Joseph. 1999. Indigeneity and the racial topography of Kant's 'Analytic of the Sublime'. In *Indigeneity: Construction and re/presentation*, ed. James N. Brown and Patricia M. Sant, 15–33. Commack: Nova Science.

Ray, Gene. 2004. Reading the Lisbon earthquake: Adorno, Lyotard, and the contemporary Sublime. *Yale Journal of Criticism* 17, no. 1: 1–18.

Roy, Ananya. 2005. To what end? *Politics and Culture* 2. http://aspen.conncoll.edu/politicsandculture/page.cfm?key=378

Schueller, Malini Johar. 2007. Techno-dominance and torturegate: The making of US imperialism. In *Exceptional state: Contemporary US culture and the new imperialism*, ed. Ashley Dawson and Malini Johar Schueller, 162–88. Durham, NC: Duke University Press.

Sheridan, Greg. 2005. There when Asia needs us. *Australian*, 6 January.

Ullman, Harlan K., and James P. Wade. 1996. *Shock and awe: Achieving rapid dominance*. Washington, DC: National Defense University Press.

Žižek, Slavoj. 2002. *Welcome to the desert of the real: Five essays on September 11 and related dates*. London: Verso.

Moving testimonies and the geography of suffering: Perils and fantasies of belonging after Katrina

Janet Walker

Department of Film and Media Studies, University of California, Santa Barbara, USA

This essay explores the use of situated testimony in documentary films and videos about belonging, displacement, and return while calling for a 'spatial turn' in trauma studies. Through an analysis of selected works about Hurricane Katrina (Spike Lee's *When the Levees Broke*, Tia Lessin and Carl Deal's *Trouble the Water*, and the activist video *New Orleans for Sale!* by Brandan Odums, Nik Richard, and the group 2-cent), this paper extrapolates from Cathy Caruth's insights about psychoanalytic 'belatedness' and critical human geography's anti-essentializing conceptions of place to expose the concomitant materiality *and* unassimilability of traumatic space. The essay questions assumptions about home and right of return, ultimately advocating what architect Eyal Weizman has called a new mode of 'practising space' in the service of social justice.

Introduction

'That china closet doesn't have no business being over here', exclaims a grief-stricken Wilhelmina Blanchard, inspecting her home for the first time since having evacuated as the hurricane bore down. Picking her way around jagged mounds of overturned furniture amid mouldy walls, she leans for support against the chest of her adult son. This sequence, which appears in Spike Lee's epic documentary *When the Levees Broke*, is one of the many heart-rending on-site testimonials that comprise, in significant part, the video footage and finished documentaries shot in New Orleans in the months after Hurricanes Katrina and Rita and the failure of flood control systems that put 80% of the city under water. Hurricane Katrina had formed over the Bahamas during the third week of August 2005, and went on to make its second landfall as a Category 3 hurricane southeast of New Orleans during the early morning hours of Monday 29 August 2005. US President George W. Bush had declared a state of emergency in selected regions two days prior, and Louisiana Governor Kathleen Blanco and New Orleans Mayor Ray Nagin had ordered mandatory evacuations that were undertaken by more than 1 million people. For those without the ability or means to evacuate, state and local authorities had designated various 'shelters of last resort', including the capacious Louisiana Superdome. In the hours following landfall, the storm surge swelled Lake Pontchartrain and the Intercoastal Waterway, overtopping the levees and breaching the floodwalls in various locations in and around the city. In the days that followed, responders in helicopters, boats, and buses finally arrived to rescue and transport out of the area the tens of thousands of people stranded at the Superdome, at the Ernest N. Morial Convention Center, on the Interstate 10 freeway, and elsewhere. At least 1836 people lost their lives in what is generally regarded as the greatest natural disaster in US history, although it has been critiqued from a social ecological perspective as eminently 'unnatural'. Investigations ensued, both of the failure of the flood control system on the Gulf Coast, a system that had been deemed grossly inadequate prior to the storm, and of the federal, state, and local preparation and response. Hurricane Rita, which made landfall on 24 September, necessitated another evacuation and caused further breaches to the compromised levee system and major re-flooding in New Orleans (Amoss 2006; Brinkley 2006; Campanella 2006; Hartman and Squires 2006; Park and Miller 2006; van Heerden and Bryan 2006).[1]

Cameras therefore captured a devastated landscape in which everything had shifted: houses lifted off foundations, or reduced to jutting piles of rubble; cars climbing the walls or weirdly conjoined, chassis to chassis; people wandering displaced, lost in the once-familiar neighbourhoods where they had been born and raised. As Spike Lee comments on the DVD commentary track, 'The foundation is not there. Your feet are not on solid ground.' The geography of the terrain – from its furnishings to its urban architecture to its ecology to its economic and racial relations – was massively altered, such that the ways and means of rehabilitation and bioremediation are an open question. And yet the bodily presence of returning residents describes a strong and tangible connection to place, community, neighbourhood, and home; an affective geography that is established and transitory, solid and imaginative.

Looking to trauma theory for insight into this dire situation, we may note the passing importance of violent acts and physical settings in Cathy Caruth's development of the psychoanalytic concept of 'belatedness', through which she theorizes trauma as a psychic structure of experience. 'The impact of a traumatic event', she writes, 'lies precisely in its belatedness, in its refusal to be simply located, in its insistent appearance outside the boundaries of any single place or time' and 'in connection with another place and time' (1995, 8–9). Indeed, Caruth's influential work has inspired a rich debate about psychic temporality and the historical truths and enigmas that traumatic experience arguably renders – but significantly less attention has been paid to the spatial aspects, present but little remarked in her writing.

Concentrating as much or more on place as on time – changing the variables to include the *where* alongside the who, what, and when – this essay will engage with the preposition in Mick Broderick and Antonio Traverso's 'Interrogating Trauma' conference call to identify 'strategies for moving "beyond" ... trauma'. Here I seek to explore the site-specific perorations and perambulations of situated testimony, both as an aspect of a proliferating documentary modality that I call the 'documentary of return', and as a manifestation of traumatic, distanced, ultimately unlocatable place within a contemporary geography of suffering.

The situated testimonies this essay seeks to witness are protests delivered mainly after Hurricane Katrina: what people say or do not, or cannot, say from their silted streets and water-ransacked homes; the meanings imported and exported with the cameras and crews who also 'return' to the scene. From the vast and growing archive of online and physically distributed testimonial works about suffering and survival after Katrina,[2] I have selected for comparative analysis three documentaries in which return is physically embodied, socially contested, and highly suggestive for critical inquiry: Spike Lee's Emmy Award winning *When the Levees Broke: A Requiem in Four Acts* (mini-series, HBO, 2006); Tia Lessin and Carl Deal's Sundance Film Festival Grand Jury Prize winner *Trouble the Water* (2008); and a brilliant one-and-a-half-minute short, *New Orleans for Sale!* (Brandan Odums, Nik Richard, and other members of the group 2-cent).[3] Each of these texts is a model of its kind—*Levees* an affecting interview-based compilation documentary;

Trouble a revealing documentary of 'shared authority' (Renov 2004; Ruby 1995; Hagedoorn 2007), part home movie and part *cinema vérité*; and *New Orleans for Sale!*, a creative performance piece. My analysis will depend on these categorical differences. But the broader agenda of this essay is to explore the distinct modes of practising space and return[4] described by each of these films, and, when grouped together, their description of the contours of a new direction in trauma studies.

Trauma and testimony

As a form of documentary direct address to filmmaker, camera, and spectator from the spot where catastrophic past events occurred, situated testimony realizes the materiality of retrospective witnessing in the power of place. Thousands of people around the world have presented their audiovisual testimonies through the pain of disastrous propinquity, because they have chosen or because they have no choice but to register their presence in a place from which they (temporarily) and loved ones and/or neighbours (permanently) have been wiped out. I am thinking here of the Rwandan digital video artists and archivists with whom Mick Broderick has worked, who speak from the school classroom near to where neighbours set against neighbours and from the grounds of the Kigali Genocide Centre, built over the mass grave of 300,000 Tutsi and moderate Hutu massacred during a one-hundred-day period (Broderick 2009). I am thinking of the *adivasi* or indigenous activists in South Asia who speak from the banks of waterways that have inundated the land that their families farmed for generations prior to the construction of massive dams for hydroelectric power (Ghosh 2009). Within the sizeable literature of testimony studies (Felman and Laub 1992; Douglass and Vogler 2003; Guerin and Hallas 2007; Langer 1991; Sarkar and Walker 2009[5]), Holocaust subject matter has held prominence. In this major diasporic testimonial paradigm, the overwhelming majority of testimonies have been delivered at a temporal and physical distance from the events they invoke. It may be that this perspective has obscured our view of situated testimony as a distinctive, affecting, performative – and extremely common – testimonial paradigm.

Situated testimonies in *When the Levees Broke* are increasingly prominent as the compilation documentary advances in broadly chronological order – and as people *can* get back to their neighbourhoods to be interviewed there.[6] On site, these interlocutors do not just verbalize but also *incarnate* the film's core problems and critique: that folks were stranded, evacuation impaired, help and rescue grievously delayed; that the government was and is at fault; that racial and economic discrimination is a factor; insurance companies are corrupt and developers are poised to profit from desperate homeowners forced to sell out cheaply; that the act of return is immeasurably difficult or impossible for the poor of whom most, in New Orleans, are black; that white gentrification is occurring; that many subsequent deaths should rightly be ascribed to the trauma of Katrina; that suffering is extending, hyperbolically into the post-evacuation phase (as one protest sign puts it, 'Katrina Survivor, FEMA victim';[7] and that the re-engineering of the levees was not achieved in the nearly 40 years after Hurricane Betsy and was by no means achieved by the date of filming (nor today).

One of the most affecting of these interviews is with Joycelynn Moses who relates her survival narrative from her ruined neighbourhood. At one point (following news footage of men wading chest deep in water to the soundtrack's solo trumpet rendition of the 'St. James Infirmary' blues), the camera travels to find her, over a red 'Danger' sign and panning right, across where the floodwaters invaded, to the landlocked barge. 'This is the barge, and when it came ... we thought we were going to die', we hear Moses recall in anguished voiceover. We see a close-up of the barge's alphanumeric markings accompanied by Moses' voiceover testimony: 'and I remember the number ING 4727'. The camera cuts to her: a slender African American woman, perhaps in late middle age, yellow hair, and bracelets on her wrists, and we are on the ground in proximity to this iconic image of upheaval. 'If they would've took this away I would've remembered the number, 'cause I wrote it down and put it in my pocketbook.' The camera follows Moses' gesturing arm and pointing finger to the settled barge, and the houses crushed beneath and in front of it. 'And the couple that live there, they couldn't get, afford to get out either.[0] They're still in there if they're still there.' The camera continues right to reveal a house that withstood the inundation, its spray-painted marking including a '0' to denote no dead bodies found within. But we know from media reports that two children and a man were sucked off a rooftop and drowned as the floodwaters in this vicinity rose and surged through the breach, arguably created by the barge's battering action (Evans 2008). Ringed by the shingles of downed roofs, Moses turns around nearly 180 degrees and stretches out her other arm. Again the camera follows. Houses and their contents smashed to smithereens. A white appliance and something yellow – perhaps a child's ride-along-toy – pop against the grey driftwood of people's former lives.[9]

> They have a man that liv[e] here. He tied hisself to beer kegs. They may still be in the yard. And he floated in the water just for three days and I just kept talking to him, telling him God gonna make a way, God gonna make a way. You goin' a make it. And he was saying, I'm so tired. I know you're tired.

Now Moses looks straight into the lens as the sequence ends with her remembered helplessness. All she could do was observe, record what she could, and, later, tell what she witnessed and felt: 'And I wanted to feed him what I had, but I couldn't get to him 'cause I didn't know how to swim.'

'Object survivors'[10] – physical reminders of what was – stop and start Moses' memories of prior habitation as they unfold vacantly in the crook of her extended arm. Riffing on the connotations of the camera 'viewfinder', Martin Lefebvre points out that views are as much framed as they are found, and, concomitantly, that 'the view itself cannot be divorced from the other experiential aspects that accompany it' (2006, xv). Turning as the camera pans, Moses delivers a kinaesthetic testimony that is a matter of sensory and cinematic movement both.

Belonging

It is against this painful and paradoxical reality of displacement-in-place that the film makes its case for return. 'New Orleanians and Louisianians are a resilient people', states a New Orleans City Council Member: 'they will rebuild their lives'. But weak and demographically uneven as it is today, recovery in New Orleans was still weaker – and certainly a struggle – during the film's shooting and post-production phases and at the time of the film's release one year after Katrina.[11] Civic groups such as ACORN (Association of Community Organizations for Reform Now) were fighting for the resources and the right to rebuild African American neighbourhoods against pressure from certain quarters, including the Urban Land Institute, to rebuild only on high ground: i.e. in the wealthier, whiter areas of the city (Crowley 2006; Carr 2005). Basic public services and infrastructure including public schools, child care, mail delivery, garbage pick-up, bus and streetcar routes took months or even years to resume in various parts of the city (Liu, Fellowes, and Mabanta 2006; Jervis 2007). There is no definitive 'after' to the brief before and extended during that are the timeframes of this film and catastrophe.

The film has adopted a number of strategies to do its part to secure the staked claim of New Orleanians, and especially African American New Orleanians, to the territory and right of return, with situated testimony both encountered (as when the crew comes upon a person who consents to be interviewed) and enacted (as with Wilhelmina Blanchard) prominent among them. Blanchard presumably would have inspected her home around that same time in any event, but this particular visit, in the company of her son, musician Terence Blanchard (who has scored several of Lee's films), his aunt, and also, off-camera, cinematographer Cliff Charles and Spike Lee (who had asked to be present for this occasion), was made in partnership with the film project. The light illuminating the interior space of the home was likely shone from a portable spotlight provided by Charles.

The flipside of the coin of situated testimony is the unsituated interview conducted against a locationally neutral backdrop: set, that is, in no place at all rather than either New Orleans or someplace else in particular. In fact this latter type is actually the film's most common type of interview, with the luminous blues and brick reds of the lit and textured backgrounds contributing its signature look. When Phyllis Montana LeBlanc explains from the steps of her FEMA trailer (finally delivered eight months after landfall) that although she and her husband are in the city they love, her mother, sisters, niece, and nephew are dispersed and unable to return because, for one thing, appropriate support services for Phyllis' nephew with autism no longer exist in the city, her words are affirmed by her sister Gina Montana's interview, out of place against its neutral background. 'With the evacuation scattering my family all over the United States, I felt like it was an ancient memory; as if we had been up on the auction block.'[12]

Oscillating, as it does, therefore, between situated testimony as an expression of territorial belonging and geographically neutral testimony as a controlled expression of outrageous dispossession, the film pauses pregnantly at the words of FEMA chief Michael Brown. Caught in news footage from the time, struggling to explain his lack of response to the tens of thousands of stranded New Orleanians, Brown stated: 'There are people that are beginning to manifest themselves out in the community that *we didn't know were there*'. Just so.

The film directs the attention of viewers – returns it in a way – not only to physical presence in this city but also to the neglect of people's needs, when public transportation out of the city was not arranged, when they were confined (as when some were turned back by armed police as they tried to self-evacuate by walking across the Crescent City connection into the demographically white city on the other side[13]), and, most of all, it returns the viewers to the apparently *alienable* belonging of the people to the place, that the film itself undertakes to rectify through enacted return, cinematographic return, and the exposure of impossible return.

Evacuating agency

Strongly as I believe in the mission and value of the uses, in *Levees*, of situated and unsituated testimony simultaneously to claim and to (dis)locate people and city through a traumatic *mise-en-scène*, I sense as well a nostalgic quality in the film's articulation of a 'longing for a home that no longer exists or [as I'll discuss] has never existed' (Boym 2001, xiii). When it comes to the would-be 'solution of return', the film's policy position that people should be allowed – and helped – to return *to the status quo* overlooks many of the social and spatial mediations of person, place, restitution, and return.

Whether trauma studies can comprehend this quandary depends on how we read the field. Here I want to acknowledge some of the limitations of existing trauma theories, a number of which have been elucidated by Susannah Radstone in her brilliant trauma scholarship over the last decade and more. One of the main criticisms levelled at trauma theory is that while the Caruthian formulation *seemingly* emphasizes the 'belatedness' or the continuously 'unexperienced nature of trauma' (Radstone 2007, 15) in fact we may discern in Caruth's work what Radstone and Ruth Leys identify, in their close readings, as an anti-mimetic tendency that conceives of trauma 'as if it were a purely external event that befalls a fully constituted subject' (Radstone 2007, 14 quoting Leys 2000, 10).

Having begun this essay teasing out of Caruth's work a suggestive, if ghostly, appearance of unassimilable space, I concur with Radstone that we stand to benefit from further analysis of Caruth's and other theories of trauma and applied trauma screen studies. With regard to this key question of the location of trauma as related to the brain function of the person and/or the field around her or him, I subscribe to a *critical* trauma studies, with the potential to recast not only the isolating framework that comprehends event and psyche as separate sovereign entities and the social science model that vacates psychic process but also any psycho-medico model of psychic process that ignores the socio-cultural aetiology of trauma.

'Events are not inherently traumatic', writes cultural trauma scholar Jeffrey Alexander, rejecting 'lay' trauma theory's 'naturalistic fallacy' in favour of a constructivist model. Rather, 'trauma is a socially mediated attribution' (Alexander 2004, 2, 8). But one might question whether Alexander's notion of social subjectively takes sufficient account of unconscious processes. Maurice Stevens' ethnocultural perspective that 'who "can be traumatized" [who has the cultural collateral, that is, to claim injury and the right to recompense] is shaped by ideas of race, class, gender and sexuality' is absolutely crucial, especially if one operates from the assumption that the 'traumatized who' her/himself is constituted within existing formations of race, class, gender and sexuality (Stevens 2005, 2006).

Surveying the field of trauma studies, I particularly appreciate Arthur Kleinman's and Veena Das's extension in their trilogy with various co-editors (Kleinman, Das, and Lock 1997; Das et al. 2000, 2001) of 'trauma' to 'social suffering', where social suffering is 'an assemblage of human problems that have their origins and consequences in the devastating injuries that social force can inflict on human experience' (Kleinman, Das, and Lock 1997, ix). Kleinman, Das, and Lock break down disciplinary boundaries around the fields of health, welfare, law, morality, and religion (ix) in order to re-establish 'the *collective and intersubjective* connections of experience' [my emphasis] and the salubrious subjectivity that social suffering damages (x).

This thoughtful, important work in critical trauma studies is, I believe, in our collective interest to sustain. But I hope this Katrina reading exemplifies the claim I offer here that trauma studies still has neglected the generative possibilities of place. What I would propose, therefore, is perhaps not so much a 'beyond' of trauma studies but a kind of spin around the cloverleaf: that is, a 'spatial turn' in trauma studies effected through the incorporation of enormously promising insights from critical human geography. It is there, in that post-positivist sub-discipline, that a materialist spatial perspective is reasserted, such that location matters, but place is not essentialized or reified as a truth-telling topography. The stones don't speak except through a kind of critical ventriloquism, yet they are more than mere inert features of a fixed terrain. In his germinal work *The Production of Space*, Henri Lefebvre delineates a particular '*object* of knowledge' that is 'the fragmented and uncertain connection' between these 'representations of space' (be they found, constructed, or both) and 'representational spaces' (including media aesthetics, institutions, and practices). He writes that this particular object of knowledge 'implies (and explains) a *subject*', notably, 'that subject in whom lived, perceived and conceived ... come together within spatial practice' (Lefebvre [1974] 1991, 230). In Edward S. Casey's terms, '[T]he lived body is coterminous with place because it is by bodily movement that I find my way in place and take up habitation there' (Casey 1987, 180).

This move and these concepts seem to me absolutely crucial both for trauma studies as an interdiscipline and for the application of trauma studies to film and media, a field that studies nothing if not the mutually formative relationship of spatial topography and being-in-the-world, or the constitution of subjectivity within and through Lefebvre's 'representation[s] of space' and 'representational spaces'.[14]

Also inspired by Lefebvre, art historian Irit Rogoff explains in *Terra Infirma* that critical human geography's 'situated knowledge' (2000, 22) enables

> a shift from a moralizing discourse of geography and location, in which we are told what ought to be, who has the right to be where and how it ought to be so, to a contingent ethics of geographical emplacement in which we might jointly puzzle out the perils of the fantasms of belonging as well as of the tragedies of not belonging. (3)

A spatial turn in trauma studies of art, film, and media would seem extremely useful for understanding trauma as the experiential displacement of place, protagonist, and, as will be discussed below, of spectator.

Returning, therefore, to the problematic of situated testimony in documentary film, and *When the Levees Broke* in particular, I would argue that, concerned as it is with the 'tragedies of not belonging', the film ignores the chance to 'puzzle out' Rogoff's 'perils of the fantasms of belonging'. While *Levees* includes frequent references to (lost) home ownership by African Americans in New Orleans, it contains few references to the long-term, intransigent problems of poverty[15] even though – as outside statistics reveal – prior to Katrina, 91.2% of the city's poor families of all races were African American and 35% of African Americans (compared with 11% of whites) were living below the poverty line (Park and Miller 2006, 13). By concentrating on immediate contingency, idealizing home and community, and embracing identity politics, *Levees* may actually inhibit the 'working through' of long-standing social malaise at the very moment when exposed racism demands a new order.

Certainly we have an ethical obligation to recognize and honour the claims of returnees to this 'fatal environment'.[16] Rooted testimonies matter. But still it behoves us to take seriously Caruth's hints about trauma's distanced 'other place', about the psychic dimensions and 'belatedness' – or profound *unassimilability* – of place and occurrence that make up the traumatic experience of which these interviewees speak. The ground of testimony-*sur-place* – like exilic space – is always, already 'other'.

Social ecology of suffering

Disenfranchisement as a kind of distancing of African Americans from their home city was already a problem of enormous historical, economic, social, and environmental consequence *before* Katrina struck. The moniker 'Katrina' alludes not only to the meteorological events of Hurricanes Katrina and Rita (including the breaches of the I-walls and canals and the overtopping of the levees) – not only to this so-called 'natural disaster'. Rather, in social ecological terms, it invokes the 'malign intersection of weather and water with a man-made social and racial topography' that we describe, all-in, as Katrina (Park and Miller 2006, 15 quoting The Brookings Institution Metropolitan Policy Program). As Yoosun Park and Joshua Miller explain, there is an unevenness of risk factors in the face of calamity such that '[t]he most disadvantaged members of the most disadvantaged communities suffer the greatest losses when disaster strikes' (10). In New Orleans specifically, '[s]ome of the most historic Black neighborhoods ....were on the lowest ground and sustained some of the most severe damage' (Crowley 2006, 141).

Park and Miller's social ecological analysis of urban landscapes reads like a location breakdown of this documentary project:

> The socially disadvantaged are more likely to live near chemical plants, landfills, and other contaminated lands. There is a greater likelihood that they will be living in more vulnerable, substandard dwellings served by older, less well-maintained infrastructures, for example, roads, sewers. They are more likely to be living in overcrowded, environmentally risky areas. Much of public housing, built during the 1950s and 1960s, tend [*sic*] to cluster in areas that are along major transportation routes, reclaimed land, or adjacent to industrial facilities. (2006, 10, citing Cutter 2005)

The location shooting of *Levees* in the devastated Ninth Ward, combined with archival footage of the stranded inhabitants, reveals a city noticeably segregated by race and income, where middle- and upper-middle-class white residents of New Orleans' 'outlying (and ... literally higher) suburban communities' are nowhere to be seen, while poor blacks wade through the toxic ooze in 'low-lying flood-prone areas' (Hartman and Squires 2006, 5).

The film's traumatic landscape was in my eye and ear when I undertook my own small trip to this environment out of which people were blown, flown, bussed, flooded, rescued, evacuated, and disappeared, about which they speak with such dignity, and to which they struggle to return, both literally and in terms of a return to structural integrity.[17] The disposition of areas of the city in April of 2008 was very much in line with what Spike Lee and those who appeared before his cameras had analysed historically and predicted two years prior: the Lafitte Avenue public housing complex, the last of the ambitious projects built in post-Second World War New Orleans by Franklin Roosevelt's Works Progress Administration, was on the verge of demolition, against public protest. The Lafitte had become notorious for criminal, especially drug-related, activity. But, 'scaled to fit within the surrounding neighborhood' and designed with wrought-iron balustrades and communal courtyards (Ouroussoff 2006), the red brick housing blocks were also home to working poor – the maids and other service workers of the city's tourism industry. The buildings had not flooded inside. Tenants were given a window of opportunity to return to New Orleans from Houston or Memphis or Atlanta or Chicago to collect their belongings. But when that metaphorical window closed so did the *actual* doors and windows of their homes, sealed up at considerable expense by the Housing Authority of New Orleans' installation of metal plates. Once opened for clearing, workers, including many Latinos new to the city, bagged up and threw away the worldly possessions of displaced African American families, in preparation for demolition.[18] This is clearly policy, not 'nature'. What with the destruction of public housing, the end of federal rental subsidies, and the recall of temporary trailers, some of New Orleans' working poor had taken up residence in tents under the I-10 freeway.[19]

Naomi Klein specifically discusses the condemning and razing of the houses of the poor in the aftermath of Katrina as an effect of the phenomenon she describes as 'disaster capitalism': a form of opportunistic corporatism that capitalizes on sudden catastrophic events to 'rai[d] the public sphere' by suspending governmental checks and balances in favour of high-stakes insider business dealings, privatization, deregulation, and drastic reduction of social spending, all of which adversely affect poor and middle-class people and any others who dissent (2007, 6). Disaster capitalism is 'fundamentalist',

Klein explains, invoking the supremacist ideology of its advocates as well as its historical and philosophical affinities with religious extremism. Within the first three paragraphs of her book *Shock Doctrine*, Klein quotes Congressman Richard Baker's chilling post-Katrina statement (also included in *Levees*): 'We finally cleaned up public housing in New Orleans. We couldn't do it, but God did.' As of March 2008, two and a half years after Katrina, New Orleans had reached only 71.8% of its pre-Katrina population of about half a million people (Russell 2006; Falk, Hunt, and Hunt 2006) with African Americans, those living in poverty, and registered Democrats as significantly overlapping demographic categories in which the rate of return is dramatically lower (Frey 2007; Powell et al. 2006; Crowley 2006; Zdenek et al. 2006).[20] The city of New Orleans, Louisiana (NOLA), it could be said, is under occupation by gentrification.

And yet the film's investment in the human rights discourse of 'right of return' may be a political, interpersonal, and geographic dead end. I hazard this statement while acknowledging: monumental negligence by the federal government and private insurance companies; disproportional capital in the hands of residential, commercial, and industrial developers; and the fact that rational people may find quite a bit of traction invoking the right of return from the standpoint of ethical commitment. But the deepest problem of 'right of return', I would argue, is not that people aren't back, but rather that the geography this discourse maps lacks potential. In a petrified topography, return may serve no purpose more fully, as Wendy Brown as argued, than to further 'reif[y] and regulat[e] the subject produced by social powers' (Brown 2000, 471).[21] It isn't safe to return to former conditions in which subjects were constrained by the economies of structural engineering and engineered race- and class-based segregation.

Trouble the Water

Kimberly and Scott Roberts, protagonists of *Trouble the Water* (2008), do return to New Orleans (like Wilhelmina Blanchard, Joycelynn Moses, and others in *Levees*), initially to survey the destruction of their neighbourhood and eventually to take up residence once again. But this film, compared with *Levees*, is less idealizing with regard to return, more open to airing the dirty laundry of monoeconomic and monoracial community, and therefore more resistant to a separatist geography that in Rogoff's terms 'bind[s] us all together under the aegis of the dominant' (2000, 110–11).

With its complicated temporal structure that begins in the middle and flashes back and forward, *Trouble*, unlike *Levees*, encompasses distinct 'before' and 'after' Katrina timeframes in which the Lower Ninth Ward neighbourhood is depicted warts and all. Here there is an active agent in the person of Kimberly Rivers Roberts who not only self-evacuates with her husband, taking along children and others who cannot help themselves, but also plans and shoots the *cinema vérité*-style home movie footage that anchors this vibrant semi-autobiographical documentary. As we hear her say to neighbours from behind the video camera she purchased just prior to the storm (Willis 2008): 'If I get some exciting shit, maybe I can sell it to the white folks.' Moreover, instead of a situated testimony here and there, this film includes an extended return trajectory in which the Robertses retrace their evacuation route, re-encountering along the way objects, obstacles, and those who would also testify.

'I'm on my way to New Orleans', we hear Kimberly Roberts say into her cell phone as she and her husband return with a friend two weeks after the storm (although released after *Levees*, *Trouble* began its post-Katrina location shooting earlier). 'Some people I met are doing a documentary; a real documentary'. And through the windows of the car, the lens of the protagonists' camera, and the lens of this 'real documentary', we see the muddied streets and downed buildings, the shocking iconography of the Katrina cycle: once she arrives, we see Kimberly and company walking and gesturing and speaking of what was: 'Everybody! This is my neighborhood ... I miss those days and it's hurt me to know that it's not going to be the same no more.'

Roberts is not only viewing the devastation but actually reconnoitering, performing inspections that had not yet been carried out by officials (even though the spray-painted markings showed they had).[22] We are with Roberts on the street when the group discovers her uncle, dead in the front room of a house where he had sought shelter, and pulls in National Guardsmen to handle the body; the odour of death suffuses the scene throughout their efforts to show respect while bearing the stench.

Kimberly and Scott Roberts and company also proactively retrace the path they had followed during their self-evacuation, returning to the stations of their self-help in the face of abandonment by the government. Unlike in *Levees*, here the territory is not deserted but rather occupied by people in authority whom they re-encounter. To take just one example, while evacuating they had been denied entrance to an abandoned naval barracks by troops with M-16s cocked and aimed. But now, upon their return, a military commander at the gate denies Scott's claim, asserting: there was 'never any hint of us using any type of force', and also, self-contradictorily, 'we had to do our job and protect the interest of the government'. Thus, although *Trouble* shares the Roberts's perspective by presenting a pathway strewn with landmarks of the group's resourcefulness and generosity (they got hold of a truck and evacuated 30 people to Alexandria, Louisiana), it also exposes the performativity of testimony and its inevitable complications as a truth-seeking mode.

Through the Roberts's down-to-earth footage of 'the before' and our own saccadic vision[23] – and in contradistinction to *Levees*' dignified narration of pre-Katrina community – we observe alcoholism, drug dealing, and combative behaviour, as when the men at a corner store challenge Roberts filming them and she snaps back, presumably alluding to the surveillance camera, 'What you looking at? You got *me* on camera.' We see snippets of a car interior while on the soundtrack Roberts' voice is heard talking with the car's occupant who is looking to buy some weed (another type of 'shit' for her to sell?); we see her uncle passed out on a well-trodden stoop in a drunken haze, prior to his death in the storm. 'Don't do that when ya'll get big', Roberts warns the children playing nearby.

In *Trouble the Water*'s orchestration of situated testimony and *cinema vérité* sequences, we hear the accusation of bias so loudly played in *Levees*, *and* the tones of self-induced damage. Scott Roberts explains that he had previously turned to drug dealing because there were no good employment options for a person with limited education. And yet, by the end of the film (perhaps 18 months later), we see the positive results of his choice to take a carpenter job. 'Now I get to rebuild my city', he exults. 'I love the smell of that sawdust.'

Near the end of the film Roberts is back in her neighbourhood, speaking warmly of the benefits of community:

> Three cars of people pass and they all know us ... If something happened to me right around here, right now, somebody's gonna do something for me 'cause they know me ... If I ain't got a ride, somebody's gonna give me a ride. And if I need some money ... they might not loan me no money, but they'll give me some conversation. So, you know, it feels good to be back home.

Yes, but. In her own footage at the beginning of the film, we had heard Roberts state that she had tried to rent a car but just 'couldn't afford the luxury' of leaving. And as the film informs us with a line of text subtitling the image of the bumper-to-bumper exodus, there was no public transportation provided for pre-storm evacuation, although Mayor Nagin did order traffic contraflow for those with wheels. Perhaps Uncle Ned too lacked a neighbourly ride out of town.

More than simply sharing *Levees*' longing for black community, *Trouble* does also suggest 'the perils of the fantasms of belonging' to a racially and economically segregated geography where neighbours lack the resources to help neighbours, and interracial strife makes hotspots of the islands and perimeters that mark out difference. And yet, where *Levees*' discourse is frustrated eloquence against injustice,[24] *Trouble* ends with an impression, however utopian, of integrated community. The 'white folks' to whom Kimberly did sell her footage (or, presumably, reach some sort of positive financial arrangement) incorporated her music as professional singer/songwriter Kold Medina amply into the film. Roberts's displacement by the storm and flood and, significantly, her co-authorship of a return narrative (living history that could be filmed and filming history that demanded to be lived) expanded Roberts's orbit beyond New Orleans: 'I'm trying to do something different. I see it now. I couldn't see it before when I was inside.'

Where is trauma?

Katrina's territory – this same and 'other' spot – is multiply inhabited with an effect of strife or benefit, as the case may be.

In the context of Israel–Palestine, Eyal Weizman has suggested that how we 'practice space' is important, especially when historical moments of evacuation offer new and humanizing possibilities for the reallocation of resources (that we would implement thoughtfully and in opposition to the 'clean slate' fundamentalism of a Richard Baker). Importing Weizman's terms, the flooded city of New Orleans could be seen to represent a moment of 'ungrounding'; undeniable disaster, yes, but still an opportunity to 'disactivate' the ills of economic and racial segregation characteristic of the pre-Katrina environment (Weizman 2008). Buildings can be repurposed, surface structures such as roadways and green spaces reorganized to connect formerly divided habitations, and the US infrastructure – as well as the levees – re-engineered in the interest of human rights. I can't but feel that such a *transformative* view of race and place – which, arguably, could include an economically, architecturally, and even racially mixed[25] housing plan along with a complete reworking of the system of resources distribution – would constitute an ethical foundation for a rebuilt New Orleans.

Levees and *Trouble* are at their most compelling when they offer a critical sense of space, as they do when their situated testimonies expose the politicized granularity of the ground below our feet and the possibilities for spatial transformation. A more explicitly activist video piece goes even further to array the complexities of shared space.

New Orleans for Sale! screened at the 2008 New Orleans International Human Rights Festival and is currently available for viewing on YouTube. I saw it on my visit to the city several days after the desire to conduct ethnographic research on 'disaster tourism' led me to take an official 'Hurricane Katrina Tour' with the Gray Line bus company. In the video, the group '2-cent' have performed a special kind of 'return' to the Ninth Ward, reoccupying the space from which many families have been expunged and registering (to disaster tourists such as me and others) the gains of carpet-bagging entrepreneurs and outsiders. Standing on roofs and sidewalks in front of damaged, vacant homes, the group members hold up hand-lettered signs that read 'America Did This' and 'This Is What You Paid To See Right' while Nik Richard asks pointedly 'It looks like there's more money to be paid in devastation than regeneration. If ya'll keep paying your money to see it, should we rebuild it?'

The video succeeds not only by virtue of the sheer power of performance but also, I contend (hoping this is considered opinion and not mere self-justification), because the tourists and 2-cent meet on common ground,[26] or, one could say, on a mobilized terrain. Shots are taken from inside as well as from the outside of passing vehicles. In identifying the boundaries of the neighbourhood while also allowing them to be breached, the video enacts an energetic encounter between those who have returned home, those who cannot return for real, and those who tour. In the spirit of engagement, I suggest the value of going and seeing and acting together; spending our money not only to visit but also to remake space as multiply inhabited community. In the Ninth Ward a number of homes designated as a Musicians' Village have been rebuilt and colourfully painted in a collaborative effort by Habitat for Humanity and local homeowners. Moreover, although the Lafitte Avenue and other housing projects were torn down rather than remodelled, the non-profit developer has made a commitment to '"one-to-one" replacement of public housing units' with a promising mix of new on-site housing and '"in-fill" development' in the surrounding neighbourhood. Existing but dilapidated homes are now being stripped back to their cypress studs, remodelled, and prepared for subsidized ownership by low-income residents (Rechdahl and Williams 2008; Sinha 2009).[27]

Where is trauma? As indicated, I support the elasticization of psycho-medico trauma models that otherwise bind up trauma as an internally psychic process. Of course, many of the survivors of Katrina were psychologically traumatized by their experiences. I was able to speak with a licensed psychologist whom the Red Cross had placed, as a volunteer, in a Dallas shelter in the weeks following the storm and flood.[28] She confirmed incredible suffering and traumatization and also the practical limits of psychological intervention when people are still missing family members and in need of medical triage. (And she blanched when I told her of our aim to 'interrogate trauma', a phrase that for her invoked an association between trauma and torture.) Matters of individual psychology notwithstanding, what I have tried to argue here is the importance, even as we empathize with or work on behalf of Katrina survivors, of theorizing the mutuality of psychosocial processes, the social ecology of disaster, and the role of situated media. Observing psychic disturbance at the medial interface, I advocate the importation of trauma models of arts and media studies we may identify as relevant, and, yes, that we interrogate trauma with all the critical acuity we can muster as a mobilized, spatialized site.

Documentary films of situated testimony and return – those I've discussed and others in the mode – comprise a limit case of the cinematic 'site-seeing' that Giuliana Bruno attributes to cinema spectating in general (2002, 15–53). However physically grounded or engaged with the affective lure of home, they still describe an 'unhomed geography' (in Rogoff's idiom) transformative with regard to rites/rights of return and porous in its ethnic, racial, generational, and economic contours. Each of the films discussed in its own way renders NOLA's 'other' space as an experientially unreachable traumatic terrain, but one for which the fullest range of reconstructive possibilities must nevertheless be imagined and explored.

Spatial trauma studies and especially, but not exclusively, these films of situated testimony have a great deal to contribute, I believe, to pressing conversations and policy work on the geopolitics of our multiply inhabited planet at a time of increasing, often forced, mobility and intense struggle for places to call home.

Acknowledgements

This essay was recast for the 'Interrogating Trauma: Arts & Media Responses to Collective Suffering' conference, and journal dossier from its original form as a chapter-in-progress for *Documentary Testimonies: Global Archives of Suffering*, ed. Bhaskar Sarkar and Janet Walker (New York: Routledge, 2009). I am grateful to Bhaskar for his astute comments on that previous version (revised and published here by permission) and to Mick Broderick, Antonio Traverso, Susannah Radstone, Felicity Collins, Suvendrini Perera, and the 'Interrogating Trauma' participants for sharing valuable insights about trauma and media. Thanks are also due to Holly Willis for introducing me to *Trouble the Water*, to Dave Cash, Liz Dunnebacke, Royce Osborn, Jennifer Peterson, Tim Ryan, and Betsy Weiss for their generous hospitality in New Orleans and to the University of California, Santa Barbara for travel funding.

Notes

1. The literature on Hurricane Katrina is voluminous and I will be citing further articles, books, and reports throughout this paper.
2. In addition to the films discussed here, see *Right to Return: Home Movies from the Lower 9th Ward* (dir. Jonathan Demme, 2008), segments of which were aired on PBS's *Tavis Smiley* in the spring of 2007; *Still Waiting: Life after Katrina* (dir. Ginny Martin and Kate Browne, 2007); *The Drive: A Documentary Tour of Post-Katrina New Orleans*, Segment one: The Lower 9th Ward (dir. Tim Ryan and Matt Wisdom, 2006); *Kamp Katrina* (dir. David Redmon and Ashley Sabin, 2007); *The Axe in the Attic* (dir. Ed Pincus and Lucia Small, 2007); *God Provides* (dir. Brian M. Cassidy and Melanie Shatzky, 2007, short); *Faubourg Tremé: The Untold Story of Black New Orleans* (dir. Dawn Logsdon, 2008); and the hybrid fictionalized feature *Low and Behold* (dir. Zachary Godshall, 2007). See also online archives including: The Hurricane Digital Memory Bank, a project of George Mason University's Center for History and New Media and the University of New Orleans, in partnership with the Smithsonian Institutions, www.hurricanearchive.org (accessed 15 August 2008); the New Orleans Video Access Center, which organized local film and videomakers to create works about Katrina that were posted online and screened throughout the country, www.novacvideo.org (accessed 15 August 2008); Alive in Truth: The New Orleans Disaster Oral History and Memory Project which collects and makes available transcripts of oral interviews, www.aliveintruth.org (accessed 15 August 2008). For a discussion of some of these and other Katrina archives, see Stein and Preuss (2006).
3. Available on 2-cent.com (accessed 4 October 2008) and YouTube.
4. Eyal Weizman used the term 'practising space' in 'Conversations', a talk presented at the REDCAT, Walt Disney Concert Hall, Los Angeles, 6 May 2008. See also Weizman (2007).
5. Bhaskar Sarkar and I discuss the extensive scholarly literature on testimony as well as the recent proliferation of audiovisual archives in our introduction ('Introduction: Moving testimonies') to *Documentary Testimonies: Global Archives of Suffering*.
6. The film's four acts (five on DVD) carry us through from immediately before to after the hurricanes (Katrina and Rita) and flood. But a finer vernier reveals a 'sort of overture', in Ernest Callenbach's phrase (2006, 6), to each act comprised in most cases of an a-chronological, associational montage set to music that includes at least one, usually more than one, aerial shot of New Orleans amongst images on the ground including a signature shot along a road narrowed by the heaped timbers and shingles of ruined homes. Each act or 'movement' (to invoke the film's rich soundtrack as well as its own titular musical reference) ends with a departure of sorts: Act II's montage of dead and bloated bodies, left floating or beached by the receding waters, is followed by a low-angle long take of poet Shelton Shakespear Alexander delivering his piercing recitation against the high arched gate of a cemetery with the sky behind. Then comes a repetition of the roadway tracking shot, and finally, over the destroyed rooftops, an indelible image of the giant barge that broke through the Industrial Canal into a residential neighbourhood in the Lower Ninth Ward. Exemplary for its epic complexity as well as sweep, the film spirals down into the maelstrom of the flooded city and yet resuscitates the bodies, voices, and ideas of people on the ground.
7. Federal Emergency Management Agency; the entity that became famous around the world for its negligence during Katrina.
8. Having listened repeatedly to this passage, I think Moses' phrase is properly transcribed. But she may have stated that the couple 'couldn't get aboard [a boat perhaps?] to get out either' rather

than 'couldn't get, afford to get out either'. Suffice it to say that financial wherewithal was an enormous factor in people's ability to evacuate safely.

9. Such objects are generative of narrative rather than mere vessels for symbolic meaning. See Jameson (1992, esp. 19).
10. This term is borrowed from its use in Holocaust museology. See Shenker (2009).
11. Less than 50% of New Orleanians had returned by the one-year anniversary, including substantially fewer African American than white former residents. See Nossiter (2006); US Census Bureau, State & County QuickFacts, http://quickfacts.census.gov/qfd/states/22/22071.htm (accessed 15 August 2008); and Wikipedia entry for New Orleans, Louisiana, sub-category 'demographics'. Other major reports on post-Katrina recovery include Liu, Fellowes, and Mabanta (2006) and Liu and Plyer (2008a).
12. An interview with public intellectual Michael Dyson is edited in here to take up Montana's reference to the history of slavery: he mocks those who would disclaim the validity of the reference: 'Oh, no, you're being hyperbolic. You're just engaging in all forms of racially inflammatory rhetoric ... ' And then concludes: 'Well, the fact is they were treating them like slaves in the ship. Families were being separated. Children were being taken from their mothers and fathers. Those more weary and those who were more likely to be vulnerable were separated from those who were stronger ... The separation of the evacuation where people lost sight and lost sound and lost sense of their loved ones ... '
13. While widely known and decried, this event *as an example of racial bias* has been denied by Gretna Mayor Ronnie Harris. A lawsuit was filed by state Senator Cleo Fields (D-Baton Rouge) and state Representative Cedric Richmond (D-New Orleans) against the city of Gretna and the Gretna Police Department. See Webster (2006).
14. For several superb film and media studies works that incorporate spatial studies see Krause and Petro (2003); Dimendberg (2004); and Lefebvre (2006).
15. There are some such references as when Calvin Mackie refers to pre-Katrina social problems including New Orleans' high murder rate, high dropout rate, and low wages.
16. I adapt the term 'fatal environment' from Slotkin (1985).
17. My friend Dave Cash in the Fair Grounds Race Course area still does not have heat upstairs because water remains in his heating ducts and neither his homeowner's insurance nor the city will take responsibility.
18. See del Barco (2005) for a report on the controversy over the arrival of Latino workers from Texas, Florida, and Mexico to undertake the strenuous cleanup work in post-Katrina New Orleans, in some cases over the protests of local residents concerned that they had been 'replaced by lower-wage Spanish-speaking workers'. See also Bearden (2007).
19. '150 people are living in tents under the I-10 overpass, 31 percent of whom are recently homeless because of the loss of federal rental assistance or their removal from temporary trailers', according to Liu and Plyer (2008b). The residents of the tent city were relocated in the summer of 2008 through the efforts of various homeless and charitable service organizations.
20. Frey indicates that 'while 64 percent of the city's pre-Katrina white population returned by July 2006, only 43 percent of black residents – and just 22 percent of black residents age 25–34 – did so'.
21. See also Brown (1995). Although space constraints preclude the development of this thought in the body of the essay, I would like to mention here that reification of black subjectivity in the case of Katrina also consists in the tendency to attribute discriminatory actions, inactions, and practices on the part of public officials to the 'fact' of blackness instead of to the failings of said officials. This point occurred to me while listening to Nessan McMillan's superb presentation, 'Bearing witness: The Rwandan genocide on the global stage', at the 'Interrogating Trauma: Arts & Media Responses to Collective Suffering' international conference.
22. 'Keeping it real', as Hot 8 Brass Band member Dinerral Shavers put it in *Levees*, gesturing toward homes bearing spray-painted marks of inspection but also barred windows and locked doors belying the graphic claim that anyone had entered ('They didn't go into none of these houses'). A prominent New Orleans musician, Shavers was shot to death while driving in a car with his wife and two children, on 28 December 2006. He was 25 years old. See Filosa (2006).
23. I write this with all due caution against overinvestment in the democratizing capabilities that André Bazin (1967) attributed to shots composed with multiple planes in sharp focus presented in long takes such that the spectator's eye, in theory, may rove at will.

24. This affective meaning with which we are left is consolidated in the ending coda. The film's credit sequence is presented as successive images of the people who have appeared, stating their names and identifying information while holding in front of their faces, or being digitally framed by, empty picture frames.
25. Any plan for racially integrated communities would need to be developed with care to maintain existing support networks while combating racist practices and policies.
26. Reference here is to Common Ground Collective, founded by Sharon Johnson, Malik Rahim, and Brandon Darby seven days after Katrina struck in order to 'rebuild the spirit of Southern Louisiana'. See www.commongroundrelief.org
27. At the time of writing, about 90 units of the Lafitte remain standing but have not been reoccupied. In fact, controversy swirls over whether the charitable and non-profit entities that are supposed to be low-income housing advocates are in fact functioning in that manner.
28. Interview with Susan Neufeldt, PhD, Goleta, California, 5 September 2008.

References

Alexander, Jeffrey C. 2004. Toward a theory of cultural trauma. In Alexander et al. 2004, 1–30.

Alexander, Jeffrey C., Ron Eyerman, Bernhard Giesen, Neil J. Smelser, and Piotr Sztompka, eds. 2004. *Cultural trauma: And collective identity*. Berkeley: University of California Press.

Amoss, Jim, ed., for the staff of *The Times-Picayune*. 2006. *The Times-Picayune Katrina: The ruin and recovery of New Orleans*. New Orleans: The Times-Picayune.

Bazin, André. 1967. The evolution of the language of cinema. In *What is cinema?* Trans. Hugh Gray, 23–40. Berkeley: University of California Press.

Bearden, Tom. 2007. New Orleans sees rise in Latino population. Online NewsHour: Report, originally broadcast 28 August. http://www.pbs.org/newshour/bb/social_issues/july-dec07/katrina_08-28.html (accessed 28 December 2008).

Boym, Svetlana. 2001. *The future of nostalgia*. New York: Basic Books.

Brinkley, Douglas. 2006. *The great deluge: Hurricane Katrina, New Orleans and the Mississippi Gulf Coast*. New York: HarperCollins.

Broderick, Mick. 2009. Mediating genocide: Producing digital survivor testimony in Rwanda. In Sarkar and Walker 2009, 215–44.

Brown, Wendy. 1995. Rights and losses. In *States of injury*. Chap. 5, 96–134. Princeton: Princeton University Press.

———. 2000. Revaluing critique: A response to Kenneth Baynes. *Political Theory* 28, no. 4: 469–79.

Bruno, Giuliana. 2002. Site-seeing: The cine city. In *Atlas of emotion: Journeys in art, architecture, and film*, 15–53. New York: Verso.

Callenbach, Ernest. 2006. *When the Levees Broke: A Requiem in Four Acts*. *Film Quarterly* 60, no. 2: 4–10.

Campanella, Richard. 2006. *Geographies of New Orleans: Urban fabrics before the storm*. Lafayette: Center for Louisiana Studies.

Carr, Martha. 2005. Rebuilding should begin on higher ground, group says. *The Times-Picaynue*, 19 November.

Caruth, Cathy, ed. 1995. *Trauma: Explorations in memory*. Baltimore: Johns Hopkins University Press.

Casey, Edward S. 1987. *Remembering: A phenomenological study*. Bloomington: Indiana University Press.
Crowley, Sheila. 2006. Where is home? Housing for low-income people after the 2005 hurricanes. In Hartman and Squires 2006, 121–66.
Cutter, S.L. 2005. *The geography of social vulnerability: Race, class and catastrophe*. http://understandingkatrina.ssrc.org/cutter/pf/
Das, Veena, Arthur Kleinman, Margaret Lock, Mamphela Ramphele, and Pamela Reynolds, eds. 2001. *Making a world: Violence, social suffering, and recovery*. Berkeley: University of California Press.
Das, Veena, Arthur Kleinman, Mamphela Ramphele, and Pamela Reynolds, eds. 2000. *Violence and subjectivity*. Berkeley: University of California Press.
del Barco, Mandalit. 2005. Katrina cleanup puts focus on Latino workers. An NPR story originally aired on 24 October. http://www.npr.org/templates/story/story.php?storyId=4972419 (accessed 28 December 2008).
Dimendberg, Edward. 2004. *Film noir and the spaces of modernity*. Cambridge, MA: Harvard University Press.
Douglass, Ana, and Thomas A. Vogler, eds. 2003. *Witness and memory: The discourse of trauma*. New York: Routledge.
Evans, Martin C. 2008. Recalling family taken by Katrina. *Newsday*, 30 August. Posted on http://xml.newsday.com/topic/ny-usmom304870424aug30,0,6469431.story (accessed 15 August 2008).
Falk, William W., Matthew O. Hunt, and Larry L. Hunt. 2006. Hurricane Katrina and New Orleanians' sense of place: Return and reconstitution or 'Gone with the Wind'. *Du Bois Review* 3, no. 1: 115–28.
Felman, Shoshana, and Dori Laub. 1992. *Testimony: Crises of witnessing in literature, psychoanalysis, and history*. New York: Routledge.
Filosa, Gwen. 2006. Two die in New Orleans shootings. *The Times-Picayune*, 29 December. http://www.nola.com/news/t-p/metro/index.ssf?/base/news-18/116737610147820.xml&coll=1 (accessed 21 July 2009).
Frey, William H. 2007. Are we 'a whole other city'? *The Times-Picayune*, 28 August. http://www.brookings.edu/opinions/2007/0828demographics_frey.aspx (accessed 21 July 2009).
Ghosh, Bishnupriya. 2009. 'We shall drown, but we shall not move': The ecologics of testimony in NBA documentaries. In Sarkar and Walker 2009, 59–82.
Guerin, Frances, and Roger Hallas, eds. 2007. *The image and the witness: Trauma, memory and visual culture*. London: Wallflower Press.
Hagedoorn, Berber. 2007. *Shared textual authority in the found footage documentary: A historical and theoretical analysis of* The Maelstrom, Grizzly Man, *and* My Architect. Research Masters diss., University of Utrecht, The Netherlands.
Hartman, Chester, and Gregory Squires, eds. 2006. *There is no such thing as a natural disaster: Race, class, and Hurricane Katrina*. New York: Routledge.
Jameson, Frederic. 1992. Introduction: Beyond landscape and Part one: Totality as conspiracy. In *The geopolitical aesthetic: Cinema and space in the world system*, 1–84. Bloomington: Indiana University Press.
Jervis, Rick. 2007. 66% are back in New Orleans, but personal services still lag. *USA Today*, 13 August. http://www.usatoday.com/news/nation/2007-08-12-neworleans_N.htm (accessed 15 August 2008).
Klein, Naomi. 2007. *The shock doctrine: The rise of disaster capitalism*. New York: Metropolitan Books.
Kleinman, Arthur, Veena Das, and Margaret Lock, eds. 1997. *Social suffering*. Berkeley: University of California Press.
Krause, Linda, and Patrice Petro, eds. 2003. *Global cities: Cinema, architecture, and urbanism in a digital age*. New Brunswick, NJ: Rutgers University Press.
Langer, Lawrence. 1991. *Holocaust testimonies: The ruins of memory*. New Haven, CT: Yale University Press.
Lefebvre, Henri. [1974] 1991. *The production of space*. Trans. Donald Nicholson-Smith. Malden, MA, Oxford and Victoria: Blackwell.
Lefebvre, Martin, ed. 2006. *Landscape and film*. New York: Routledge.
Leys, Ruth. 2000. *Trauma: A genealogy*. Chicago: University of Chicago Press.

Liu, Amy, and Allison Plyer. 2008a. The New Orleans index anniversary edition: Tracking the recovery of New Orleans and the metro area. The Brookings Institution. http://www.brookings.edu/experts/liua.aspx?more=rc&filter=topic&sortTopic=new+orleans (accessed 22 October 2008).

———. 2008b. Executive summary: State of policy & progress, April 2008: Two years, eight months since Katrina made landfall. *The New Orleans Index*. The Brookings Institution Metropolitan Policy Program & Greater New Orleans Community Data Center. www.gnocdc.org (accessed 22 October 2008).

Liu, Amy, Matt Fellowes, and Mia Mabanta. 2006. Special edition of the Katrina index: A one-year review of key indicators of recovery in post-storm New Orleans. The Brookings Institution. http://www.brookings.edu/experts/liua.aspx?more=rc&filter=topic&sortTopic=new+orleans (accessed 22 October 2008).

McMillan, Nessan. 2008. Bearing witness: The Rwandan genocide on the global stage. Paper presented at the 'Interrogating Trauma: Arts & Media Responses to Collective Suffering' international conference, November, in Perth, Australia.

Nossiter, Adam. 2006. New Orleans population is reduced nearly 60%. *New York Times*, 7 October. http://www.nytimes.com/2006/10/07/us/07population.htm (accessed 15 August 2008).

Oursoussoff, Nicolai. 2006. Architecture: All fall down. *New York Times*, 19 November. http://www.nytimes.com/2006/11/19/weekinreview/19ouroussof.htm (accessed 28 December 2008).

Park, Yoosun, and Joshua Miller. 2006. The social ecology of Hurricane Katrina: Re-writing the discourse of 'natural' disasters. *Smith College Studies in Social Work* 76, no. 3: 9–24.

Powell, John A., Hasan Kwame Jeffries, Daniel W. Newhart, and Eric Stiens. 2006. Towards a transformative view of race: The crisis and opportunity of Katrina. In Hartman and Squires 2006, 59–84.

Radstone, Susannah. 2007. Trauma theory: Contexts, politics, ethics. *Paragraph* 30, no. 1: 9–29.

Rechdahl, Katy, and Leslie Williams. 2008. Lafitte revival to encompass neighbourhood. *The Times-Picayune*, 21 August. Posted on http://www.nola.com/news/index.ssf/2008/08/meeting_tonight_on_lafitte_off.html (accessed 21 September 2008).

Renov, Michael. 2004. Domestic ethnography and the construction of the 'other' self. *The subject of documentary*. Minneapolis: University of Minnesota Press.

Rogoff, Irit. 2000. *Terra infirma: Geography's visual culture*. London: Routledge.

Ruby, Jay. 1995. The moral burden of authorship in ethnographic film. *Visual Anthropology Review* 11, no. 2: 1–6.

Russell, Gordon. 2006. New population statistics gloomy – rate of return to area down dramatically. *The Times-Picayune*, 8 August. http://www.nola.com/news/t-p/frontpage/index.ssf?/base/news-6/1155016899280970.xml&coll=1 (accessed 21 July 2009).

Sarkar, Bhaskar, and Janet Walker, eds. 2009. *Documentary testimonies: Global archives of suffering*. New York: Routledge.

Shenker, Noah. 2009. Embodied memory: The institutional mediation of survivor testimony in the United States Holocaust Memorial Museum. In Sarkar and Walker 2009, 35–58.

Sinha, Anita. 2009. Damaged roots in the fight for public housing. *San Francisco Bay View: National Black Newspaper*, 11 May. http://www.sfbayview.com/2009/damaged-roots-in-the-fight-for-public-housing/ (accessed 18 July 2009).

Slotkin, Richard. 1985. *The fatal environment: The frontier in the age of industrialization, 1800–1890*. New York: Atheneum.

Stein, Alan H., and Gene B. Preuss. 2006. Oral history, folklore, and Katrina. In Hartman and Squires 2006, 37–58.

Stevens, Maurice. 2005. Department of Comparative Studies, Ohio State University, Critical theories of trauma: Institutional practices and theoretical reflections. Kirwan Small Grants Proposal (unpublished), submitted in support of the 'Critical Trauma Studies' conference held at Ohio State University, May 2005.

———. 2006. From the Deluge: Traumatic iconography and emergent visions of nation in Katrina's wake. *English Language Notes* 44, no. 2: 217–22.

van Heerden, Ivor, and Mike Bryan. 2006. *The storm: What went wrong and why during Hurricane Katrina – the inside story from one Louisiana scientist*. New York: Viking.

Webster, Richard. 2006. Gretna police blocking passage of New Orleanians seeking refuge. *New Orleans CityBusiness*, 9 October. http://findarticles.com/p/articles/mi_qn4200/is_20060009/ai_n16769340 (accessed 4 August 2008).
Weizman, Eyal. 2007. *Hollow land: Israel's architecture of occupation*. London: Verso.
———. 2008. Conversations. Public talk presented at the REDCAT, Walt Disney Concert Hall, 6 May, in Los Angeles.
Willis, Holly. 2008. The political becomes personal: Docs use real people to make big issues easier to tackle. Sundance Film Festival, Focus on Film, 22 January. http://www.sundance.org/festival/insider/2008-01-22-FOF-political-personal.asp (accessed 23 January 2008).
Zdenek, Robert O., Ralph Scott, Jane Malone, and Brian Gumm. 2006. Reclaiming New Orleans' working-class communities. In Hartman and Squires 2006, 167–84.

After the apology: Reframing violence and suffering in *First Australians*, *Australia*, and *Samson and Delilah*

Felicity Collins

School of Communication and Critical Enquiry, La Trobe University, Melbourne, Australia

This article explores the cinematic reframing of media images that normalize violence and suffering in remote Aboriginal communities. It proposes that, in the light of the 2007 Northern Territory Emergency Response and the 2008 apology to the Stolen Generations, the archival history series *First Australians*, the postmodern blockbuster *Australia*, and the arthouse drama *Samson and Delilah* contribute to an anti-colonial politics by creating cinematic spaces for affective and ethical response to issues of 'bare life' that tend to be exhausted, rather than worked through, in media temporality.

After the apology

Media images of chronic violence and suffering in remote Aboriginal communities haunt present-day relations between Indigenous and settler Australians. Far from being hidden, these images of 'bare life' (Agamben 1998) have become a routine part of our media diet, making only passing claims upon our attention. But the flood of responses to the release of an archival history series, *First Australians* (Rachel Perkins, 2008), a postmodern blockbuster, *Australia* (Baz Luhrmann, 2008), and an auteurist arthouse drama, *Samson and Delilah* (Warwick Thornton, 2009), suggests that cinematic events that address Indigenous–settler relations do have the capacity to galvanize public attention, under certain conditions.[1]

The potential of these cinematic texts[2] to provoke an ethical response to media images which normalize Aboriginal deprivation and otherness is contingent upon a belated but history-making event: the apology by the newly elected Labor government to the Stolen Generations, broadcast nationwide from Parliament House in Canberra on 13 February 2008. For the many Australians who stopped work to gather in front of public screens and witness this event, Prime Minister Rudd's apology marked a long overdue shift in the politics of reconciliation, a politics which had been ably exploited by the conservative Howard government to shore up its three terms in office. This belated apology (first mooted in the 1997 *Bringing them Home* report on the removal of Aboriginal and Torres Strait Islander children from their families) opened the way for the reinvigoration and renewal of an anti-colonial politics of subjectivity.

However, the apology to the Stolen Generations is not the only event to shape the public response to *First Australians*, *Australia* and *Samson and Delilah*. Since 2006 there has been a surfeit of writing and media commentary by journalists, public intellectuals and activists on endemic violence in remote Aboriginal communities. Although such violence has been investigated, documented and reported in the media since the late 1970s (Langton

2008/2009, 29–35), the most recent attention to the issue was sparked by the revelation, on ABC Television's *Lateline* in May 2006, of horrific cases of sexual abuse of women and children in town camps in Central Australia. The public outcry in response to the allegations made by Magistrate Nanette Rogers – on the use of customary law to protect Aboriginal offenders against criminal charges and penalties – led directly to the *Little Children are Sacred* report, released on 15 June 2007. The report was used to justify the contentious Northern Territory National Emergency Response, announced on 21 June 2007, as the last televisual policy initiative of the Howard government. It entailed the suspension of the anti-discrimination act and the spectacular despatch of 600 soldiers, along with teams of bureaucrats and health professionals, to remote communities.

The case for an emergency intervention in the Northern Territory was legitimized by press, radio and television coverage of atrocious 'Third World' living conditions in Aboriginal communities, exemplified by the Melbourne *Age*'s agenda-setting photo-journalism campaign which continues to this day. An unprecedented flood of books and essays by artists, activists and intellectuals is another measure of the widespread impact of the 2006 *Lateline* report. The most prominent of these include: playwright Louis Nowra's soul-searching *Bad Dreaming: Aboriginal Men's Violence against Women and Children* (2007); Chloe Hooper's award-winning *The Tall Man* (2008) on the court hearings that followed a brutal death in custody and subsequent riot against Queensland police on Palm Island; Brian Toohey's hardboiled *Quarterly Essay* 'Last drinks' (2008) on the politics of the Northern Territory intervention; Marcia Langton's brave essay on 'The end of "big men" politics' in Aboriginal communities (2008/2009); Germaine Greer's provocative public lecture on rage (2008); and, most recently, Peter Sutton's account of the end of the liberal consensus on Indigenous policy in *The Politics of Suffering* (2009). This vigorous public debate is driven by the ethical imperative to speak up about the suffering of others. But the ethos of the debate is marked by a growing reluctance to blame 'lateral violence' in Aboriginal communities on the traumatic afterwardsness (or *nachtraglichkeit*) of colonial dispossession.[3] Instead, many commentators have followed the lead of Cape York activist Noel Pearson, questioning left-liberal policies of self-determination that have failed to mitigate the effects of 'lateral' and 'vertical' violence in Aboriginal communities (Langton 2008/2009).

This highly politicized discourse on violence and intervention can make film analysis seem trivial, but in the remainder of this article I want to make a case for the affective and ethical politics of working through such issues in cinema. In brief, I argue that the flow of media images of 'bare life' in remote Aboriginal communities evokes regular pinpricks of shock, shame and moral outrage; but at the same time media temporality exhausts the initial shock of these images, normalizing the very violence and suffering that activist-intellectuals and policy makers seek to ameliorate.[4] Cinema, under these circumstances, has the capacity to narrativize and reframe media images, and to draw a broader constituency into an anti-colonial response.

Trauma cinema

> [W]hether and how we respond to the suffering of others, how we formulate moral criticisms, how we articulate political analyses, depends upon a certain field of perceptible reality having already been established. (Butler 2009, 64)

Before looking more closely at how cinema might reframe 'a certain field of perceptible reality' already established by archival, publicity and news images, I will briefly reprise trauma theory's long-standing suspicion of empathy and affect, seen by many as obstacles to ethical-political response.

Much work on trauma cinema highlights the use of material traces such as family photographs, home movies, archival footage and witness testimony to reach some sort of accommodation, not so much with the event itself but with its symptomatic aftermath. In this view, trauma cinema is defined by a modernist desire to fracture subjectivity as the only adequate response to the overwhelming, traumatic aftermath of holocaustal events. Trauma films, in this view, deal with 'world-shattering events' in a non-realist mode and disturb the spectator's empathetic identification with characters (Walker 2005, 19–20). Miriam Hansen, however, has pointed to the limits of a binary opposition between self-reflexive modernism and illusionistic realism, reminding us that, 'like it or not, the predominant vehicles of public memory are the media of technical re/production and mass consumption', particularly film and television (2001, 213). Thomas Elsaesser goes further, arguing that 'the cinematic resources of drama, melodrama, suspense and violence are legitimate means' of investing history with feelings (1996, 149). While advocates of a modernist trauma cinema concede the power of popular media to invest history with feeling, they continue to harbour an ingrained suspicion of 'too much' empathy and affect. A case in point is Tony Hughes D'aeth's conclusion to his critique of *Rabbit-proof Fence*:

> One can recognize and celebrate the vision of the makers of *Rabbit-proof fence* who have brought the issue of the Stolen Generations into the most affectively powerful and demographically penetrating of media, particularly in a political context that is grounded in denial. A friend described how she saw fellow passengers weeping on the Qantas flight on which it was screening. There must be a value in this [...]
> But ... [t]he empathetic investment on which the film is so heavily reliant constitutes in my view something of a Trojan Horse. (Hughes D'aeth 2002)

This distrust of 'empathetic investment' as the Trojan Horse of assimilation (through 'immersive identification' with the other) is a recurring refrain in the reception of Australian films dealing with Indigenous–settler violence. But if we accept that there is a limit to both popular *and* modernist techniques for articulating traumatic subjectivity, under what conditions might a national screen culture have the potential to elicit *Betroffenheit* – an affect which 'covers empathy and identification, but in an active, radical sense of being "stung into action"' (Elsaesser 1996, 173–4)?

Acting out, working through

It has become a truism of 'trauma culture' that it is imperative to 'work through' trauma by communicating or 'translating' its pain in the arts or media (Kaplan 2005, 19). But what interests me in this project is the possibility of realigning empathetic investment with an ethical working through of trauma. I begin with Dominick LaCapra's insistence that 'it's via working through that one acquires the possibility of being an ethical and political agent' (2001, 144). I then discuss Judith Butler's rigorous working through of 'what it means to become ethically responsive' in the face of the Abu Ghraib photographs (2009, 63). For LaCapra and Butler, the critical distance of working through is tempered by empathy and affect, both of which are necessary to ethical response.

LaCapra's emphasis on the political and ethical agency of 'working through' derives from his definition of historiography as a dialogic exchange with the past, entailing affect, empathy and questions of value in a process that 'does not eliminate hyperbole for the sake of a middling reasonableness or complacency' (2001, 35). He suggests that 'acting out', or reliving the past, may well be a necessary part of the dialectic of working through, in so far as hyperbolic acting out resists closure, cure and mastery (144–5). However, it is the critical distance of 'working through' that enables responsibility – understood as the ethical capacity to respond to and reactivate unfulfilled possibilities 'that lost out in the past' (148). But, LaCapra warns that unchecked identification with the other is an impediment to responsibility: someone possessed vicariously by the past 'may be tragically incapable of acting responsibly or behaving in an ethical manner involving consideration for others as others' (28). Empathy must be tempered by recognition that emotional response does not authorize one to speak in the other's voice or take the other's place as surrogate victim or perpetrator (27, fn. 31). However LaCapra's modernist-literary template for new subject positions beyond identification and objectification (179 80) has limits for critics interested in the media's unruly articulation of trauma in images that circulate as multiplatform events.[5]

Butler's work on the widely circulated Abu Ghraib photographs offers a way of deciphering moments when the digital circulation of the photographic image might provoke an ethical response to the suffering of others. Butler begins her critique of the Abu Ghraib photographs by taking issue with Susan Sontag's view 'that contemporary photography tended to aestheticize suffering for the purposes of satisfying a consumer demand – this last function making it inimical to ethical responsiveness and political interpretation alike' (Butler 2009, 69). Unlike the *momentary* pathos relayed by the photograph, in Sontag's assessment, the 'pathos conveyed by narrative forms "does not wear out"' (qtd in Butler 2009, 69). For Butler, however, photographs can and do prompt an ethical response if we pay attention to the frame. This is because social norms of who counts as human 'arrive in visual form' and 'it is the face of the other that demands from us an ethical response' (77). The norm of who counts as human is embedded in the frame:

> There are ways of framing that will bring the human into view in its frailty and precariousness, that will allow us ... to react with outrage when lives are degraded or eviscerated without regard for their value as lives. And then there are frames that foreclose responsiveness ... (77)

While Sontag commands the 'atrocious image' to haunt us, she maintains her position that photographs lack the temporality essential to narrative interpretation and political response (Butler 2009, 96). In contrast, Butler's focus on the *frame* grants the photograph an *enduring* temporality. Taking her lead from Barthes, Butler argues that the photograph installs and solicits 'a perspective on the absolute pastness of a life' in a double temporality of 'what has been' and 'what will have been' (97). A photograph that anticipates the future loss of a life establishes that life as grievable. But there is a further temporality which allows us to interpret and respond to the photograph: when the photograph is taken up by the media it goes into indefinite circulation and, 'thanks to these images, the event has not stopped happening' (85–6). Butler concludes that when the image circulates 'outside the scene of its production' we have the chance to see the dehumanizing norm encrypted in the photographic frame (100).

Ethical encounters

LaCapra draws our attention to the necessity of a hyperbolic working through of traumatic histories in order to become ethical agents. Butler (2009) draws our attention to the 'affective and interpretive' reframing of images (98) in a media temporality of indefinite circulation, and reminds us that a key condition for an ethical encounter with others is the 'mediating forms and frames that make responsiveness possible' (180). How, then, might a robust ethical response to the spectacle of dehumanized or 'bare' lives in Aboriginal communities be elicited by cinematic frames that operate within a media temporality of indefinite circulation? I have written elsewhere on the media as an intersubjective space of ethical encounter (Collins 2008, 2009) and will not reiterate those arguments here, except to say that our relations with others are determined by social and media norms that designate some as 'familiar' and some as 'strange' others, and that our exposure to the vulnerability of others in the media can make an ethical claim upon us by unsettling our subjectivity and calling our self-sufficiency into question.[6]

In the remainder of this article I focus on cinematic 'forms and frames' that engage with and recirculate archival (*First Australians*), publicity (*Australia*) and photojournalist (*Samson and Delilah*) images. These documentary, blockbuster and arthouse forms of cinema make different kinds of empathetic and affective (or sensory) claims on the spectator, but what they have in common is an interest in reframing the violence of the past and soliciting ethical and anti-colonial responses to the violence of the present.[7]

First Australians

It took producer-writer-director-narrator Rachel Perkins six years (with co-producer Darren Dale, co-writer Louis Nowra and co-director Beck Cole) to create the seven-part television history *First Australians*, broadcast on SBS in 2008. The 'Shakespearean' challenge for Perkins and her collaborators was to envision Australian history from an Indigenous perspective for a national television audience and for the educational DVD market. Each episode was filmed in a different region of Australia, with an overlapping chronology between episodes. Taking her cue from *The Civil War* (Ken Burns, 1990), Perkins made the decision to eschew re-enactments in favour of the pictorial record, landscape shots, interviews, diary extracts and voiceover narration. Wrestling with a vast archive (of 7000 images), Perkins decided to focus on 'stories of resilience' embodied by key characters in each episode: 'There were a lot of challenges in uncovering characters who had a voice that carried through time and into the records, who could be represented visually, and whose lives we could piece together', but the real challenge was to engage the television audience in a reframing of national history that required a discomfiting shift in empathy: 'We knew we couldn't tell a story that was just a trail of horror but we knew it was that story as well' (Perkins, qtd in George 2008, 20–1).

This dilemma, of reframing the nation's origins in colonial violence while keeping Indigenous and settler audiences on side, was resolved by embedding the 'trail of horror' in personal, character-based stories set in the past and narrated through written and visual sources that survive mostly as traces of settler perspectives on the past. These archival sources are framed by present-day commentary in two forms: interviews with talking heads, clearly identified as Indigenous or settler experts in the field; and Perkins' voiceover narration that works to contain the surfeit of visual material and the surfeit of feeling expressed by the talking heads.

How does this strategy – of reframing national history in terms of violent yet intimate encounters between Indigenous and settler characters *and* commentators – create a space for affective engagement and ethical response to the violence of the present? LaCapra's support for a historiography which refuses to 'eliminate hyperbole' is pertinent here: 'Hyperbole enacts stylistically the fact that one is affected by excess and trauma, but one can be excessive in many ways ... including ... unearned judiciousness that harmonizes problems and may even signal a numbing insensitivity to their import' (2001, 35). The 'trail of horror', given little or no weight in settler histories, is registered in *First Australians* through an unceasing flow of images and documents, turning points and calamities – an excess of images and events that challenge the perception that Australia's founding history, as taught in schools, was a dull and parochial affair.

In Episode 1 of *First Australians*, the inaugural site of hyperbole is the nexus between intimacy and violence embedded in the fraught relationships between Bennelong and Governor Arthur Phillip, Patyegarang and Lieutenant William Dawes, and Windradyne and William Suttor. Each potential friendship is shadowed by violence, including the kidnapping of Bennelong, the payback spearing of the Governor, the armed resistance of Pemulwuy, and the massacre of Windradyne's family for the sake of a few potatoes. The ethical norm of the entire series is embedded in the reframing of archival images which testify to the lost potential of these first intimate encounters.

The other site of excess in this episode is the nexus between hyperbolic feeling and judicious reasonableness, evident in the clash of views espoused by Professor Marcia Langton, Yiman/Bidiara Nation, and Inga Clendinnen, Emeritus Professor of History. The sequence dealing with the smallpox epidemic of 1789 is a case in point. While the image track assembles a mix of paintings and landscape images to depict the calamity and decimation of smallpox as it spread through Aboriginal tribes, Langton and Clendinnen take opposing positions on the germ warfare theory that smallpox was deliberately 'let loose by the British'. Langton admits, 'we can't say definitively', but nonetheless declares emphatically, 'in my own mind it came with the First Fleet'. Clendinnen protests, 'I simply can't comprehend that notion at all. In all the [British] accounts there is bewilderment, despair, horror.' The weight of archival evidence mounts up against Langton (as it must when the historical record is established by the victors) but the surfeit of feeling on both sides is what makes the sequence strangely affective. Working through and reclaiming the lost potential of the past in such hyperbolic moments reopens history's wounds.

What space for affective and ethical response, then, does the series create for viewers who might well be averse to feeling and responding to the wounds of history? Online responses to *First Australians* demonstrate the dialectic between pinpricks of shock and the rapid onset of boredom, typical of media temporality.[8] On the one hand, the SBS website for *First Australians* in November 2008 contained pages of unsurprising responses based on identification with and objectification of the other: the series was said to be enlightening, it showed 'us' the truth 'we' did not know, it made 'me' cry (with shame), it made 'me' proud, it made 'me' feel so sorry for 'them'. These remarks in turn opened up a space for commentary on how self-regarding empathy (whether of pride, shame or sorrow) objectifies Indigenous Australians and reinforces 'white' subjectivity as the norm. At the other end of the spectrum, students, forced by their teachers to review the series, had no truck with such 'responsible' views. They took the opportunity to express their resentment of the task in hyperbolic terms: 'this thing is sumtymz interesting but boring ... its soo boring ... im dying already' and 'I am seriously going to die of boredom.'

The significance of intimate relations between colonizers and natives, as a possibility for the present, is easily lost in the hyperbolic flow of archival material whose very excess can exhaust the viewer's capacity to respond. Digital technologies might, however, open up one prospect for redeeming such material for an anti-colonial politics. For viewers who download an episode from the SBS website or buy the series on DVD, the possibility arises of pausing the flow of images: to look long and hard at one image; to listen to a voice again; to replay a sequence; or to fast forward to a half-remembered story or character in order to follow its visual and verbal rhetoric more closely – as I did to understand the structure and argument behind the compelling affect of the smallpox sequence, encountering again those discomfiting interviews steeped in feeling. In this practice of re-viewing – of pausing the flow, slowing the pace, becoming immersed in the material – the viewer is drawn into the indefinite circulation of images from the archive. Through selective immersion, something more enduring than a self-regarding or bored response becomes possible. For the immersed viewer, the colonial past in all its otherness – in its newly arranged televisual form – becomes a virtual space in which multiple encounters with anti-colonial subjectivities might yet take place.

Australia

Released just after *First Australians* went to air, Baz Luhrmann's *Australia* (2008) is a different kind of hyperbolic event in national screen culture. As a postmodern paean to cinematic storytelling, it exploits the profit-maximizing commodity form of the Hollywood blockbuster. As an allegorical reframing of Australia colonial history it can be interpreted as an anti-colonial or *philoxenic* invitation for whitefellas to become 'as good as black'.[9] Yet early reviews of the film failed to recognize either its postmodern revel in 'unoriginality' or its allegorical reframing of Australian film history to retell the colonial story. In 'Gone with the wind: An Australian fiasco', British-based expatriate Peter Conrad laments the failure of *Australia* as an 'historical epic'. He takes the film to task for portraying 'us as timid, imitative colonials' and for failing to signal 'our proud national independence' (2009, 30). Conrad's response to the film – which assumed white subjectivity as the norm – was widespread but not universal. Citing Germaine Greer's equally 'castigating and misleading' review of the film, Langton positions *Australia* squarely within an anti-colonial politics of subjectivity: 'nine months after the apology to the stolen generations by Prime Minister Kevin Rudd, I was thrilled with Luhrmann's compassion and good humour, and his visionary way of overcoming the guilt complex that poisons our national debate' (2008, 11).

There is, however, an argument to be made that Luhrmann's hyperbolic pastiche of film genres and styles commodifies the history of the Stolen Generations. In this view, the sensory immersion of the spectator in computer-generated storybook images aestheticizes frontier violence, evoking momentary pathos rather than sustained ethical response. But it can also be said that the blockbuster film is a commodity form designed for multiple viewings (in cinema, then on DVD with commentary tracks, extra features, the director's cut, anniversary editions) – a mode of immersed *and* critical spectatorship over time – that has become the norm in the digital era. As Hudson and Zimmerman argue, this new cinephiliac mode of spectatorship – invited by postmodern pastiche and enabled by digital technologies – can either commodify or politicize the past. It can commodify history 'by immobilizing images and psychic imaginaries within the confines of a past that is always only a rarefied object caught within unfulfilled desires'; or it can open the past 'to the multiple vectors of recirculation for new connections and new meanings' (2009, 139). There are myriad ways in which *Australia*, as a highly orchestrated event in national screen culture and world cinema, commodifies the past, not least through advertising tie-ins to tourism. But there are also ways in which *Australia* politicizes the past by pastiching film history and putting new images into circulation – enabling cinephiliac viewers to invest an imaginary past with new connections and anti-colonial meanings.

Here, I restrict my discussion to two publicity images to show how *Australia*, understood as a blockbuster marketing event, participates in the indefinite circulation and reframing of the pathos of 'the Aboriginal' torn between two worlds. The first is a portrait of Brandon Walters, the charismatic young actor whose character, Nullah, is the film's central figure of empathetic investment – as the storyteller negotiating two cultures. The portrait was named 'Brandon' and can be seen as a continuation of the 'brand' *Australia*. The artist Vincent Fantauzzo was introduced to Walters and his family by Luhrmann, but the initial project of painting Walters *with* his family was put aside in favour of a larger-than-life, widescreen close-up of Brandon's face. As winner of the People's Choice award in the 2009 Archibald Prize, a *photograph* of the portrait was widely circulated in a newspaper advertising campaign promoting the touring Archibald exhibition, coinciding with the DVD release of *Australia*. The photograph provoked fleeting recognition, but the portrait holds the gaze by magnifying two flaws. What arrests the attention in the portrait is the diagonal band of light that draws the gaze to the dry, cracked lips and a mark on the nose. The pathos of authenticity evoked by these flaws 'reveals' the person behind the image – only to confirm the marketability and vulnerability of 'Brandon' as the embodiment of Nullah, whom we already 'know' from the film.

The second intersection of the film with the publicity image is a newspaper photograph of David Gulpilil and Brandon Walters in a line-up of *Australia*'s stars, notably Nicole Kidman and Hugh Jackman who carried the bulk of the film's promotion. Like the film it promotes, this publicity photograph can be reframed as a politicized image of anti-colonial affiliation – a point I expand below. The source of the photograph was a press conference where it was noted in passing that *Australia* would be Gulpilil's last film. But what arrests my attention in this photograph is the shock of Gulpilil's long grey hair and beard. This transformed image of the fresh young actor who made his film debut in *Walkabout* (1971) elicits the shock of time having suddenly passed. This suddenness anticipates a time when Gulpilil, himself, will have disappeared from the frame, not only of national cinema, but of life itself. There is a pathos here, but one that might politicize rather than commodify Gulpilil's last film role.

The issue that arises from these images is whether, as Sontag insists, the pathos of the publicity photograph merely 'haunts' us while only the sustained temporality of narrative leads to understanding and ethical response. In the context of the apology and Prime Minister Rudd's promise 'to close the gap' between Indigenous and settler Australians, the portrait, 'Brandon', invites objectification and self-regarding empathy – expressed as anxiety by Nicole Kidman and Germaine Greer about the 'already' doomed future of Walters as a young, male member of a remote Aboriginal community. But the publicity photograph of Gulpilil with his co-stars provokes something else, an affect layered in media temporality. I argue elsewhere that in his role as a star-celebrity Gulpilil has repeatedly acted as a host-friend – inviting the whitefella to the Aboriginal world. But this invitation has gone unrecognized as a form of resistance to colonial norms of Aboriginality embedded in Gulpilil's objectification as a strange-other tragically divided between two worlds (Collins 2009). However for those familiar with Gulpilil's oft-repeated invitation to share his culture and language, recorded in a vast archive of media interviews over four decades, the pathos of non-recognition is far from momentary.

I want to propose that one of the issues that *Australia* works through is the dilemma that Gulpilil embodies as a star-celebrity, 'divided between two worlds'. This dilemma dates back to the pathos and unfulfilled potential of those initial colonial encounters featured in *First Australians* – with the intimacy and violence between Bennelong and Governor Phillip as the prototype. In this framework, Gulpilil's long-standing offer of anti-colonial friendship requires an ethical response from settler Australia. It is fitting, then, that this offer, and the need for a response, is allegorized in the final scene of *Australia*. In his last performance of Aboriginality for a white director, Gulpilil is no longer cast in the role of an intermediary between two worlds. He maintains his language and culture throughout the film and stands apart from the action. At the end of the film, summoning his grandson, Nullah (Brandon Walters), he keeps his distance from Missus Boss (Nicole Kidman) and Drover (Hugh Jackman) and says, in language, 'You have been on a journey, now we are heading home, to my country, to our country.' The full weight and pathos of this speech – rescinding the open invitation to whitefellas to become guest-like in *his* country – can only be felt if we recognize in this scene Gulpilil's act of walking away from the role assigned him in Australian national cinema.

When Gulpilil, allegorically speaking, turns his back on white Australia and returns to his country, the ethical invitation to anti-colonial affiliation becomes Nullah's responsibility. He makes a farewell promise to Missus Boss: 'I will sing you to me, Missus.' When she responds, 'And I will hear you', we could say that Missus Boss makes an ethical response on behalf of settler Australia, accepting Nullah's invitation to join him in becoming neither black nor white, but minor.[10] This invitation to anti-colonial subjectivity is heralded by critics such as Langton, but is ignored by critics like Conrad who long for a commodified 'epic history'. What Luhrmann's pastiche of the colonial past offers is not mastery or closure but an ethical reframing of publicity images and cinematic genres through which we encounter each other and the past. Rather than 'respectful distance', this amicable reframing offers 'close encounters' that 'establish an alliance through the process of being unsettled' (Ahmed 2000, 18).

Samson and Delilah

Arguably, an even more unsettling encounter, located firmly in the present, is offered by Warwick Thornton's first feature film, *Samson and Delilah*. In a stark contrast to the hyperbolic visuality of both *First Australians* and *Australia*, Thornton adopted the measured realism of arthouse drama to reframe media images of 'bare life' and 'lateral violence' in Central Australia. After a long apprenticeship working in the Central Australian Aboriginal media and making short films, Thornton set out to make a love story for 'his mob' about two kids:

> One is a [petrol] sniffer and one is not. It was designed for Central Australia because we do write these kids off there. Not only in town, where the newspapers every second day is about 'the problem' [. . .] Elders in Aboriginal communities . . . are writing these kids off as well [. . .] I wanted to show two incredibly beautiful children who have fought all their lives just to breathe . . . I wanted to show that to Central Australia, and if the rest of Australia or the world get involved that's fantastic. (Thornton 2009)

The reception of *Samson and Delilah*, after winning the Palme d'Or in May 2009, involved a circular exchange between media and cinema publics. This exchange is evident in the unprecedented amount of media discussion of the 'honest', 'brave' and 'confronting' way that *Samson and Delilah* deals with young lives already 'written off' by the media and by Aboriginal elders. The exchange is also evident in the way the film itself can be seen as an affective and ethical reframing of the intense media coverage of Aboriginal violence and suffering, reported 'every second day' by the newspapers.

To show how *Samson and Delilah* creates a cinematic space for affective and ethical response to the incessant flow of media reports on violence in Aboriginal lives, I want to focus on three instances of photojournalism, each of which constitutes a horizon of public response to the film. The first is the campaign photograph, specifically the hundreds of news images put into circulation since Nanette Rogers went public on the overwhelming number of extreme cases of sexual abuse and violence coming before the courts in Central Australia. The campaign photograph is connected to investigative journalism and entails an ethical commitment to keep the issue before the public until government intervention ameliorates the problem. One such photograph, framed by the headline, 'Child abuse six times higher for Aborigines', appeared in *The Age* on 3 July 2009. The full-colour photograph dominates the page. What is striking but typical is the expanse of red earth that occupies most of the visual field. Silhouetted against this redness are a young man lying prone in the foreground, two younger children moving through the middle ground, and in the background, the silhouettes of four tiny figures. On the horizon, framed by trees, we see two tin-roofed houses, some rubble, and what might be a water tank standing high above the treeline. No reference is made to the photograph in the two-column report, and the place and people in the photograph remain unidentified. It is a generic photograph of an impoverished community where children are framed as vulnerable figures in an iconic outback landscape. The left-hand side of the photograph displays two columns of statistics under the title 'Worlds Apart', comparing life expectancy, child abuse/neglect, imprisonment, home ownership, education and income for 'Indigenous' and 'rest of population'. The source of the photograph is the government report *Overcoming Indigenous Disadvantage 2009*, acknowledged in tiny print in the corner of the image.

The second instance is the widely circulated myth-making publicity photograph of the director and stars of *Samson and Delilah* hovering on the red carpet at the Cannes Film Festival, nervously acknowledging the cameras. The third is the myth-busting, front page, full-colour shot of the actor Rowan McNamara (Samson) at home in the privacy of his own room, in a town camp outside Alice Springs, far from the glamour of Cannes, but also far from the anonymity of 'indigenous disadvantage'. Coming across these two images, after viewing *Samson and Delilah* at my local arthouse cinema, I realize that the film and its publicity images 'blast' the generic campaign photograph out of its newspaper context, giving names, faces and a place to the anonymous figures used to illustrate 'indigenous disadvantage' in a never-ending flow of government and media reports.

But if my own experience, supported by online accounts, is anything to go by, *Samson and Delilah* does more than rehumanize generic images of 'bare lives' reduced to violence and suffering. The film makes these lives human and grievable. The experience of seeing the film with a receptive and responsive audience lingers as a powerful bodily affect long after the initial viewing. One name for this lingering affect is grief but another might be the haunting temporality of utter devastation that requires an ethical response. This lingering affect is the residue of the film's evocation of cinematic time – of life, slowed down to a walking and sitting and lying-down pace. As online blogs indicate (negatively and sometimes positively), nothing much happens in this film. Action is reduced to the bare essentials of movement between spaces in a steady rhythm, disrupted by violent activations of offscreen space. The slow build towards a culminating violence takes place *as if* before our eyes, but is driven by something that is just out of frame.

At one level it is as if those anonymous figures silhouetted against the red ochre in the generic news photograph have come alive in cinematic time, as endangered lives which must, *not yet*, be written off. Rather than the photograph's 'absolute pastness' of a life, this arthouse drama reframes news photographs of non-lives riven through by violence – a violence that originated before these *particular* lives and will continue beyond them. The film's devastating intimation of something like the ontological reality of a formative violence – that cannot be articulated in media reports of *acts* of violence, nor understood simply as the residue or afterlife of colonial violence – is what haunts us in this circular exchange between cinematic and news images. By reframing 'bare lives' as vulnerable and grievable lives, the film provokes an ethical response that has been numbed by the hyperbolic flow of media images, government reports and expert debate. It is this, I think, that accounts for the film's extraordinary success as a media and cinematic event.

Reframing violence and suffering

Some readers may object to my discussion of an archival history series, a blockbuster film and a low-budget drama as if they evoke the same kinds of experiences and responses despite their distinct styles, modes of address and ideological projects. My point is that, unlike most Australian feature films and documentary series which attract neither media nor public interest, these three products of a publicly funded, national screen culture sparked extensive media and public attention precisely because they speak (in different ways) to the politics of reconciliation after the apology, *and* to the sense of urgency and crisis generated by media preoccupation with violence in remote Aboriginal communities.

Within their different generic forms, each of these films arrived on our screens as an event in national screen culture. As such, they generated media talk, but they also created occasions for pausing the flow of media temporality. This is not to re-establish modernist contemplation over media distraction, self-reflexivity over hyperstimulus, fractured subjectivity over immersion in storytelling. Rather, the post-apology films reframe a familiar iconography so that what is lost or ignored in the incessant flow of media temporality is precisely what invites an affective and ethical response in cinematic spaces. Digital modes of recirculating and reviewing cinematic and media texts have complicated any claims that might be made about how and when an ethical response to images and narratives of violence and suffering might produce anti-colonial affiliations as a norm of Australian subjectivity. But the multiplatform reception of *First Australians*, *Australia* and *Samson and Delilah* rehearses this possibility.

Notes

1. The opening episode of *First Australians* was broadcast on a public screen in Taylor's Square in Sydney in October 2008; the advertising campaign itself became an issue of public debate and media commentary on history and truth; the websites promoting *First Australians* and *Australia* were cross-linked; the Human Rights Arts and Film Festival organized a panel of health and other experts to discuss *Samson and Delilah* at the Nova arthouse cinema complex in Melbourne in May 2009; the Lacanian journal *Analysis* has put out a call for contributions to a collective series of notes on *Samson and Delilah*; a conference on Baz Luhrmann's *Australia* at Australian National University was held in December 2009; and one-day events have been held on the films under the rubrics of history and postcolonialism. All three have defied the industry truism that Aboriginal themes ensure box office failure.
2. I refer to *First Australians*, *Australia* and *Samson and Delilah* as cinematic texts and events because they are high-quality audiovisual texts that are promoted and recognized as special events within national screen culture. *First Australians* is a documentary series broadcast on public television. Like *Australia* and *Samson and Delilah*, it attracted funding from public film agencies such as Screen Australia, it enjoyed a high profile in print, broadcast and online media, and it went straight to DVD after its initial release. Although national screen culture is both cinematic and televisual, I use cinematic here in order to denote a space within media temporality for certain kinds of feature films, documentaries and drama series that demand a more sustained and less distracted attention from the viewer, whether in the cinema or in front of a television or computer screen.
3. On *nachtraglichkeit* as a mode of temporality involving deferred revision of memory traces in relation to events that return as trauma, see Laplanche in Caruth (2001) and Radstone (2007, 77–8; 2000, 85–6).
4. On the condensation, displacement, repetition and exhaustion of social issues and historical events in media temporality, see Ellis (1999) and Schwarz (2004).
5. I refer here to the promotion and consumption of audiovisual texts across a variety of platforms, including public screens, televisions, home theatres, personal computers and hand-held devices.
6. My understanding of cinema as an intersubjective space of affective and ethical encounter is indebted to Langton (1993), Ahmed (2000), Butler (2005) and Gandhi (2006).
7. For a phenomenological approach to film spectatorship as a sensory mode of ethical engagement, see Stadler (2008). For a cognitive theory of narrative cinema's formal structures of sympathetic alignment, moral allegiance, and devices of empathetic simulation and affective mimicry, see Smith (1995, 73–106).

8. The posting of opinions as part of a routinely orchestrated response to the online promotion of *First Australians*, *Australia* and *Samson and Delilah* produces a new digital resource for media critics, one that challenges the conclusions that might be drawn from textual analysis of spectator positions. Here, I only touch on this resource, noting that the pattern and range of opinions is remarkably similar in all three cases.
9. See Gandhi (26–32) for a distinction between *homophilic* citizenship based on sameness and *philoxenic* solidarities based on anti-colonial affiliations.
10. See Healy (2008) for a cultural history of encounters with Aboriginality as a space of negotiation, entailing both European and Aboriginal subjects 'becoming minor'.

References

Agamben, Giorgio. 1998. *Homo sacer: Sovereign power in bare life*. Palo Alto: Stanford University Press.

Ahmed, Sara. 2000. *Strange encounters: Embodied others in post-coloniality*. London and New York: Routledge.

Butler, Judith. 2005. *Giving an account of oneself*. New York: Fordham University Press.

———. 2009. *Frames of war: When is life grievable?* London: Verso.

Caruth, Cathy. 2001. An interview with Jean Laplanche. *Postmodern Culture* 11, no. 2. http://muse.jhu/edu/journals/postmodern_culture/vol11/11.2caruth.html (accessed 23 January 2004).

Collins, Felicity. 2008. The ethical violence of celebrity chat: Russell Crowe and David Gulpilil. *Social Semiotics* 18, no. 2: 191–204.

———. 2009. Resisting the ethical violence of coercive Aboriginality: David Gulpilil. In *Celebrity colonialism*, ed. Robert Clarke, 189–208. Newcastle upon Tyne: Cambridge Scholars.

Conrad, Peter. 2009. Gone with the wind: An Australian fiasco. *The Monthly*, February, 30–6.

Ellis, John. 1999. Television as working-through. In *Television and common knowledge*, ed. Jostein Gripsrud, 55–70. London: Routledge.

Elsaesser, Thomas. 1996. Subject positions, speaking positions: From *Holocaust, Our Hitler*, and *Heimat* to *Shoah* and *Schindler's List*. In *The persistence of history: Cinema, television, and the modern event*, ed. Vivien Sobchack, 145–83. New York: Routledge.

Gandhi, Leela. 2006. *Affective communities: Anticolonial thought, fin-de-siècle radicalism, and the politics of friendship*. Durham, NC and London: Duke University Press.

George, Sandy. 2008. [Re]writing history. *Australian Writers Guild: In Focus*, November, 20–2.

Greer, Germaine. 2008. *On rage*. Melbourne: Melbourne University Press.

Hansen, Miriam. 2001. *Schindler's List* is not *Shoah*: The second commandment, popular modernism, and public memory. In *The historical film: History and memory in media*, ed. Marcia Landy, 201–17. New Brunswick, NJ: Rutgers University Press.

Healy, Chris. 2008. *Forgetting Aborigines*. Sydney: UNSW Press.

Hooper, Chloe. 2008. *The tall man: Death and life on Palm Island*. Camberwell, Vic: Hamish Hamilton.

Hudson, Dale, and Patricia R. Zimmerman. 2009. Cinephilia, technophilia and collaborative remix zones. *Screen* 50, no. 1: 135–46.

Hughes D'aeth, Tony. 2002. Which rabbit-proof fence? Empathy, assimilation, Hollywood. *Australian Humanities Review* 27. http://www.australianhumanitiesreview.org/archive/Issue-September-2002/hughesdaeth.html (accessed 25 August 2009).

Kaplan, E. Ann. 2005. *Trauma culture: The politics of terror and loss in media and literature*. New Brunswick, NJ: Rutgers University Press.

LaCapra, Dominick. 2001. *Writing history, writing trauma*. Baltimore and London: Johns Hopkins University Press.

Langton, Marcia. 1993. *Well, I heard it on the radio and I saw it on the television ... an essay for the Australian Film Commission on the politics and aesthetics of filmmaking by and about Aboriginal people and things*. Sydney: Australian Film Commission.
———. 2008. Why Greer is wrong on Australia. *The Age*, 23 December, 11.
———. 2008/2009. The end of 'big men' politics. *Griffith Review* 22: 13–38.
Nowra, Louis. 2007. *Bad dreaming: Aboriginal men's violence against women and children*. North Melbourne: Pluto Press.
Radstone, Susannah. 2000. Screening trauma: *Forrest Gump*, film and memory. In *Memory and methodology*, ed. Susannah Radstone, 79–107. New York: Berg.
———. 2007. *The sexual politics of time*. Abingdon: Routledge.
Schwarz, Bill. 2004. Media times/historical times. *Screen* 45, no. 2: 93–105.
Smith, Murray. 1995. *Engaging characters: Fiction, emotion, and the cinema*. Oxford: Clarendon Press.
Stadler, Jane. 2008. *Pulling focus: Intersubjective experience, narrative film and ethics*. London: Continuum.
Sutton, Peter. 2009. *The politics of suffering: Indigenous Australia and the end of the liberal consensus*. Melbourne: Melbourne University Press.
Thornton, Warwick. 2009. Interview with Luke Buckmaster, 12 May. http://blogs.crikey.com.au/cinetology/2009/05/12/interview-with-warwick-thornton-writerdirector-of-samson-delilah/ (accessed 25 June 2009).
Toohey, Brian. 2008. Last drinks: The impact of the Northern Territory intervention. *Quarterly Essay* 30: 1–97.
Walker, Janet. 2005. *Trauma cinema: Documenting incest and the holocaust*. Berkeley: University of California Press.

Confronting 'choiceless choices' in Holocaust videotestimonies: Judgement, 'privileged' Jews, and the role of the interviewer

Adam Brown

School of History, Heritage and Society, Faculty of Arts and Education, Deakin University, Geelong, Australia

'Privileged' Jews include those prisoners in the camps and ghettos who held positions which gave them access to material and other benefits. Subject to extreme levels of coercion, these victims were compelled to act in ways that have been judged as both self-serving and harmful to fellow inmates. Such situations, which exemplify what influential theorist Lawrence Langer terms 'choiceless choices', are the chief concern of Primo Levi's paradigmatic essay on the 'grey zone'. In light of these key conceptualizations of the ethical dilemmas of Holocaust victims, the paper analyses the representation of 'privileged' Jews in several videotestimonies recorded at the Jewish Holocaust Museum and Research Centre (JHMRC) in Melbourne, Australia. It will be shown that judgements of victims *in extremis* cause considerable problems for attempts to testify to the complex situations and experiences of 'privileged' Jews. The role of the interviewer is a crucial factor in this, particularly when interviewers are themselves Holocaust survivors. The paper reveals that while it might be argued that moral evaluations of 'privileged' Jews should be suspended, judgements are often imposed on Holocaust testimonies in various ways and have a significant impact on their content.

Introduction

'Privileged' Jews include those prisoners in the camps and ghettos who held positions which gave them access to material and other benefits. Subject to extreme levels of coercion, these victims were compelled to act in ways that have been judged as both self-serving and harmful to fellow inmates. Lawrence Langer's concept of 'choiceless choices' and Primo Levi's notion of the 'grey zone' provide particularly valuable insights into the ethical dilemmas confronted by 'privileged' Jews during the Holocaust and the problems faced by those who attempt to represent these liminal figures. Despite the crucial importance of 'privileged' Jews during the event and their ongoing significance to its legacies, limited scholarly attention has been granted to this complex and sensitive issue.

This paper will analyse the representation and judgement of 'privileged' Jews in several survivor videotestimonies recorded at the Jewish Holocaust Museum and Research Centre (JHMRC) in Melbourne, Australia. The JHMRC offers a unique collection of over 1300 videotestimonies, as Holocaust survivors were instrumental in both initiating the videotestimony project and often taking part in it as interviewers themselves. It will be revealed that while Levi and Langer suggest that one should suspend judgement of 'privileged' Jews when confronted with their traumatic experiences, moral evaluations often play an important role in the construction of firsthand accounts. Indeed, judgement plays a crucial part in the interview process, and the relationship between interviewer and interviewee is often a site of tension. An exploration of these complex situations contributes much to the already burgeoning field of oral history.

The 'choiceless choices' of 'privileged' Jews and the problem of judgement

A key premise of Jewish religious thought, and indeed most classical European philosophy, is that human actions are governed by free will (Herring 2006, 155). In short, one chooses how one behaves; hence one can be held responsible for one's actions (Peperzak 2004, 188, 197). However, the ethical dilemmas encountered by 'privileged' Jews during the Holocaust render issues of agency and accountability highly problematic. Without choice and subsequent responsibility, the faculty of moral judgement is threatened. The impossible scenarios that confronted 'privileged' Jews can be seen to exemplify what Langer terms 'choiceless choices', although these dilemmas are not limited in Langer's work to victims in 'privileged' positions. In his study *Versions of Survival: The Holocaust and the Human Spirit*, Langer defines 'choiceless choices' as 'crucial decisions [that] did not reflect options between life and death, but between one form of abnormal response and another, both imposed by a situation that was in no way of the victim's own choosing' (1982, 72). The notion of a 'choiceless choice' has been popularized in William Styron's novel *Sophie's Choice* (1979), in which a mother is forced to choose by a Nazi officer which of her two children will be killed. Langer argues that, due to their unresolvable quality, 'choiceless choices' are not even to be considered matters of deciding between a 'greater' or 'lesser' evil. Jewish behaviour under Nazi persecution took place in an environment constructed by the perpetrators not of immorality but of 'non-morality'; an environment 'beyond good and evil' (1982, 72).

While 'privileged' Jews might be seen to have acted at the expense of fellow prisoners in various ways, for various reasons and under varying levels of coercion, given the distance of time and experience (and arguably even without this distance), it is problematic for anyone to evaluate the consequences, motivations and personal autonomy that were in play during the events in question. If it is the case that, as Slavoj Žižek succinctly puts it, 'only a free choice is morally binding' (2001, 74), then it might be argued that 'privileged' Jews should not be judged for their behaviour *in extremis*. Some scholars, such as Irene Kajon, optimistically contend that Auschwitz is 'capable of showing us essential aspects of the human spirit, and hence of bringing our knowledge of good and evil into sharper focus' (2000, 192). Positioning himself against this view, Langer draws heavily on survivor testimony to describe the 'optionless anguish of the deathcamp' and points to its implications for judgement and representation (1982, 74). Considering 'choiceless choices' to be a defining feature of the Holocaust, Langer stresses the inappropriateness of pre-existing categories of morality and representation when attempting to come to terms with the event. Langer stresses that conventional notions of 'dignity', 'courage', 'sacrifice', 'heroism', 'freedom' and 'choice' are among the long 'list of free words that died in Auschwitz, leaving no successors' (95). Heavily influenced by Levi's early Holocaust memoirs, Langer highlights the problems of representation and judgement that confront attempts to understand the traumatic experiences of Jews. He writes:

> Choiceless choices are perversions of power and will; they proclaim the impotence of the victim, who contaminates his future by the very compulsion to survive in which his oppressors seek to drown his moral nature. (146)

Persecuted Jews' 'decisions', if they can be called that, were made under extreme duress, and the notions of intent or volition, which Risa Sodi (1990, 10) identifies in her discussion of Levi's writings as central to most concepts of justice and judgement, are impossible to evaluate. Indeed, Langer's concept of 'choiceless choices' is frequently connected by scholars to Levi's 'grey zone' (Leys 2007, 18–24; Melson 2005).

Levi's pivotal essay entitled 'The grey zone' was published in his final book, *The Drowned and the Saved* (1986), just one year before he died. Echoing many of Langer's sentiments regarding the ethical dilemmas facing Jews, Levi narrows his focus to those victims in so-called privileged positions. He concentrates on the extreme situations of the *Kapos* ('chiefs') of forced labour squads in the camps, the members of the *Sonderkommandos* ('special squads') forced to work in the Auschwitz crematoria, and of Chaim Rumkowski, the much-criticized leader of the *Judenrat* (Jewish Council) of the Lodz Ghetto. While Levi emphasizes that the perpetrators of Holocaust atrocities must be held accountable for their actions, he points out that judging the behaviour of 'privileged' Jews is considerably more problematic: 'The condition of the offended does not exclude culpability, and this is often objectively serious, but I know of no human tribunal to which one could delegate the judgement' (1986, 29). Levi positions these liminal figures at the core of the 'grey zone', a metaphorical realm of moral ambiguity that he characterizes as having 'an incredibly complicated internal structure, [which] contains within itself enough to confuse our need to judge' (27). Reflecting on the Auschwitz *Sonderkommandos*, which were liquidated and replaced approximately every four months, Levi declares that 'our need and ability to judge falters', and stresses that we should 'let a judgement of them be suspended' (41). Levi's call to suspend moral judgement when representing Jews *in extremis* is mirrored in Langer's discussion of 'choiceless choices'. Reflecting on the 'dismal fate' of the *Sonderkommandos* forced to perform such ghastly activities before an inevitable death, Langer declares: 'We reserve judgment for the authors of that fate, not its victims' (1982, 97).

Levi and Langer focus primarily on Auschwitz, although the associated problems of judgement and representation also apply to the ghettos. Contemporary philosopher Zygmunt Bauman states that *Judenrat* officials and Jewish police played 'a crucial mediating role in the incapacitation of the Jews', although he also meditates on their lack of 'choice' (1989, 129). In what parallels Langer's argument regarding 'choiceless choices', Bauman writes of the high level of coercion and minimal 'options' created by the Nazi authorities, forcing the *Judenräte* to partake in the 'save what you can' game – a game of acting *rationally* on good intentions that invariably resulted in death for the many and survival (albeit temporarily) for the few' (129). Indeed, Levi clearly states that the same *impotentia judicandi* that arises from the situation of the *Sonderkommandos* 'paralyses' us when considering Rumkowski's activities in the Lodz Ghetto (1986, 43). While we should not condemn the controversial *Judenrat* leader, Levi writes, we cannot 'absolve him on the moral plane' either (49). Paradoxically, however, Levi himself cannot abstain from judging those he argues should not be judged, as has been discussed elsewhere (Brown 2007, 2008). It might therefore be the case that if passing judgement on 'privileged' Jews is inappropriate, it is also inevitable.

Significantly, Levi criticizes the simplifying effects he perceives in certain forms of Holocaust representations, namely history and film – effects that are caused by a 'Manichean tendency which shuns half-tints and complexities', and resorts to the black and white binary opposition(s) of 'friend' and 'enemy', 'good' and 'evil' (1986, 22). While Levi stresses that it is of fundamental importance that the distinction between perpetrators and their victims not be undermined, he holds that an adoption of ethical Manicheanisms only trivializes the complexity of Holocaust experiences, particularly the morally ambiguous behaviour of 'privileged' Jews. Likewise, Langer warns against 'formulas and single truths', and argues that 'those who attempt to generate such truths ... sacrifice ambiguity for the sake of coherence, seeking to construct a possible future from the debris of an impossible past' (1982, 4). The paucity of language, or what Langer describes as 'the inadequate mediating efforts of the world' (5), is particularly evident in attempts to (re)construct the ethical dilemmas of 'privileged' Jews. The interrelated problems of judgement and representation are evident in the interview process in survivor videotestimonies.

Holocaust videotestimonies and the relationship between interviewer and interviewee

> Holocaust testimony, in whatever medium, confronts the dilemma of finding the right registers to connect meaningfully with past trauma and encode it. Given that any testimony is reliant upon language, the question of emplotment and the adequacy of language surface as points of inquiry and intense debate. (Maclean, Abramovich, and Langfield 2008, 8)

While a considerable critical literature has been preoccupied with the (un)representability of the 'Holocaust experience' (Friedlander 1992; Kaplan 2007; Weissman 2004; Eisenstein 2003; Fridman 2000; Cole 1999; Schwarz 1999), little explicit attention has been given to the role of moral judgement in representations of Jews, particularly those in 'privileged' positions. Similarly, only brief and infrequent mention is made of these figures in the large number of publications focusing on the genre of Holocaust testimony (Waxman 2006; Bigsby 2006; Miller and Tougaw 2002; Bernard-Donals and Glejzer 2001; Patterson 1998; Felman and Laub 1992). However, perhaps owing partly to the belated establishment of the various projects aiming to collect survivor videotestimonies around the world, studies drawing on these audiovisual sources are now beginning to appear with greater frequency (Stier, 2003; Maclean, Abramovich, and Langfield 2008). The value of videotestimonies, which, like written testimonies, individualize victims and their suffering, rests not only in their inclusion of verbal text but also in the exposure of the image through the camera, necessitating a consideration of facial expression, body language and so on. In his study *Traumatic Realism: The Demands of Holocaust Representation*, Michael Rothberg stresses the importance of acknowledging the specificities of oral testimony as a 'representational medium that is mediated and governed by conventions' (2000, 118). Mapping the series of conventions that govern videotestimonies will always be a far from comprehensive exercise, not least because of the dissimilarities between different testimony-gathering projects. Nonetheless, practically all videotestimonies share some core components. In his analysis of the 'structural context' that 'frames' the content of a testimony, Oren Stier highlights the interviewer as an integral mediatory figure (2003, 75).

Dominick LaCapra aptly notes that the importance of the role of the interviewer in survivor videotestimonies goes well beyond their contribution to the historical record. He points out that the relationship between interviewers and interviewees may place immense pressures on the act of witnessing, having 'more general implications for historical research, especially with respect to highly sensitive, emotionally laden, and evaluatively significant issues' (2001, 86–7). One such issue might be seen to be the complex 'choiceless choices' confronting 'privileged' Jews, which have been a somewhat tabooed subject in popular and scholarly discourse (Brown 2009). It hardly needs to be mentioned that interviewers will, consciously or otherwise, bring their own agenda to the construction of videotestimonies. Interruptions, interjections and insistent redirections of the topic of discussion on the part of interviewers may complicate the act of bearing witness. Indeed, this possibility in the interview process has significant implications, as the active participation of the interviewer in the construction of a Holocaust videotestimony 'can facilitate or impede the outcome' (Langfield and Maclean 2009, 200–1).

In prescriptive texts on how to conduct oral history interviews, strong warnings against the intrusion of a testimony by interviewers are commonplace (Yow 2005, 98; Thompson 1978, 165). Paul Thompson writes that interviewers 'who cannot stop talking themselves, or [cannot] resist the temptation to contradict or push an informant with their own ideas, will take away information which is either useless or positively misleading' (165). It must be emphasized here that the purpose of this paper is not to criticize any interviewing practices exhibited in the JHMRC videotestimonies or to 'judge' the individuals (whether interviewers or interviewees) for any judgements they appear to make, but to explore *how* the problem of judgement affects representations of 'privileged' Jews in the genre. Of course, it should also be noted that this discussion does not preclude other factors influencing the interview process, such as the interview protocols and parameters constructed by the institution in question.

As will become clear below, the problems of judgement and representation clearly impinge on attempts to represent 'privileged' Jews in survivor videotestimonies. One major point to be considered here is that the vast majority of 'privileged' Jews have left no testimony of their own, as very few victims (with or without 'privileged' positions) survived the war. The scarcity of accounts by 'privileged' Jews raises the question of how others can represent their experiences. Annette Wieviorka suggests that 'certain categories of survivors' have tended to abstain from recalling their experiences, and points to 'privileged' Jews as a case in point (2006, 18). Nonetheless, those holding 'privileged' positions in the camps and ghettos make frequent appearances in survivor testimonies and other modes of representation. Evaluations of the general attitude of 'non-privileged' survivors towards 'privileged' Jews are not always consistent. Alan Mintz describes Jewish 'collaboration' as 'rife and the object of deep and implacable hatred on the part of Jews who were its victims' (2001, 184), while Aaron Hass argues that most Holocaust survivors are reluctant to condemn 'Jewish collaborators' due to the pressures they were put under to survive (1988, 172). In the field of life writing, G. Couser emphasizes the ethical obligations an author has when 'representing vulnerable subjects', who 'are unable to represent themselves in writing or to offer meaningful consent to their representation by someone else' (2004, xii). This dilemma also applies to genres other than life writing and is of particular relevance to the extreme situations of 'privileged' Jews, whose predicament arguably contributes to what has been termed the 'empathetic incomprehensibility' of the Holocaust (Magurshak 1988, 422–5). Therefore, since they often perished along with other victims of the Holocaust, it is important to examine representations of 'privileged' Jews with a critical eye. Moreover, since former 'privileged' Jews have sometimes been willing and able to record their experiences in videotestimonies, representation is further problematized. Indeed, the impact of judgements relating to the theme of 'privilege' is particularly striking when the interviewee is a former 'privileged' Jew.

Former 'privileged' Jews as interviewees

The almost oxymoronic categorization of 'privileged' Jews is exemplified in the case of Thea Kimla, who survived her incarceration in Auschwitz while her entire family perished during the Holocaust. Kimla, who recorded her videotestimony at the JHMRC in 1993, was a frequent member of resistance organizations against the Nazi authorities. Upon arrival at the camp, 'privileged' political prisoners who knew of Kimla's previous resistance activities allocated her a position in the 'Canada' work group in order to give her, in Kimla's words, 'a chance to survive'. Kimla describes 'Canada' as 'a commando of two thousand women which worked twelve hour shifts sorting out the satchels ... of the people which were gas-chambered [*sic*]'. As exemplified in the well-known fiction of Tadeusz Borowski (1959), the 'Canada' prisoners had access to additional goods that could be bartered for extra rations. Volunteering information regarding her somewhat 'privileged' status, Kimla acknowledges that 'being at that job, of course, I could again pinch a lot of things'. Significantly, Kimla notes that she often gave extra items of clothing to fellow prisoners and begins to point out that she joined the Auschwitz underground resistance movement. Interrupting Kimla's narrative with what appears to be a subtle judgement, the interviewer inquires whether her food allocation was better than other prisoners not from the 'Canada' commando. The survivor replies: 'No, no, my food condition was better because I *pinched* things, and I "organised" things, and I could *exchange* things for a piece of bread or for something.' Kimla's tone sharpens noticeably as she clarifies the nature of her 'privileges', her head nodding aggressively as she enunciates the word 'pinched' and 'exchange'. This is one of several instances throughout the videotestimony when Kimla appears slightly frustrated with the interviewer, a non-survivor, who occasionally needs Kimla to reiterate what she has said in order to understand. Importantly, while reflecting on her time in 'Canada', Kimla notes that the prisoner in charge of her barrack – the *Blockälteste* ('Block Eldest') – was Frances Tack-Kousal, who survived Auschwitz and was also interviewed at the JHMRC when she emigrated to Australia.

The issue of 'privilege' plays a more prominent role in the videotestimony of Tack-Kousal (1993), a Czech Jew who was deported to Auschwitz in mid-1942, early in the camp's existence. The subject of Kousal's 'privileged' status is raised within the first 15 minutes of the three-hour testimony. When Kousal explains with some difficulty how, on her third day in the camp, she obtained her first 'privileged' position as a *Stubenälteste* ('Room Eldest'), the interviewer is actively involved in the narrative:

> Interviewer: Do you know for what reason they picked these ten girls?
> Kousal: That's what I said. They picked us out to be *Stubenälteste*.
> Interviewer: I know. I mean why you – why these ten girls?

Kousal, who was given this position at 20 years of age, responds to the repeated question with a shrug of her shoulders, while the interviewer comments, 'You don't know.' Kousal then explains at length what she views as a possible reason for being singled out; namely, that she had perhaps been more 'Aryan' in appearance in the eyes of the SS. Even after Kousal has given this plausible interpretation and commented that 'in a way we were the very lucky ones', the interviewer returns to the subject, reiterating her question: 'So you were just picked out of the column ... "You and you and you and you"?' After wincing in confusion, Kousal again confirms this enthusiastically while the interviewer quietly notes in a seemingly disbelieving voice: 'Really? Mmm ...' As in the aforementioned videotestimony of Kimla, a notable interest in the issue of 'privilege' on the part of the interviewer impacts on the direction the testimony takes. The influence of the interviewer's judgement is again evident when Kousal's reminiscences have shifted to the living conditions of the prisoners. Spontaneously, the interviewer once more returns to Kousal's allocation of a 'privileged' position: 'Can I ask something else. When you were selected – the ten girls – to be *Stubenälteste*, were you told what your job would be, what you had to do?' While the preface to this question is seemingly constructed to obtain new information, Kousal can only confirm the duties she has already mentioned, including the supply of rations and cleaning of the barrack.

The interviewer's retrospective judgement also seems to play a role when the subject of the daily roll calls is mentioned. When Kousal explains that it was her responsibility to ensure that prisoners from her room were assembled, the interviewer's corresponding comment attaches negative connotations to the activity. With a strong measure of irony, the interviewer asks: 'It was your job to say "*Raus, raus, raus*!" was it? To wake up people in the morning?' Kousal, who is perhaps aware of the implications of these words given the well-known phrasing used by the SS, hesitates before affirming this was the case. Interestingly, however, Kousal goes on to explain to the interviewer that roll calls were not as severe in Auschwitz I (the main administrative camp) as they later were in Birkenau (Auschwitz II). After the interviewer interrupts with, 'I'm sorry, I don't follow', Kousal looks upwards and notes, 'Yes, that's what people don't understand.' The survivor then emphasizes that without the threat of 'selections' for the gas chambers, prisoners did not fear roll calls at that time. Interestingly, because of Kousal's constant struggle with expressing herself in English, the specific words that the interviewer employs in observations and questions impact directly on the survivor's narrative and often become part of the testimony itself. When the interviewer asks what other activities occupied Kousal during the day when other prisoners were engaged in forced labour, she suggests that those with 'privileged' positions had an 'easy time'. As a result, Kousal, grasping for words, uses the same phrase as the interviewer to describe her situation. The notion of 'privileged' Jews having an 'easy time' in Auschwitz misrepresents their status as victims of Nazi oppression and the extreme pressures they were forced to endure. Additionally, as in Kimla's videotestimony, the interviewer inquires whether Kousal obtained a larger food ration as a result of her position, to which Kousal also replies in the negative: 'No, at that time we didn't ... We had all the same [*sic*].' The issue of 'privilege', particularly in terms of Kousal's later status as a *Blockälteste*, is continually returned to throughout the interview, invariably as a result of the prompting of the interviewer.

These examples reveal that the construction of a firsthand account in videotestimonies given by former 'privileged' Jews can be an emotionally fraught process. To add an extra dimension to this already complicated situation, the individuals questioning survivors for the JHMRC, as noted above, may also be survivors of the Holocaust. This, of course, is not to suggest that there is something exceptional about survivor interviewers making judgements. All interviewers bring their own individual contexts, incorporating their views, values and perspectives, to the interview. The influential Holocaust scholar Geoffrey Hartman, who points to the unpredictability of the relationship between interviewer and interviewee, maintains that '[c]are has to be taken to neutralize any personal agenda of the interviewers' (2004, 211). Nonetheless, neither 'objective' witnessing nor 'objective' interviewing is possible. The personal backgrounds of survivor interviewers are perhaps even more likely to influence the way in which they approach the interview process, and not necessarily with problematic results. Indeed, Michele Langfield and Pam Maclean note in their discussion of the JHMRC videotestimonies that the interaction between interviewee and interviewer, when both roles are occupied by survivors, has considerable potential for enhanced empathy and understanding (2009, 200–1). On the other hand, interactions of this kind can also have considerable implications for the judgement of 'privileged' Jews.

Holocaust survivors as interviewers

The influence of a survivor interviewer on the interview process can be seen in the videotestimony of Pola Lumby (1994), who was incarcerated in the Benzin Ghetto in

Poland before escaping the 'Final Solution'. While Lumby did not hold a so-called privileged position, the interviewer changes the topic of discussion to 'privileged' Jews several times in a seemingly strong attempt to invoke the interviewee's moral evaluation of these figures. Significantly, the interviewer reveals at the beginning of the interview that both survivors lived in Benzin, and hence both share some similar memories of specific places and people. It might be assumed that this circumstance would provide a rich contextual layer for the narrative to unfold in, and this is often the case; however, it also opens up the possibility of disagreements during the interview regarding certain details or perceptions. Early in the interview, while Lumby is recalling conditions and experiences in the Benzin Ghetto, the survivor interviewer guides her towards the subject of the community's *Judenrat* and Jewish police. After Lumby describes passive resistance undertaken in the Ghetto in the form of educating Jewish children, the survivor interviewer poses a question directly relating to the judgement of 'privileged' Jews: 'So you remember when the *Judenrat*, when the Council of Jewish Elders, got organised [...] what was your feelings and what was your perception at that time, not now, at that time? [*sic*]' In explicitly seeking a moral judgement, the interviewer tellingly assumes Lumby will have a negative opinion of the *Judenrat* in retrospect, even before she expresses any views on the subject. When Lumby begins to answer, her interviewer interrupts with: 'What did you think of it?' Lumby replies, 'Well, we thought it was a necessity. I myself thought it was a necessity', thus contradicting the implicit judgement being made by the interviewer.

Lumby then proceeds to explain how the *Judenrat* had to collect money and possessions from the Ghetto population, while the survivor interviewer grimly inquires: 'What for? What for?' Lumby seems to display no anger whatsoever towards the Council officials for their actions, instead holding the perpetrators solely responsible for the expropriation of Jewish belongings. The discussion that immediately follows Lumby's claim that it was the Germans who collected Jewish valuables reveals an atypical involvement of the interviewer in Lumby's narrative:

> Interviewer: So when the order came for the Jews to give silver and radios and so on –
> Lumby: Yeah.
> Interviewer: – it was the *Judenrat* that collected them?
> Lumby: Yes.
> Interviewer: Am I right?
> Lumby: Yes.
> Interviewer: Yes. Not the Germans.
> Lumby: No. But they were there – they were there – watching what's coming in.
> Interviewer: Yes. Sure.

The number of interjections, questions and comments on the part of the survivor interviewer highlights the volatility of the issue of 'privileged' Jews. When the interviewer stresses that it was the *Judenrat* that confiscated the valuables and 'not the Germans', Lumby's reply continues to show a seemingly non-judgemental stance towards the Jewish Council. While far from aggressive, this exchange gives a clear sense of a subtle disagreement between the survivors, one that does not seem capable of being readily resolved. When the interviewer goes on to ask what other Council activities Lumby remembers from her time in the Ghetto, further implicit judgements are revealed to be at work in the interview process. Crucially, it is uncertain whether the issue of 'privileged' Jews, which becomes a significant part of Lumby's comparatively short, one-and-a-half-hour videotestimony, would have been raised at all without the insistence of the interviewer.

The impact the survivor interviewer can have on the representation of 'privileged' Jews is even more evident in cases where interviewees are former 'privileged' Jews, as can be seen in the videotestimony of Magda Blau (1994). Deported from Czechoslovakia to Auschwitz early in the camp's existence, Blau survived three and a half years in Auschwitz I and Birkenau, at one point being made responsible for 30,000 women as *Lagerälteste* ['Camp Eldest'] of the Women's Camp. Blau's JHMRC videotestimony and her recent, self-published memoir, *From Childhood to Auschwitz Birkenau* (2003), provides a detailed account of her incarceration before and during her 'privileged' period. Barely surviving both malaria and paratyphus, Blau narrowly escaped several 'selections' and was even pulled from a line heading for the gas chamber. During the almost six-hour-long videotestimony Blau recorded over a period of two days for the JHMRC, she represents herself as consistently generous, self-sacrificing and protective of others. Nonetheless, the queries and comments of her interviewers, one of whom is another Jewish survivor of several concentration camps, express moral judgements throughout Blau's videotestimony.

Implicit judgements become apparent when the discussion turns to the notorious SS overseer Irme Griese. Blau states that 'I called her Irma even when she was *Lagerführer* ["Camp Leader"]'. Reverting to an ironic tone, the survivor interviewer replies: 'You were Jewish ... and you had such a personal contact with her.' The comment is not positioned as a question, although it does evoke a justification from Blau, who emphasizes her sense of duty to others: 'Yes, because ... I was saying to myself: "Only once you're going to the chimney, but until you go in, your duty is [to] help, help where you can. And to help you can only – when you stand up to yourself, when you don't show fright [*sic*]."' Additionally, after Blau's position as Block Commander of a 'Prominent' barrack has been discussed, the interviewer returns to it in order to clarify what tasks the position involved. As Blau lists these, including food distribution, counting prisoners, and supplying prisoners for sterilization, the interviewer repeats each answer after her. This is the only time this happens during Blau's testimony. As in the videotestimonies of Kimla and Kousal, the subject of specific benefits afforded to 'privileged' Jews is broached on several occasions, such as when the interviewer asks Blau: 'The people who were privileged in the previous barrack, did they get better food or bigger rations of food or ... ?'

Later in the interview, the survivor interviewer asks Blau whether there were any Jewish *Blockältester* other than her, a question that is again intended to return Blau's discussion to the behaviour of 'privileged' Jews. While it is difficult to ascertain whether Blau senses any latent judgements impinging on the interview process, she nonetheless directly addresses the issue of judgement, testifying to the 'choiceless choices' confronting an individual in a 'privileged' position:

> Oh, yes, there was, there was. But, you see, I tell you what, because there are some voices that the *Blockältester* was this or that, err, different opinion. But I tell you that imagine a sixteen–seventeen year old girl to be responsible for a thousand, thousand two hundred hungry, sick, hard-working women, to make them to stand there at the roll call, to get them out from bed [*sic*].

The quiet repetition of 'yes' on the part of the other survivor in the room while Blau makes this statement serves to remind the viewer of the influence the interviewer has on the content of the narrative being recounted.

Hence the process of judgement can be seen to influence the roles and perceptions of those involved in all three of what Dori Laub has characterized as the

> separate, distinct levels of witnessing in relation to the Holocaust experience: the level of being a witness to oneself within the experience, the level of being a witness to the testimonies of others, and the level of being a witness to the process of witnessing itself. (1995, 61)

In short, the interviewee, the interviewer and the viewer(s) of the interview may all be affected in some way by the passing of moral judgement on 'privileged' Jews. As with Lumby's videotestimony, it may be that without the direct and indirect prompting of the survivor interviewer, the issue of 'privileged' Jews would have featured little in Blau's account, and thus not been thrust upon the viewer at frequent intervals.

Conclusion: Approaching liminal figures

> Conventional vocabulary limps through a situation that allows no heroic response, no acceptable gesture of protest [. . .] This predatory profile of survival, when fear of such death, not affirmation of a basic human dignity, drives men and women to behavior they would not consider under normal circumstances, confirms another moment when reality defeats both a language of judgment and a mode of moral behavior. (Langer 1982, 146)

Exploring the traumatic experiences of 'privileged' Jews would seem to be a crucial facet of ongoing attempts to come to terms with the Holocaust. Situating the sensitive issues of moral ambiguity and 'compromise' within a discourse that views the Holocaust as (with)holding a universal meaning, Levi claims that such issues are essential to attempts to understand the human condition. He writes that the 'grey zone' is 'indispensable to know if we want to know the human species, if we want to know how to defend our souls when a similar test should once more loom before us' (1986, 25–6). At the same time, however, the unprecedented ethical dilemmas confronting victims defy a straightforward interpretation that gestures at the event's perceived 'universality'. The specificity of Holocaust experiences, not least of all those of 'privileged' Jews in the camps and ghettos, seems to exist beyond pre-existing moral frameworks, evading traditional notions of 'heroism', 'dignity' and 'choice'. Judgement is threatened, if not undermined, by the 'choiceless choices' imposed on Jewish victims. However, this paper has suggested that if moral judgements of 'privileged' Jews are inappropriate, they may also be unavoidable.

The challenges posed to language by the Holocaust are considerable and the genre of videotestimony reveals many obstacles to efforts to construct and record firsthand accounts. The examples of survivor videotestimonies from the Jewish Holocaust Museum and Research Centre reveal that judgements of 'privileged' Jews affect the content of the act of witnessing in various ways. Frequently, contrasting perspectives on the behaviour of 'privileged' Jews are manifest in the direct interaction between interviewees and interviewers. The implications of judgement are particularly evident when the witness is a former 'privileged' Jew, or the interviewer is also a Holocaust survivor. Significantly, the controversial issue of 'privilege' often arises in the testimonial narrative only when the interviewer directs the witness to this subject. This raises the curious question of whether judgement may itself have at times been *necessary* to engage with the issue in the first place, in spite of the problematic implications contained in this judgement. Explorations of the ethical dilemmas of 'privileged' Jews will undoubtedly continue to play a part in attempts to come to terms with the Holocaust. It is here, perhaps, that instances of extreme trauma pose insurmountable obstacles to representation and expose the fragility of human judgement when confronted with a morally liminal situation. As Pam Maclean, Dvir Abramovich and Michele Langfield note in their introduction to a recent volume focusing on the JHMRC collection, 'if one conclusion can be drawn from the study of Holocaust testimony, it is that the ethics and impact of remembering the Holocaust cannot be taken for granted' (2008, 23).

References

Bauman, Zygmunt. 1989. *Modernity and the Holocaust*. Ithaca, NY: Cornell University Press.

Bernard-Donals, Michael, and Richard Glejzer. 2001. *Between witness and testimony: The Holocaust and the limits of representation*. Albany: State University of New York Press.

Bigsby, Christopher. 2006. *Remembering and imagining: The chain of memory*. Cambridge: Cambridge University Press.

Blau, Magda. 2003. *From childhood to Auschwitz Birkenau*. Melbourne: self-published.

Borowski, Tadeusz. 1959. *This way for the gas, ladies and gentlemen*. Trans. Barbara Vedder. Harmondsworth: Penguin.

Brown, Adam. 2007. The trauma of 'choiceless choices': The paradox of judgement in Primo Levi's 'grey zone'. In *Trauma, historicity, philosophy*, ed. Matthew Sharpe, Murray Noonan, and Jason Freddi, 121–40. Newcastle upon Tyne: Cambridge Scholars Press.

———. 2008. Traumatic memory and Holocaust testimony: Passing judgement in representations of Chaim Rumkowski. *Colloquy: Text, Theory, Critique* 15: 128–44.

———. 2009. Marginalising the marginal in Holocaust films: Fictional representations of Jewish policemen. *Limina: A Journal of Historical and Cultural Studies* 15. http://www.limina.arts.uwa.edu.au/current/ibpcommended.

Cole, Tim. 1999. *Selling the Holocaust: From Auschwitz to Schindler: How history is bought, packaged, and sold*. New York: Routledge.

Couser, G. Thomas. 2004. *Vulnerable subjects: Ethics and life writing*. Ithaca, NY: Cornell University Press.

Eisenstein, Paul. 2003. *Traumatic encounters: Holocaust representation and the Hegelian subject*. Albany: State University of New York Press.

Felman, Shoshana, and Dori Laub, eds. 1992. *Testimony: Crises of witnessing in literature, psychoanalysis, and history*. New York and London: Routledge.

Fridman, Lea Warnick. 2000. *Words and witness: Narrative and aesthetic strategies in the representation of the Holocaust*. Albany: State University of New York Press.

Friedlander, Saul, ed. 1992. *Probing the limits of representation: Nazism and the 'Final Solution'*. Cambridge, MA: Harvard University Press.

Haas, Peter J. 1988. *Morality after Auschwitz: The radical challenge of the Nazi ethic*. Philadelphia: Fortress.

Hartman, Geoffrey. 2004. Audio and video testimony and Holocaust studies. In *Teaching the representation of the Holocaust*, ed. Marianne Hirsch and Irene Kacandes, 205–19. New York: Modern Language Association of America.

Herring, Basil. 2006. Choice-diminished behavior and religious-communal policy. In *Judaism, science, and moral responsibility*, ed. Yitzhak Berger and David Shatz, 155–68. Lanham, MD: Rowman & Littlefield.

Kajon, Irene. 2000. Auschwitz as crucial experiment: The Lord's suffering servant in the interpretation of André Neher and Emmanuel Levinas. In *Good and evil after Auschwitz: Ethical implications for today*, ed. Jack Bemporad, John T. Pawlikowski, and Joseph Sievers, 191–9. Hoboken, NJ: KTAV.

Kaplan, Brett Ashley. 2007. *Unwanted beauty: Aesthetic pleasure in Holocaust representation*. Urbana and Chicago: University of Illinois Press.

LaCapra, Dominick. 2001. *Writing history, writing trauma*. Baltimore and London: Johns Hopkins University Press.

Langer, Lawrence L. 1982. *Versions of survival: The Holocaust and the human spirit*. Albany: State University of New York Press.

Langfield, Michele, and Pam Maclean. 2009. Multiple framings: Survivor and non-survivor interviewers in Holocaust videotestimony. In *Memories of mass repression: Narrating life stories in the aftermath of atrocity*, ed. Nanci Adler, Selma Leydesdorff, Mary Chamberlain, and Leyla Neyzi, 199–218. New Brunswick and London: Transaction.

Laub, Dori. 1995. Truth and testimony: The process and the struggle. In *Trauma: Explorations in memory*, ed. Cathy Caruth, 61–75. Baltimore and London: Johns Hopkins University Press.

Levi, Primo. 1986. *The drowned and the saved*. Trans. Raymond Rosenthal. London: Michael Joseph.

Leys, Ruth. 2007. *From guilt to shame: Auschwitz and after*. Princeton: Princeton University Press.
Maclean, Pam, Dvir Abramovich, and Michele Langfield. 2008. Remembering afresh? Videotestimonies held in the Jewish Holocaust Museum and Research Centre (JHMRC) in Melbourne. In *Testifying to the Holocaust*, ed. Pam Maclean, Michele Langfield, and Dvir Abramovich, 3–28. Sydney: Australian Association of Jewish Studies.
Magurshak, Dan. 1988. The 'incomprehensibility' of the Holocaust: Tightening up some loose usage. In *Echoes from the Holocaust: Philosophical reflections on a dark time*, ed. Alan Rosenberg and Gerald E. Myers, 421–31. Philadelphia: Temple University Press.
Melson, Robert. 2005. Choiceless choices: Surviving on false papers on the 'Aryan' side. In *Gray zones: Ambiguity and compromise in the Holocaust and its aftermath*, ed. Jonathan Petropoulos and John K. Roth, 97–106. New York: Berghahn.
Miller, Nancy K., and Jason Tougaw, eds. 2002. *Extremities: Trauma, testimony, and community*. Urbana and Chicago: University of Illinois Press.
Mintz, Alan. 2001. *Popular culture and the shaping of Holocaust memory in America*. Seattle and London: University of Washington Press.
Patterson, David. 1998. *Sun turned to darkness: Memory and recovery in the Holocaust memoir*. Syracuse: Syracuse University Press.
Peperzak, Adriaan T. 2004. *Elements of ethics*. Stanford: Stanford University Press.
Rothberg, Michael. 2000. *Traumatic realism: The demands of Holocaust representation*. Minneapolis: University of Minnesota Press.
Schwarz, Daniel R. 1999. *Imagining the Holocaust*. New York: St. Martin's Press.
Sodi, Risa. 1990. *A Dante of our time: Primo Levi and Auschwitz*. New York: Peter Lang.
Stier, Oren Baruch. 2003. *Committed to memory: Cultural mediations of the Holocaust*. Amherst and Boston: University of Massachusetts Press.
Styron, William. 1979. *Sophie's choice*. New York: Random House.
Thompson, Paul. 1978. *The voice of the past: Oral history*. Oxford and New York: Oxford University Press.
Waxman, Zoë Vania. 2006. *Writing the Holocaust: Identity, testimony, representation*. Oxford: Oxford University Press.
Weissman, Gary. 2004. *Fantasies of witnessing postwar efforts to experience the Holocaust*. Ithaca, NY and London: Cornell University Press.
Wieviorka, Annette. 2006. *The era of the witness*. Trans. Jared Stark. Ithaca, NY and London: Cornell University Press.
Yow, Valerie Raleigh. 2005. *Recording oral history: A guide for the humanities and social sciences*. Walnut Creek, CA: Rowman & Littlefield.
Žižek, Slavoj. 2001. *Did somebody say Totalitarianism? Five interventions on the (mis)use of a notion*. London: Verso.

Films and videotestimonies

Blau, Magda. 1994. JHMRC Videotestimony No. 459, 30 January and 2 February. DVD.
Kimla, Thea. 1993. JHMRC Videotestimony No. 257, 13 January. DVD.
Lumby, Pola. 1994. JHMRC Videotestimony No. 463, 8 February. DVD.
Tack-Kousal, Frances. 1993. JHMRC Videotestimony No. 570, 11 February. DVD.

The guilt zone: Trauma, masochism and the ethics of spectatorship in Brian De Palma's *Redacted* (2007)

Mark Straw

Department of American and Canadian Studies, University of Birmingham, Birmingham, UK

The main question of this paper is the fraught psychological realm of the combat veteran or soldier in the Brian De Palma film *Redacted*. This will explore how a traumatic male subjectivity is constructed and is rendered explicitly in the staging and dramatization of the film. It will also explore how this trauma impacts on the communities inscribed in the film and the implied community of the films' spectators. This paper will therefore deal with the issue of how war is memorialized, processed and critiqued through deploying traumatized male subjectivity in cinema. I will deal with this question by referring to a now well-established critical discourse of 'trauma cinema', influenced especially by E. Ann Kaplan and Ban Wang, Janet Walker, and Thomas Elsaesser, and also to Deleuze's model of masochism. I intend to argue that (as mentioned previously) masochistic male subjectivity is deployed in films in which the central male protagonist is ostensibly traumatized. I also argue that, given the recent 'turn to ethics' in film studies, this masochistic subjectivity has important implications for the spectatorship of catastrophe and suffering. *Redacted*, in particular, seems to be aware of its ethical position through its reflexivity and forced collision with genuine images of death. The value of this is to show how spectators are sited in relationship to film images of death and suffering and to point out the ethical complexities of 'consuming trauma'. It is also of use in that the position of masochistic spectatorship offers a route out of the binding power relations which inflict inaction and passivity on consumers of contemporary visual culture.

Redacted (De Palma, 2007) has been perhaps one of the most polarizing films of recent years. The film won a 'Silver Lion' ('best director') award at the Venice Film Festival, and yet those who have actually seen the film remain a privileged few, since it has been denied general release in most regions of the world and was for a comparatively long time unavailable on Region 2 DVD.[1] Roger Ebert proclaimed the film to be 'a ferocious argument against the engagement in Iraq' (2007) and Marjorie Baumgarten in *The Austin Chronicle* praised the film for its 'combustible energy' and found that 'despite its shortcomings, *Redacted* is a film brimming with spontaneity and fury'. Other reviews were less complimentary; Joe Morgenstern in the *Wall Street Journal* bluntly described it as a 'work of propaganda' and 'an awful aberration', whereas Desson Thomson, writing in the *Washington Post*, criticized the film for its implication of the audience and US society, declaring that this is the 'same old Brian enjoying the peeping, bringing us into the guilt zone, then saying shame on all of us' (2007).

So who or what is the 'same old Brian'? If we look at his directorial career we see it is hallmarked by numerous films that explore the act of watching and the passive state that goes hand in hand with this act: *Body Double* (1984), *Dressed to Kill* (1980) and *Blow Out* (1981) all contain themes of voyeurism, whilst other films display an engagement with the idea of watching and its relationship to power and powerlessness – for example, Tony Montana's paranoid surveillance of the security cameras around his mansion via a bank of video monitors in *Scarface* (1983) and the helpless situation of the protagonist in *Casualties of War* (1989). In particular it is this last film, *Casualties of War*, that bears the most similarities to *Redacted*, since they are both war films with comparable thematic concerns. *Redacted* is concerned with a fictional take on a factual event, the Al-Mahmudiyah killings of 12 March 2006. In real life, this involved the gang rape and murder of a young Iraqi girl named Abeer Qasim Hamza al-Janabi, and the subsequent murder of her parents and sister. In the film, one of the characters seeks to expose the behaviour of his fellow soldiers in the hope of bringing the perpetrators of this heinous crime to justice. Similarly, *Casualties of War* is based on events from 1966 during the Vietnam War, and describes the kidnap, rape and murder of a young Vietnamese girl by a squad of American soldiers, and the attempts of one of the squad members to resist the violence and degradation meted out to the girl. Marita Sturken (1997) has commented that the problem with *Casualties of War* is that its 'real focus is the rift in morality among the Americans and their own victimization' (106). It could also be argued that this same problem pervades *Redacted*, since, as we shall see, the majority of the narrative investment is in the tensions, arguments, disputes and social interplay between the American soldiers. The effect of this is to temper the account of Iraqi victimhood with a disproportionate focus on American suffering.

Returning to Desson Thomson's comments regarding *Redacted*, it is intriguing that the concept of 'peeping' is incited, especially considering spectatorial engagement with the film and how the film goes about constructing the various subjectivities populating its narrative and audience reception. To this end, I argue that *Redacted* seems to site spectators in an implicated, 'guilty' position of inactivity in relationship to film images of death and suffering and to point out the ethical complexities of consuming what are ostensibly images of bodily and psychological trauma.

As already mentioned, *Redacted* is concerned with fictionally inscribing the Al-Mahmudiyah killings of 12 March 2006. Five US Army soldiers from the 502nd Infantry Regiment were charged in relation to this brutal incident. On 11 July 2006, the Mujahideen Shura Council released graphic video footage of their proclaimed retaliation for this incident: the bodies of two soldiers kidnapped from the same unit as the accused. Four of the five soldiers were convicted of the crimes through courts-martial and were sentenced to between 27 months and 110 years' imprisonment as punishment. The fifth soldier accused had left the army by the time the crimes were discovered and was therefore tried in a federal court. He was convicted in May 2009 and was sentenced to life without parole in September 2009.

The reason for giving the above sketch of the real-life events is not to invoke a comparison between events in the film and factual occurrences but rather to give background to the critical reception of the film and the manner in which it is consumed as a media product. The film consists of pastiches[2] of numerous media/visual sources which include a soldier's video diary, a professional documentary made by a French production team, 'ATV' (probably meant to signify Al-Jazeera) journalist reports, video footage of US Army psychological evaluations, Islamic extremist Internet sites with embedded video, a video blog from a soldier's wife, and video on a 'YouTube'-style website.

However, since the film depends on rapidly shifting styles and aesthetics, and on numerous disparate media forms in order to convey its narrative, this has an effect on the manner in which the text is consumed. The effect of using contrasting and eclectic media styles in order to produce a text should pose a challenge to authoritative coherent discourse and narration. However, since the different visual styles are all imitations, and are all under the supervision of the assembling eye of De Palma, coherence is maintained. We are provided with the illusion of actively culling the narrative from a multiplicity of sources, when in fact we are manipulated into this position through the 'fictional documentary' style. However, it must be emphasized that this auteurist account of *Redacted* is not a definitive component of my framework. The intention is to demonstrate that the complex issues of subjectivity, victimhood, trauma, ethics and masculinity that haunt this film are *in some part* accountable to the manner in which the film is presented as an audiovisual document. Therefore, to refer back to Thomson's opinions regarding *Redacted*, it seems that we are quite deliberately manipulated into a position of guilt and shame. In fact, this seems to be the very sine qua non of the film; passivity and inaction are dramatized as being as destructive as the hegemony and tyranny of US military aggression and belligerence, and the locus of this inaction is the mode of post-modern, virtualized and abstracted spectatorship which is dominant in US culture. The protocol of 'watching', whether this be through rolling news channels, websites like 'YouTube', Hollywood war films, or military strategy video games, is bound up with a masochistic subjectivity in which spectators desire to repeat feelings of unpleasure, guilt, pain, and self-beratement. More will be said about this below, but for now let us look at how masculinity, trauma and subjectivity are constructed in the film.

The narrative of *Redacted* is initially focalized through the character of a private named Angel Salazar who incessantly films army life in Iraq with his digital video camera. His initial justification for this is that he hopes to get into film school; the army will be paying his college fees post-service. He also explicitly and self-consciously declares that he is making a 'war film' with 'no logical narrative'. Obviously, these comments have to be sited within the context of *Redacted* as a work of (partial) fiction, and the product of a Hollywood director. The character of Salazar is in some ways used to signal De Palma's intent: the director mentioned in an interview with Simon Hattenstone (2008) in *The Guardian*: 'When you have a terrible crime, you want to know how these boys were brought to do this, and that's what the movie shows.' Therefore, the private embodies a distinct authorial voice in the film. Since he is marked out as 'the film-maker' we have a screened body onto which we can project our emotional investment in our spectatorial relationship to the film image. Also, in order to aid identifications and empathize with this 'film-maker' character, his 'everyman' credentials must be promoted (much in the same way Swofford in *Jarhead* is presented to us as a convincing 'everyman' for emotional investment). To this end, he barely exists as a unique character in the film. Occasionally, he turns his video camera on himself to address the audience, but rarely says anything of note beyond a few clichéd platitudes, and is unable to provide witty retorts to the ribbing he receives from his buddies – during one of his close-up face-to-camera shots, someone brandishing a squeaky toy rubber duck makes it 'kiss' his face, and someone wafts a toothbrush in front of his mouth. This blank persona seems to be designed to enable a multitude of identifications and draw the spectator into empathizing with his subject position. Ultimately, however, we shall see how Salazar's position of 'film-maker' and focalizing agent/spectator par excellence is ruinous and in turn implicates the passive mode of spectatorship and the inert nature of contemporary Western society. This indirect critique reflects on the atrocities of the Iraq War and their role in sustaining and reinforcing

US hegemony. In a way, this passive spectatorship is implicated as a means by which US strategic aims are secured and the occupation and exploitation of Iraq are legitimized.

There is another reference here. The characters in the film man a car checkpoint and their vulnerability and exposure, when allied with their constant sense of impending doom, takes its mental toll and produces many of the early dramatic diegetic conflicts. Early on in the film, one of the soldier-characters Salazar so incessantly films compares his situation to that of the hapless Dante in *Clerks* (Smith, 1994), by commenting on the oft-repeated line in that particular film: 'I'm not even supposed to be here today'. This not only functions as an ironic comment on the US Army's 'stop loss' policy[3] but also, through affording us a glimpse of inter-textuality, De Palma may be pointing out the contradictions and oppositions upon which our spectatorial investment in the truth is predicated. In his use of pastiche, and making the film-maker our focal subject, De Palma is signalling the problematic nature of authenticating experience, and perhaps showing us ultimately that the moving image is a cipher, a sign without signification, and, in the words of Thomas Elsaesser (2001), 'traumatic'. Elsaesser declares that film is a means of 'authenticating experience', since there is a power of immediacy associated with it; it gives a texture and a voice to 'everyday history'. Therefore it is capable of 'faking' authenticity through its editing, narrational and aesthetic techniques, all of which confirm that the moving image is a 'symptom without a cause' or 'an event without a trace' (2001, 197). This hollowness at the centre of film, which can be comparable to trauma, is a product of its own constructed nature due to the techniques of classic narrative, which produce the illusion of intimacy and immediacy. Ultimately, Elsaesser leads the reader to the claim that trauma theory is an attempt to deal with 'recovered referentiality', and in this light tends to perform its own temporal regression by positioning itself 'behind postmodernism'. The benefit of this move is that the theorist is able to 'chart [trauma theory's] political blockages (and) implicitly acknowledge [...] the fact that the grand narratives have been exhausted' (201). In this sense, there is an inherent recognition that the cultural fields of modernism and post-modernism are at play here. This is especially so when one considers that the initial association with trauma is that of modernity (Kaplan and Wang 2004, 2) and so a relationship exists between trauma and the modernist urban experience. Modernism with its typical 'hyper-subjective viewpoints' was a 'response to the traumas of urbanization and industrialization' (Hirsch 2004, 23) and so in a sense is partly responsible for the confused and chaotic depictions of subjectivity one finds in war films, horror films and the like. Obviously, trauma and war film have long associations stretching back to the flashbacks and traumatic memory portrayed in films such as *The Best Years of Our Lives* (William Wyler, 1946), and the post-First World War concerns surrounding corporeal trauma as evinced in films such as *The Cabinet of Dr. Caligari* (Robert Wiene, 1920) and *The Unknown* (Tod Browning, 1927).[4] So it may be the case that the berserk style and aesthetics of war cinema may be attributed to cultural forces beyond the specificity of trauma and may connect with the grander fields of modernism and post-modernism. Therefore, trauma theory at once positions itself 'behind' post-modernism in that it is antipathetic towards grand narratives, but at the same time it activates and depends upon the precepts of these narratives. The mode of film-making De Palma appears to be espousing in this case is one which declares its own fractured relationship to 'authenticating experience'; using pastiche to highlight how 'real' it *can* be, but using post-modern inter-textuality and trauma in order to flag the constructed and 'hollow' nature of the process.

Not only is the textual image in itself traumatic but so is the effect of the media industry on the subject. Through presenting us with a multiplicity of sources and visual styles,

De Palma is emphasizing the almost hysterical relationship one can possess towards contemporary media. Assaulted by a multiplicity of media forms and a constant babble of voices and images, the subject becomes hystericized and undone. Andreas Huyssen has even posited that contemporary fascination with studies of memory and trauma are an 'attempt to slow down information processing, to resist the dissolution of time [...], to recover a mode of contemplation outside the universe of stimulation and fast-speed information and cable networks' (1995, 7). This dismantlement, in effect, becomes a fantasy, and the spectator (in a manoeuvre identified and described by Lynne Kirby [1993, 67–84] in her discussion of spectatorship and early cinema) starts to desire this assault, this penetration, this *pleasurable sensual assault.* Therefore, the contemporary media image, literalized by De Palma as one of his many pastiches, lacks referentiality, and so is traumatic, and also carries with it a hystericizing potential. As Thomson's film review accidentally implicates, according to a masochistic account of spectatorship, viewers desire the self-abasement and shame imposed by *Redacted.* However, in this viewing position the radical political message of the film is internalized, but instead of political or cultural transformation, a position of radical pleasure emerges. Politics of culture and the state rapidly slide into a politics of masochism whereby the spectator's compulsion to repeat scenarios of guilt, self-abasement and pain is made pleasurable through the relationship to the moving image.

Further, the proximity of pleasure and pain and questions of male subjectivity are raised within the plot of the film. In response to the above-mentioned complaints regarding the soldiers and their 'stop loss' status, the black duty sergeant, Sergeant Sweet (his race is relevant to one of my later arguments) screams that they all need to accept their position and 'stand the fuck up and be a fucking man about it!' He also impels them to 'drive on with a fucking hard on!' Manliness, the erect penis, and robustness are all conflated in these proclamations. The soldiers are supposed to embrace their subjection to military authority, and accept their 'sitting duck' position of extreme vulnerability manning the checkpoint. This subjection is accompanied with sexual arousal, which in a way 'proves' their robust 'impenetrable' manhood. Few could deny the masochistic connotations of this dynamic of sexuality, suffering and masculinity.[5]

In another scene, over a game of cards using a pornographic picture deck, a character called Private Rush[6] contemplates, 'is it wrong to fall in love with the king of clubs?'[7] to much mirth and amusement. This phrase seems to articulate the ambivalent nature of how masculinity is performed in the film, and also provides a masochistic subtext to proceedings, the implication being that of the subject forming a romantic (and possibly sexual) attachment through desiring to be beaten by a dominant symbol of patriarchy. It seems relevant here to bring in one of Freud's later theories of masochism, contained in his essay 'A child is being beaten', originally published in 1919.

In this essay Freud isolates the commonalities between descriptions of beating fantasies related to him by clinical case studies. He then establishes that 'the first fantasies of the kind were entertained very early in life' and 'when the child was at school and saw other children being beaten by the teacher, then, if the phantasies had become dormant, this experience called them up again' (1995, 159). Freud goes on to make clear that for the masochistic 'perversion' to arise, the subject must experience pleasure in *watching others* being beaten, for this primarily indicates that pleasurable fantasies attached to being beaten by one's father are being repressed and turned outwards in this scenario. Specifically, guilt is mentioned as the determining factor in the masochistic structure, since the beating scenario registers as a scene of punishment and degradation.

However, what is interesting regarding Freud's investigations of the masochistic complex from the perspective of film studies and visual culture is the fact that the fantasy depends crucially on *watching* a child (or substitute) being beaten, and so it is reliant on *passive spectatorship* of someone else's pain. The structure of looking and witnessing is noted by Freud when he adds that, 'here the child who produces the phantasy appears almost as a spectator' (1995, 169). An economy of the visual, pleasure, and pain is established in the masochistic scenario, and therefore masochism has specific links to traumatic vision.

Indeed, masochism and trauma contain numerous commonalities. They are both characterized by repetition compulsion, oscillation between mastery and submission, and, as Freud delineates above, a spectatorial scene of pain. Susannah Radstone (2000) discusses this sense of repetition and engagement with various national myths of memory in an essay on trauma and cinema, which specifically refers to one of the more aesthetically post-modern texts of 1990s film, *Forrest Gump*. She states that the traumatic state goes against a linear narrative conception of cause and effect, in which the past comes to shape the present experience. Radstone theorizes the spectatorship involved in trauma cinema as involving the spectator being 'caught between an initial "looking away" and the beginnings of remembrance' (99). In other words, in contemporary Western culture, a convergence exists of 'fantasies of innocent victimhood with fantasies of omnipotence' (101), and the viewer of films which attempt to make contact with history is caught oscillating between fantasies of omnipotence and powerlessness; this doubleness drives spectatorship of trauma cinema. It is this doubleness revolving around suspense and disavowal that also characterizes the masochistic contract, according to Gilles Deleuze (1991, 134).

Accounts of trauma and trauma cinema stress the victimized and self-abated bodily and psychological formations of subjectivity, and there seems to be something curiously masochistic about this. Indeed, since we are dealing with war cinema, one might say that this is all too apparent in the narrative focus of these films, since we witness soldiers who have forsaken all claims to individuated subjectivity and have subjected themselves totally to military and patriarchal authority. This wilful submission is accompanied with extremities of pain, pleasure and violence. It is clear then that my account of trauma cinema incorporates masochism and masochistic subjectivity, not just in terms of the aesthetics and narrative content of war films but also in terms of the spectators' relationship to these films too.

Rush's desire to be beaten by a master, contextualized within the framework of pornography and the desiring male gaze, seems to subtly mirror the conditions the soldiers are provided for 'coping' with their extended deployment on the checkpoint. They must sexualize their pain and turn it into the primal condition of their 'dependable manliness'. But as is the case with 'driving on with a fucking hard on', this sexuality is totally onanistic. There is no externalization of their sexual desire, just masochistic internalization and reconfiguration of the pain of re-deployment, and the unreturned gaze of pornography.

Significantly, it is the character of Private Rush together with a character called Private Flake who instigate the idea of raping the 15-year-old Iraqi girl. In the lead-up to this event, Rush complains in graphic terms about his lack of 'action' and melodramatically and comically describes the ruination of his sexual organs as a result of this neglect in lurid, puerile detail. The male penis rears its ugly head again. Aside from the obvious parallels where one can see that the film is clearly setting up US military power and non-consensual sexual domination/violence as analogous, it is possible to argue that the film posits the masochistic position of the soldiers as unviable and leading to a pathology of aberrant, violent sexuality. However, that would mark the character of Private Rush as representative, when it is clear that he is the exception rather than the rule. What emerges, therefore, are differing types of masochistic military subjectivity which manifest themselves in different forms. This characterization could even imply that the repulsive character of Rush, who bullies, cajoles and browbeats his way through military life, is unable to adopt the radical psycho-sexual position of masochism and instead resists through recourse to extreme sadism. Gilles Deleuze has commented that masochism and sadism are from very different, perhaps opposing, economies of pain and pleasure (1991, 104). Steven Shaviro has also stated that those who resist the pleasures of self-abandonment and the masochistic subject position are involved in maintaining what is essentially an illusion of wholeness and coherency, as opposed to the dissolution and fragmentation associated with masochism (1993, 196). Rush's sadism is therefore representative of US foreign policy and is analogous to the mainstream desires of normative culture to impose coherency and meaning on experience and to give credence to the lie of fixity and wholeness. He aims to 'repair' his ailing manhood through violent sexual assault, and so enacts – on behalf of the US nation – a brutal restitution of phallic authority. The hysterical, paranoid, threatening atmospherics of their checkpoint duty are compensated for by vicious re-masculinization.

We must compare this male subjectivity to four other characters in the film; the aforementioned Salazar, Flake, Lawyer McCoy (not actually a lawyer, it's his name), and Gabe Blix. But first, we must contextualize the rape scene. Throughout the first part of the film, the character of Sergeant Sweet (the duty sergeant mentioned above) consistently warns the other characters about the risks posed by IEDs (improvised explosive devices), left by roadsides and in innocuous positions by 'the enemy' (who this enemy is, we are never quite sure). It comes to pass that in the wake of Private Flake's indolent and negligent soldiering, Sergeant Sweet gets blown to pieces by an IED. This moment is captured on Salazar's video camera. Framing this sequence we see footage from embedded video on a militant Islamic extremist website showing the planting of the IED. A few scenes later, the US Army unit are depicted via an 'Embedded Journalist Exclusive Report' conducting a night time raid on an Iraqi home where they erroneously believe the perpetrators of the planting of the IED live. The soldiers treat the occupants of the house brutally and confiscate documents claiming they are 'evidence' when none of them can read their contents. The madness of this whole spurious operation is highlighted by the persistent questioning by the 'embedded journalist'. It is later on in the film, after the aforementioned card game, when the players are highly charged with alcohol, that the rape is conceived and carried out.

The rape scene is played out in night vision, courtesy of Salazar's video camera. The night vision counter-intuitively serves to expose the horrific intensity of the crime. It does not distance the spectator, but rather draws one in, purely through dint of the blurry, pixellated, digital images and the distorted and sharp green/black/white colour scheme. The impenetrable but oddly stark nature of the images provides visual intrigue and produces a fascination with the texture of the images, a desire to decipher the sometimes oblique nature of the imagery, and also creates a state of transfixed horror, courtesy of the immediacy and austerity of the visual text.

The four soldiers in attendance are Salazar, McCoy, Rush, and Flake. Flake subdues the rest of the girl's family through violent force as Rush commences the horrible act, bending her over and lifting up her dress whilst the girl cries and protests. McCoy, who is superior in rank to the other soldiers, objects in strong terms, but McCoy has a gun put to his head and he, along with Salazar, is bullied and threatened into leaving the house under the pretence of going on 'faggot watch' outside. The manner in which they are bullied and threatened is by questioning where their 'balls' are. Once again, male sexuality, pleasure and domination become conflated, and a lack of adherence to this aggressive sadistic regime is equated to homosexuality. 'Watching' seems not only to be analogous to inaction but also to a deprival of normative hegemonic masculinity. Once outside, McCoy explodes with rage at Salazar, staring directly into the camera, his rage intensified by the night vision colouring, the pupils of his eyes burning a brilliant white, transforming his face into an alien, predatory snarl. He spills his invective in an undeviating fashion, proclaiming Salazar to be no better than 'a fucking jackal ripping pieces of meat off a fucking carcass' for not trying to interfere and object. It is at this moment we have an explicit condemnation emerging from the film's discourse of a regime of passive, inactive spectatorship witnessing atrocities, and spectatorship is likened to corporeal dissolution and an explicitly 'homosexual' position.

We shall stay with the character of Salazar now, since he is the one vehemently identified with this inactive spectatorship. One of the film's scenes is a video recording of Salazar's psychological evaluation. It shows him grappling with some of the outward and inward signs of post-traumatic stress disorder (PTSD). He has developed certain nervous tics and he describes vividly his recurring nightmares involving 'her burnt body', which he swiftly corrects to 'his'. It is clear from this moment that what has traumatized him is the guilt he feels through not intervening, just watching and filming the rape and the brutal violence meted out to the girl and her family. Echoing real life, the soldiers burn the girl's body after the rape and murder. However, Salazar claims that what is really troubling him (no one has disclosed the military brutality at this point) is the dramatic and sudden death of Sergeant Sweet. We therefore witness a sudden transformation in the character of Salazar; he goes from being the possessor of an assaultive, almost sadistic, gaze in the form of his prying 'documentary' video camera, to a position of weakness and victimhood, to a troubled and a traumatic neurosis. He fiercely proclaims at one point that he is deeply troubled by the concept of 'people watching and doing fuck-all', an intense self-criticism, but, like McCoy's 'jackal' comment, it is seemingly levelled at the audience in order to include us within the film's economy of guilt and implication. The question of one's ethical engagement with images and 'watching' them is highlighted by the fact this sequence is supposedly filmed from a remote video camera and therefore there is no interjecting subjectivity governing the framing or movement of the camera image. The lack of direct control over the video images of Salazar's grief and pain gives us raw, unmediated access to what is supposedly 'real'; there is no one calling the shots, and so therefore the only ones 'watching and doing fuck-all' are us, the external audience. However, Salazar is able to disavow and suspend his guilt, at least in enunciative terms (he never admits the deeper concerns he possesses), by linguistically covering it over with the dismembered black body of Sergeant Sweet. Blackness and the nightmare of dissolution disguise his guilt, and his refusal to come clean about what he has witnessed, although to some degree due to being scared of the possible recriminations from Rush, is also possibly due to a desire to preserve his state of self-torment. The disassembled black body is used to cover over guilt, pain and self-recrimination.

In this context it is interesting that the rape of the young Iraqi girl is depicted as occurring from behind, since this has the potential to be coded as anal rape.[8] As Klaus Theweleit (1989) has argued, 'the anus is identified as a site of aggression precisely because of its potential to produce vast deterritorialization' (160). Therefore, we can see that issues of domination, power, and then wresting illusory control of that power are involved in the rape sequence, where penetration means 'loss of ego, injury and death' (Yosef 2004, 67). The soldiers must go to great lengths to secure their sense of fixed/whole male subjectivity by avoiding the emasculating and disassembling potential of penetration, and instead becoming the penetrators. Violent sexual domination and its equivalence to US military aggression may therefore be coded as a closeted homosexual desire hidden beneath the sadism. This is especially pertinent considering the actions of Rush and the manner in which he mocks and belittles Gabe, Blix and McCoy. Blix is shown to have an interest in literature: he comments regarding the pornographic playing cards that 'this one is my favourite, she looks nice' (in the definite sense of being a nice *person*), and his spectacles and slight frame mark him out as far from the dominant image of hyper-masculine military identity. McCoy, in the introductory sequences, also disparagingly comments about '"don't ask don't tell"[9] here' and when Rush is warning him not to squeal regarding the rape, he manhandles him, holding him uncomfortably close in a tight grip before Blix acquiesces and Rush signals his approval by commenting, 'good boy'. The naming of Blix echoes the name of the UN weapons inspector, and hence this entire scene can be read as US domination of international law, and using its aggressive, over-sexualized, hyper-masculine presence as a weapon to ride roughshod over global diplomacy and convention.

This questioning of Blix's sexuality and his accompanying emasculation/infantilization shows a sadistic desire to dominate on the part of Rush and insist on a 'female' coding for those he dominates. His desire to penetrate extends beyond the rape, but the desire for masculine and military 'wholeness' and the 'vast deterritorialization' (Theweleit 1989, 319) produced by anal penetration can be linked to the nightmare of dissolution enacted by Sweet's body being blown to bits. It is the 'enemy' which is penetrated, whereas the so-called homosocial bonds between the men of the US Army unit mean that, under the threat of penetration in the sadistic and violent guise of forces which desire the restoration of an illusory wholeness and fixity, there is in fact only dissolution: of bodies courtesy of IEDs; of minds courtesy of PTSD; of aesthetic regimes courtesy of ever-changing subject positions and media forms deployed in the film; and, as mentioned above, through dissolution of subject matter, since by implication we are 'ripping pieces of meat off a carcass'.

Let us now return to the character of Salazar. In the wake of his video psychological evaluation he is depicted filming himself on patrol on the streets of Samarra, when after laying down his (still-filming) video camera, he is kidnapped and bundled into a van by several Iraqis. The story of what happens to him is then conveyed through various extremist websites with embedded video depicting his decapitation (in a scene visually reminiscent of the numerous harrowing filmed executions of citizens and soldiers of coalition countries that emerged in the wake of the US-led invasion and occupation of Iraq) and then the laying of his body in a farmer's field for discovery.

In a way, it seems that Salazar is 'punished' for his regime of inactive watching through the fate that befalls him and acts as a condemnation of passive spectatorship. But it also seems that Salazar is folded into the film's discursive engagement with contemporary visual geopolitical culture. Through evoking the images of filmed execution, he becomes part of the awful iconography of the 'war on terror', and therefore passive spectatorship becomes mythologized and codified as a component of this contemporary geopolitical epoch. Inaction and passivity, therefore, become both subject and object of the gaze, indicating the self-perpetuating and reflexive nature of this regime of contemporary visual culture.

Let us return to the issues of masochistic male subjectivity haunting this film. We have already discussed how the film presents images which conflate sexual arousal and scenarios of pain and suspense. The film also presents characters who are deeply traumatized, and hence embody a compulsion to repeat. The character of McCoy is depicted in the final scene of the film, back home, in a bar, with a jacket and open neck shirt, in the company of his wife, family, and friends. The scene is captured by his father filming his homecoming party on a video camera. In response to a request that he tells some 'war stories', he breaks down, and visibly upset and shaken, he laments straight into the lens of the camera that 'I have these snapshots in my brain that are burnt in there forever, and I don't know what I am gonna do about them.' This stands in marked contrast to what Sturken has described as the 'irretrievability' (1997, 23) of historical images. In McCoy's case it is indelibility, perpetuity, and helplessness which mark his traumatic memory. He is the ultimate victim, unable to control his punishment and pain, and yet the forced and unbearably emotionally constipated veneer of 'celebration' which is lent to the proceedings in the bar by his father's insistence on a round of applause and cheers for his son, seems to lend a masquerade of pleasure to the scenario.

Despite this proximity of emotional pain and false bonhomie, the film leaves us with characters abandoned in melancholic, unresolved states, which offer the spectator no re-entry into the dominant fiction. We are left in the margins, suffering and miserable; Salazar is dead in the wake of his PTSD, McCoy is left crying and staring blankly into the video camera, Flake and Rush left facing investigation by the military police. The film refuses closure and healing; we have no idea regarding the fates of many of the characters, and no attempt is made to 'explain' or 'work through' the effect of US militarism. There is no reconstruction of male subjectivity either; the emotional masochism and damage depicted in the film through Salazar's PTSD and McCoy's and Blix's melancholic state in the wake of the rape is not healed by simply 'talking'. 'Talking' doesn't help Rush or Flake either, as their statements to the military police reveal their psychotic sadistic pathologies and entrap them in the investigative process. Accompanying this emotional destruction is also corporeal destruction; Salazar is decapitated, and Sweet is blown to pieces. It seems that De Palma is being careful not to leave any chance of the restitution of patriarchal military subjectivity.

That this refusal of closure and healing is deliberate on De Palma's part is signalled by a brief, but significant scene towards the end of the film. Via a pastiche of a 'YouTube'-style website, we see a video clip of a female teenager ranting directly into the camera.[10] She is the female voice of protest in this film and articulates a violent revenge on the patriarchal abuses of power embodied and popularized in Hollywood war films. She mocks and blames Vietnam movies in particular for mythologizing loose cannon violence ('let's torch the whole fuckin' village!' she sarcastically proclaims in a faux grunt snarl) and for perpetuating the notion that 'We are the über-race! Sieg Heil, motherfucker!' This is De Palma acknowledging his own role in constructing these mythologies and providing 'closure' and 'healing' through his Hollywood Vietnam War effort, *Casualties of War* (1989). This self-reflexive process is significant since it sees De Palma shifting his authorial subjectivity onto the body of this protesting woman, and with her nose ring, tattoo, and poster of Che Guevara it implies De Palma's correlation with the iconography of contemporary counter-culture. If this is the case, then De Palma is carefully acknowledging his film as a 'rant' and a riposte to the glamorization and valorization of American exceptionalism and the physical horror of combat. As mentioned at the start of this paper, Marita Sturken (1997) has commented that the problem with *Casualties of War* is that its 'real focus is the rift in morality among the Americans and their own victimization' (106), and this idea of concentrating on the 'rift in morality' and the Americans' victimization infuses *Redacted.* There is a rift in the unit and a rift in the film's aesthetics and narrative due to the numerous enunciative subject positions adopted. Also, the victim status of the soldiers is emphasized by the final scene depicting McCoy's emotional breakdown, and our emotional attachment to Salazar and his subsequent mental and corporeal ruination. Scenes where we 'see the bombs from below', i.e. witness Iraqi victimhood, are sometimes refracted through the subjectivity of US militarism; the rape scene is conveyed through Salazar's passive video gaze and McCoy's seeming greater concern with Salazar's inactivity than with the rape itself. The moments when Iraqi victimhood is not refracted through US military subjectivity are courtesy of the 'ATV' sequences. In one of these, featuring the rape victim's father being interviewed, his words and feelings are enunciated and translated clearly. Nevertheless, an uneasy relationship still exists between victimhood and the film's predominant empathies, embodied by the final sequence of the film, entitled 'Collateral damage, actual photographs from the Iraq War'.

After we leave McCoy staring blankly and grimly into the video camera, we are greeted with the aforementioned title, which is followed by a montage of still images of the death and destruction of Iraqi people. The phrase 'collateral damage' seems to me to ironically echo the title of the terrorism-themed Arnold Schwarzenegger vehicle of the same name that had its release date pushed back in the wake of the 9/11 attacks. In making this subtle reference, De Palma is continuing his critique established in the 'ranting teen' sequence, whereby Hollywood's fetishizing of combat violence and American exceptionalism is credited with perpetuating myths of US hegemony and neo-imperial hostility. The photographs themselves are horrific, featuring images of bodies severely wounded by bullets and bombs, numerous corpses, and the remains of Abeer Qasim Hamza al-Janabi. At this point it seems appropriate to turn to how this sequence and the film overall impact on spectatorship.

If we return to Desson Thomson's comments regarding the film 'bringing us into the guilt zone', then the 'collateral damage' sequence seems designed purely for this purpose. But throughout the film there has existed an undercurrent of masochistic subjectivity, so is this applicable to the mode of spectatorship demanded of this film? Yosef (2004) has stated that the masochist 'stands guilt on its head by making punishment into a condition that makes possible the forbidden pleasure' (76). Therefore, as spectators, we are implicated in the ruinous regime of passivity invoked by Salazar, and yet we still remain safely inured in our outlying spectator positions, undoubtedly taking a degree of visual pleasure from the process of watching the film. As Sturken (1997) points out, 'the film camera's inherent tendency to fetishize its subject matter is compounded [...] by the spectacular nature of the war' (107). When we come to *Redacted*, the technology of war has progressed to the extent that proliferated media formats become encompassed in this regime of fetishizing filmic subject matter. The very means by which our visual culture is mobilized – websites, rolling news reports, documentaries – become the objects of glamorization, and so perhaps *Redacted* perpetuates the passive distant gazes which bring the spectator 'into the guilt zone'. We adopt the victimized, assaulted subject position constructed in the film, but rather than being assigned a traumatic/melancholy sense of guilt in order to mirror the characters of McCoy and Salazar we are in the privileged position of being able to disavow our guilt and ethical investment in the film image. The 'collateral damage' sequence offers a 'cathartic absolution of guilt' (Sturken 1997, 106) since it exists outside of the main narrative of the film. This separation between narrative and photo-journalism draws attention to the constructed nature of the film and hence shatters any remaining notions of wholeness, coherency and fixity one might have possessed whilst watching the main body of the film. In a sense, this invokes a pure masochistic subjectivity, since we are presented with a closing scene without closure, and we are assured suspense and irresolution ad infinitum as narrative is jettisoned entirely and we are presented with real images of bodily dissolution. Moreover, fantasies of self-abandonment and fragmentation are fulfilled, since across the film we are constantly manipulated into an intersubjective, victimized position crossing boundaries of race and gender, owing to the constantly varying sites of narrative perspective.

The 'collateral damage' sequence opens up the question of ethics and spectatorship. As Michele Aaron has argued, ethical film-making must make us think about our position, culpability, or complicity as a spectator (2008, 114). *Redacted* posits numerous compelling questions to its audience regarding the question of inactive and passive spectatorship, and to an extent implicates the spectator as complicit in this regime. De Palma also ethically self-questions his position of film-maker, through projecting his authorial presence, using pastiches of media forms, and critiquing cinematic history. However, the 'collateral damage' sequence troubles this ethic. This is because despite the multifarious media forms imitated, photo-journalism holds a different power, due to its reliance on still images, and the lack of complementary sensory information, such as sound. Aaron suggests, in discussing Susan Sontag's (2003) writings on photographs of atrocity, emotive reactions to images of atrocity and suffering disavow us of any potential *responsibility for those images.* Our externally displayed emotions and our emotive reactions are 'our bit' in the economy of spectatorship and visual culture; in a sense, we relinquish ethical investment by shedding tears (Aaron 2008, 117).

On the one hand, the emotive reaction intended by the photographic montage 'collateral damage' undoes the ethical position engendered by the film's reflexivity, but on the other, it could work to reinforce its ethical position through drawing a continuous line through film-making practice and photo-journalism. The politics of masochistic subjectivity and spectatorship go some way to addressing this. The confluence of pain and pleasure in the bodies of US male militarism and filmic spectators betrays the crucial role of psycho-sexual fantasy in the economy of contemporary visual culture. Masochism, in its contractual[11] acceptance of pain and self-abasement, accords the masochist with great political subversive power. Part of this power is the ability to cast off desire for cohesiveness and fixity, and so to be penetrated and assaulted, perhaps even emotionally wounded by images of atrocity, bestows enormous cultural and political capital on this spectator. Ultimately, it would seem that *Redacted* makes us more than aware of how we are accountable 'to what we have consented to' (Aaron 2008, 120); firstly by implicating inactive and passive spectatorship, and then through highlighting the radical pleasures to be found in the shattered identities and bodies, and the self-abasement and pleasure associated with war cinema, and contemporary visual culture. The condition of inactivity is diagnosed, and we are provided with the empowering cure through the radical subversion of patriarchal power to be found in the masochistic subject position.

To conclude, it is worth briefly considering the role of one piece of classical music deployed towards the end of the film. The piece in question is 'E lucevan le stelle' from Act Three of Puccini's *Tosca*. The piece concerns Mario Cavaradossi (Tosca's lover) awaiting execution, and can be read, in the context of the film, in three ways. Firstly, it subtly indicates that the implicated soldiers, Rush and Flake, will be punished for their actions, and hence may suggest some form of closure and healing. Secondly, it could represent a message of tragic fate for US operations in Iraq. Or there is a slightly more complex third reading in which we see this piece of music as romanticizing the soldiers' suffering and valorizing their depiction as victims, only this time in the context of high culture and sexual longing. Sexuality and a scenario of entrapment demonstrate the masochistic underpinnings to militarized male subjectivity. The traumatic nature of the militarized male subjectivity of Salazar, in his 'Ulysses tied to the mast'[12] scenario of inactive spectatorship, shows how trauma and masochistic subjectivity are inherently linked and dramatizes the ethical problems behind bringing spectators into 'the guilt zone'.

Notes

1. Could it possibly be the case that films which are vehemently 'anti-war' or attempt to unsettle the dominant fiction of the United States as exceptional and victimized are subject to extraordinary levels of marginalization, especially when the forms of narrative and symbolic signification deployed in the film are complex and do not conform to the standard Hollywood pattern of 'crisis and resolution'? See the cold critical and economic reception given to films such as *In The Valley of Elah* (Paul Haggis, 2007) and *Battle for Haditha* (Nick Broomfield, 2007), which have been dubbed 'Bin Laden cinema' (Hattenstone 2008).
2. Richard Dyer (2007) establishes pastiche in film, literature, and visual culture as a knowing allusion to, or invocation of, preceding texts. The implication is that we are conscious of the foundations and basis for these allusional and invocatory texts.
3. The controversial policy by which US soldiers can have their dates of service involuntarily extended beyond what they originally signed up for is intriguingly explored by Kimberley Peirce in her film *Stop Loss* (2008).
4. For an intriguing account of disfigurement and post-First World War film please see Karen Randell (2003).
5. Raz Yosef (2004, 51) uses the writings of Klaus Theweleit to discuss the role of masochism in producing and maintaining the imaginary hard, irreducible body of the soldier. Specifically, Yosef discusses the thought that it is this imagined hard body which is the soldier's defence against being absorbed into a nightmare world of dissolution and the 'menacing liquidity associated with women and the enemy'; his pent up 'floods of energy' contained within his hardened periphery are, in effect, displaced onto external agents. In Theweleit's (1989, 244) words, the soldier asserts his hard identity and the fixity of his peripheral boundaries through 'a kind of sustained erection of the whole body'.
6. Many of the film review critics mentioned in the opening paragraph speculate whether he is named after the right-wing radio shock-jockey Rush Limbaugh. They certainly both share a corpulent repulsiveness and a taste for unsavoury bigoted views.
7. As a matter of interest, the 'King of Clubs' in the 'personality identification playing cards', otherwise known as the 'Most-Wanted Iraqi Playing Cards', was Izzat Ibrahim ad-Douri, Vice-President of the RCC and essentially the 'Most Wanted' member of the former Ba'athist regime, as of writing.
8. Also, Flake demands of Rush, 'where are your balls?', to which he disgustingly replies, 'nearly in her ass'.
9. Referring to the controversial military policy of disdainful sublimation of recruits' sexuality.
10. She is one of the few female voices in the film, which in itself speaks of an interesting perpetuation of a significant marginalization within popular war films. The only other female characters who are given significant speaking roles are the ATV journalist and McCoy's wife, who imparts her story via her video blog entitled 'Just A Soldier's Wife'. The self-definition purely in terms of the 'other' of her soldiering husband and the marginal simplicity in the deployment of the word 'just' speak volumes.
11. Deleuze (1991, 91–102) establishes that the relationship between victim and aggressor in the masochistic performance is always a contractual one: each accepts their role in the symbolic economy of masochism, the point being to emphasize the severity of the law and power rather than to jointly revel in the conflation of pain and pleasure.
12. Gaylyn Studlar (1988), taking Jean Laplanche as her psychoanalytical guide, discusses the 'primal scene' which the infant must bear witness to, like 'Ulysses tied to the mast or Tantalus on whom is imposed the spectacle of parental intercourse', and therefore posits masochistic subjectivity as bound up with spectacle, desire and fantasy.

References

Aaron, Michele. 2008. *Spectatorship: The power of looking on*. London: Wallflower Press.
Baumgarten, Marjorie. 2008. Review of *Redacted*. *The Austin Chronicle*, 4 January. http://www.austinchronicle.com/gyrobase/Calendar/Film?Film=oid%3A577014
Deleuze, Gilles. 1991. *Masochism: Coldness and cruelty*. New York: Zone Books.
Dyer, Richard. 2007. *Pastiche*. London: Routledge.
Ebert, Roger. 2007. *Redacted*. rogerebert.com, 16 November. http://rogerebert.suntimes.com/apps/pbcs.dll/article?AID=/20071115/REVIEWS/711150303/1023
Elsaesser, T. 2001. Postmodernism as mourning work. *Screen* 42, no. 2: 193–201.
Freud, Sigmund. 1995. 'A child is being beaten': A contribution to the study of the origin of sexual perversions. In *Essential papers on masochism*, ed. Margaret Ann Fitzpatrick Hanly, 159–81. New York and London: New York University Press.
Hattenstone, Simon. 2008. No one wants to know. *The Guardian*, 8 March. http://www.guardian.co.uk/film/2008/mar/08/features.iraqandthemedia
Hirsch, Joshuah. 2004. *Afterimage: Film, trauma, and the Holocaust*. London: Eurospan.
Huyssen, Andreas. 1995. *Twilight memories: Marking time in a culture of amnesia*. London: Routledge.
Kaplan, E. Ann, and Ban Wang. 2004. *Trauma and cinema: Cross cultural explorations*. Hong Kong: Hong Kong University Press.
Kirby, Lynne. 1993. Male hysteria and early cinema. In *Male trouble*, ed. Constance Penley and Sharon Willis, 67–84. London: University of Minnesota Press.
Morgenstern, Joe. 2007. Old English goes new Hollywood in epic *Beowulf*. High-tech wizardry makes classic sing; *Redacted* is dismal. *Wall Street Journal*, 16 November. http://online.wsj.com/article/SB119517337319395051.html?mod=2_1168_1
Radstone, Susannah. 2000. Screening trauma: *Forrest Gump*, film and memory. In *Memory and methodology*, ed. Susannah Radstone, 79–108. Oxford: Berg.
Randell, Karen. 2003. Masking the horror of trauma: The hysterical body of Lon Chaney. *Screen* 44, no. 2: 216–21.
Shaviro, Steven. 1993. *The cinematic body*. Minneapolis and London: University of Minnesota Press.
Sontag, Susan. 2003. *Regarding the pain of others*. London: Hamish Hamilton.
Studlar, Gaylyn. 1988. *In the realm of pleasure: Von Sternberg, Dietrich and the masochistic aesthetic*. New York: Columbia University Press.
Sturken, Marita. 1997. *Tangled memories: The Vietnam War, the AIDS epidemic, and the politics of remembering*. Berkeley: University of California Press.
Theweleit, Klaus. 1989. *Male fantasies II: Male bodies: psychoanalyzing the white terror*. Cambridge: Polity Press.
Thomson, Desson. 2007. Review of *Redacted*. *Washington Post*, 16 November. http://www.washingtonpost.com/wp-dyn/content/article/2007/11/15/AR2007111502452.html
Walker, Janet. 2005. *Trauma cinema: Documenting incest and the Holocaust*. Berkeley and Los Angeles: University of California Press.
Yosef, Raz. 2004. *Cannon fodder: Queer masculinities and nationalism in Israeli cinema*. New Brunswick, NJ: Rutgers University Press.

Filmography

Battle for Haditha. Directed by Nick Broomfield. UK: Channel Four Films, 2007.
The Best Years of Our Lives. Directed by William Wyler. USA: RKO Radio Pictures, 1946.
Blow Out. Directed by Brian De Palma. USA: Filmways, 1981.
Body Double. Directed by Brian De Palma. USA: Columbia Pictures, 1984.
The Cabinet of Dr. Caligari. Directed by Robert Wiene. Germany: Decla-Bioscop, 1920.
Casualties of War. Directed by Brian De Palma. USA: Columbia Pictures, 1989.
Clerks. Directed by Kevin Smith. USA: View Askew Productions, 1994.

Dressed to Kill. Directed by Brian De Palma. USA: Filmways, 1980.
In the Valley of Elah. Directed by Paul Haggis. USA: Blackfriars Bridge Films, 2007.
Redacted. Directed by Brian De Palma. USA: The Film Farm, 2007.
Scarface. Directed by Brian De Palma. USA: Universal Pictures, 1983.
Stop Loss. Directed by Kimberley Peirce. USA: Paramount Pictures, 2008.
The Unknown. Directed by Tod Browning. USA: Metro-Goldwyn-Mayer, 1927.

When places have agency: Roadside shrines as traumascapes

Catherine Ann Collins[a] and Alexandra Opie[b]

[a]*Rhetoric and Media Studies, Willamette University, Salem, OR, USA;* [b]*Art and Art History, Willamette University, Salem, OR, USA*

This essay focuses on roadside shrines as places where time seems to replay itself and the experiences of loss are continuously re-experienced – what Foucault would term heterochronias where the evocation of the initial trauma leaves the past open in the present, constraining individual agency while giving agency to place. The located memorials are also symbolic spaces when adorned with ceremonial, domestic, and personal artefacts that sacralize them. These traumascapes help the pilgrim negotiate the chaotic and traumatic event of the past and hold out the possibility of a bearable future.

Introduction

Drive the back roads of Oregon, or any other state in the United States, and you will encounter what have been termed roadside shrines, vernacular memorials, or sites of pilgrimage. These are natural landscapes that temporarily are transformed from profane to sacred space because they are sites of memory. As Pierre Nora notes: 'memory attaches itself to sites, whereas history attaches itself to events' (1989, 22). They are most often places for remembering lives lost in traffic accidents, but occasionally they commemorate deaths from drive-by shootings or other violent acts. Roadside shrines are as close to the actual site of the violence as possible; representing the boundary between life and death, they are distinctive for memory work. They are not sequestered from daily life, as are cemeteries. Located beside busy highways, or erected along back roads without space for cars to pull over, their accessibility is often limited, even though they may remain visually pronounced. Sites of violent and unexpected death are transformed by family and friends who feel the need to remember, grieve, and to give temporary order to chaotic memories. They are not formal sites for memory like cemeteries but rather personal places that change the cultural space.

The culture of roadside shrines in the US tradition began in the eighteenth century in the south-west, although it has become more visible throughout the country in the last 20 years. At times the memorial crosses and embellishments have been officially sanctioned: in the 1940s and 1950s, Arizona's Highway Patrol erected white crosses at the site of traffic fatalities (Durbin 2003, 26). This paper, however, focuses on vernacular shrines erected by family and friends of the victims. These spontaneous shrines change dramatically over time and vary markedly from one site to the next because they are highly personalized spaces.

This essay and Alexandra Opie's art installation that accompanied it at the 'Interrogating Trauma: Arts & Media Responses to Collective Suffering' international conference (2–4 December 2008) are the culmination of our joint research into the intersection of trauma, temporality, memory and place. We focus on vernacular memorials that embody the search for symbolic spaces to make visible the grief and trauma that these deaths bring about. Multidisciplinary scholarship defines trauma broadly. Writing from a psychological perspective, Cathy Caruth argues that trauma is not defined by the nature of the event but 'solely in the *structure of the experience* or repetition' (1995, 4). The traumatic response occurs belatedly, endures long after the incident, and destabilizes the person. Trauma is present when the individual cannot control his or her memories of an event, nor find closure for the experience. Kirby Farrell's discussion of post-traumatic culture wherein trauma is described as 'belated, epiphenomenal, the outcome of cumulative stresses' (1998, 3) acknowledges the characteristic structure of the experience of trauma, but points to broad cultural disasters that may accumulate to give rise to the traumatic response. Where Caruth addresses the survivor of a disaster, Farrell's approach to trauma includes any member of a culture for whom the accumulated stress results in a shattering of the individual's sense of order. The traumatic response as conceived in this essay includes family and friends of a victim – even of something as common as a traffic fatality – if the nature of their grieving following a tragedy meets the *structure of the experience* that Caruth and Farrell both assume. What might be seen as a tragic auto accident to one person could be a traumatic incident for another person.

Our interest in roadside shrines developed from personal interaction with family members of accident victims who seemed unable – in one case for more than a year – to find closure to their grief. Frequent visits to the site and constant improvements and cultivation of the shrine, along with repeated reference to the still unresolved nature of the accident, suggested a traumatic response to the death of a family member. In this essay, roadside shrines are interrogated as special places for memory work, memorializing, and recuperation from trauma. Erected for private grieving but located in public space, roadside shrines are performative acts. Negotiating the borders between the private and the public, they mark death and grant a space for working through the loss. As such, they are a form of visual rhetoric meriting scholarly attention.

The intended meaning for a monument or memorial is always subject to reinterpretation because, as James Young argues, they 'take on lives of their own, often stubbornly resistant to the state's original intentions' (1993, 3). Memorializing seeks to bridge the past we remember and the future we desire by providing closure to painful events. The same impetus inheres with vernacular memorials. For some individuals the site of death evokes verbal and visual memorialization in an effort to obviate the trauma.

There is growing multidisciplinary interest in roadside shrines as vernacular memorials. Geographers including Cynthia Henzel (1995) have focused on the presence and distribution of crosses marking traffic fatalities; anthropologists such as Sylvia Grider (2006) have detailed the characteristics and terminology of vernacular shrines; and scholars in fine arts such as Erika Doss (2002) have turned to an exploration of how and why commemoration develops in response to grief and how it is expressed in the public sphere. Furthermore, sociologists such as Jeffrey Durbin (2003) explore the material culture of mass grief and mourning, including the tradition of erecting crosses at the site of automobile accidents. Elizabethada Wright links Foucault's concept of heterotopian space to two cemeteries in New England to argue that cemeteries are rhetorical memory places: 'what is remembered is directly connected to where it is remembered. A memory must have a place where a memory can crystallize and secrete itself; it must deliver the rhetorical goods' (2005, 55). Extending this multidisciplinary research, this essay will focus primarily on the ideas advanced by Michel Foucault, Rebecca Kennerly, and

Kenneth Burke to attend to the importance of place in the process of grieving, recovering from trauma, and memorializing. We argue that roadside shrines, as temporary, vernacular heterotopian spaces, are sites of memory that in endowing the visitor with agency facilitate mourning and are a necessary step toward trauma recovery. The term traumascapes in the title of this essay is borrowed from Maria Tumarkin (2005) to reference sites of trauma that evoke 'legacies of violence, suffering and loss' (12). She argues that trauma occurs to survivors when the 'ways in which they usually experience the world and make sense of their own place in it are effectively shattered' (2005, 11). Where public memorials evoke mythic stories to structure national memories and help a nation move on, these localized traumascapes, while reflecting cultural icons – flags on the 4th of July, for example – are individualized spaces used to come to terms with a death that seems unexplainable. While in the case of roadside shrines the victims are not survivors of the event but the relatives and friends of the dead person, what is important to both is the singularity of the place for the process of working through trauma.

Part one of this essay borrows Foucault's term 'heterotopia' (1998) and approaches these sites as heterotopian space and place. These are not authorized sites of commemoration; they lack permanence and official sanctioning and reflect the efforts of ordinary people making sense of their own private pain. The argument here is that when an individual assumes agency in creating a site and returns to the site for memory work, he or she is working through the chaos that remains in the wake of a loved one's death. Too often they are the kinds of places neglected in the scholarship in favour of the official, the grand, the historically significant event being commemorated. As Everett concludes about other forms of spontaneous shrines, these are places generally recognized as within the public domain that get used for 'private and public mourning, as spaces in which to negotiate meaning' (2002, 3). Sidewalks, fences, lampposts, and the verges along roads, whether private or public, become placeholders of memory, or in Marita Sturken's terms (1997), a technology of memory, a place to go to work through grief.

Part two focuses on the site as a space for negotiating memory, for both remembering and forgetting. The analysis extends the research of Kennerly (2002) on the performative dimension of such memorial sites to include the physical site and the offerings that symbolically and metonymically preserve the memory of the person and the loss that is felt. To aid in the memory process, friends and family bring offerings to the site: something the dead person treasured, a favourite object of the visitor, or a more traditional symbol of commemoration such as flowers or crosses. The offerings are detailed in part three by attending to the form of spontaneous shrines to discover shared symbolic representations. If, as Kenneth Burke notes, form is the 'arousing and fulfillment of desires' (1968, 24), attention to the form of these shrines may offer insight into the way they function rhetorically – as symbolic acts.

Roadside memorials as heterotopian space/place

Foucault's concept of heterotopian space frames our discussion of how the site of roadside shrines facilitates a working through of trauma. Foucault defines heterotopias as atypical emplacements in that they 'suspend, neutralize, or reverse the set of relations that are designated, reflected, or represented [*réflechis*] by them' (1998, 178). He explains that heterotopias 'have a function in relation to the remaining space' in this case 'creating a different space, a different real space as perfect, as meticulous, as well-arranged as ours is disorganized, badly arranged, and muddled' (184). The order brought by creating, maintaining, or even visually acknowledging the site by looking and seeing it differently – not as the place of violent death but as space for remembering and honouring – offers relief from the chaos of traumatic memory and grief. Grooming the site, adding seasonal displays, and creating a sense of permanence in the construction of the shrine are all acts that reflect agency rather than victimage. The very possibility of such agency is often absent in the trauma victim. One simple but powerful way to gain agency is to take a profane and tragic space and make it sacred. In separating out a small part of the larger landscape, in adding symbolic offerings, in grounding the space with ceremonial and domestic objects, the site becomes sanctified. Sacred space offers time and place for engagement in the traumatic memories.

Foucault argues that heterotopian space also displaces time. Temporal discontinuities bring the past to bear on the present and future. He uses the example of a cemetery to explain:

> the heterotopia begins to function fully when men are in a kind of absolute break with their traditional time; thus the cemetery is indeed a highly heterotopian place, seeing that the cemetery begins with the strange heterochronia that loss of life constitutes for an individual, and that quasi eternity in which he perpetually dissolves and fades away. (Foucault 1998, 182)

At roadside shrines time seems to replay itself and the experiences of loss are continuously re-experienced. Although the site evokes pain, it is also a space in which to re-experience the time and place of death in order to make sense of the loss. The present and past collapse; the evocation of the initial trauma leaves the past open in the present, constraining individual agency while giving agency to place. Just as the site stripped agency from the person who died, it controls those who mourn, as it continually returns the mourner to the moment of loss. Herein lies the contradictory nature of memorials. If agency is given over to the site, how does the individual gain control? We argue that the ability to give some order to the chaos of memory helps assuage the traumatic response. Constructing the site, bringing offerings, choosing to visit the shrine while knowing that doing so may evoke the traumatic memory are all acts that gain agency for the petitioner. In so doing, healing may begin.

The space created for memory work is outside of time in another way as well; vernacular memorials are often transitory, that is *momentarily* out of time. For a short time, neutral community space is transformed into memorial place/space. An example is a roadside shrine in Silverton, Oregon, erected after the death of a young man from Ireland. The site saw major development in the days following his death but was completely removed in less than a month. Although vernacular memorials are not physically there to eternally suggest memory work, while they are in place, visitors to the site are encouraged to reflect on the loss of life and to confront the social suffering this loss engenders. Although this temporary memorial lasted less than a month, without this dedicated display the public's attention to the death would have been much briefer. The visual power of the flowers, letters, posters, and candles on display forced the viewer to break time and commemorate. In this way, even a temporary memorial manipulates time for individual and community memory work. The first step to recovery is to engage the mourning process.

Yet even when memorials are not removed, time can change them in curious ways. Some roadside shrines are carefully and continually maintained: fresh flowers and objects appropriate to the season are placed at the memorial sites – pumpkins before Halloween and wreaths and Christmas ornaments in December (see Figure 1).

For many, however, the memorial is frozen in time past. The disjuncture is less due to the gap between the past and future and more a result of a present lack of care for the memorial and the expectation for maintenance that the act of memorializing begs.

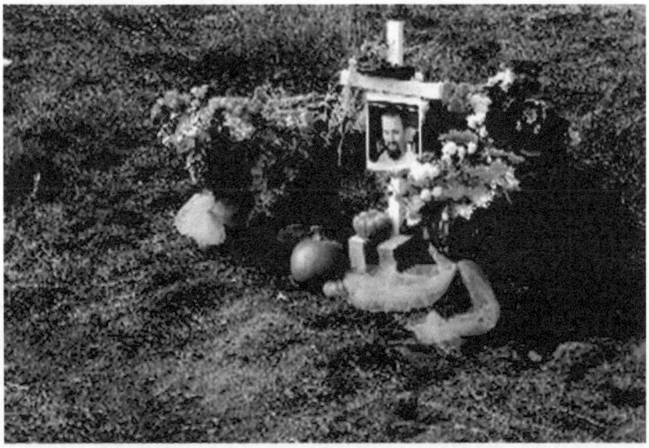

Figure 1. Located on Wallace Road, north-west of Salem, Oregon.

Numerous shrines along the Oregon roadsides appear to have been untended for a long time. Silk flowers are faded, live potted plants are overturned and long dead, painted and printed signage is faded beyond easy recognition, and photographs have lost all detail. At a memorial to a young man who died at 18, an official document, cocooned in plastic, remains pinned to the light post. Whether the object was a licence, identity tag or photo is now indeterminate.

In addition to displacements in space and time, Foucault notes, 'heterotopias always presuppose a system of opening and closing that isolates them and makes them penetrable at the same time' (1998, 183). Entrance to the space may be restricted or demand ritual to accompany the transition from outside to inside. When driving past such shrines, one can have a glimpse of a memorial and recognize its form, but in order to access the specifics of the site one must stop and enter the space. In doing so one encounters the personalized offerings that are less visible to the cars passing by – letters, photos, and occasionally grieving family and friends. Messages are there but remain locked away until one fully uncovers the letters or unfurls the flag on which a message has been inscribed. Even discovering the date of death may entail temporarily removing some of the adornments. In several sites wreaths left over from Christmases past obscure the text.

Foucault's argument that heterotopian space is closed to easy access is apparent when considering the relationship between the space for the shrine and the vehicle that brings the mourner close to the site. Without a break in time, without fully entering the site and participating with its objects, the casual observer is excluded from the space. The presence of a memorial may remind a driver of the dangers of the road, while triggering a response to the death of another traveller, but the space for negotiating memory is closed. For a casual observer, the roadside shrine is not a traumascape; it is a largely empty, albeit acknowledged, memorial site.

As a site for memory work, roadside shrines epitomize heterotopias. In giving materiality to the memory of loss and creating sacred space, if only temporarily, these sites reflect the contested and subverted nature of memory. In Foucault's terms the space/place is both real and unreal fantasy at the same time; it facilitates memory as it simultaneously allows for the inversion of memory. Thus some scholars argue that once a monument is established, the hard work of memory is taken out of the memorializing process, buried 'beneath layers of national myths and explanations' that give the memory a sense of completion rather than demanding contemplation and engagement (Young 1993, 5). But until they are abandoned and while they are actively created and visited, roadside shrines allow individuals to gain some agency, and thereby some relief, from the chaos of traumatic memory.

Memory and identity

Marita Sturken begins *Tangled Memories* by noting: 'Memory gives meaning to the present, as each moment is constituted by the past. As the means by which we remember who we are, memory provides the very core of identity' (1997, 1). Sturken and others who study cultural memory argue that it is contested and changeable. Thus our national identity changes with memories of the Vietnam War, 9/11, or the presence of AIDS or other traumatic events. The same is true of memories of an individual. The individuals who grieve a person's death tell the story of that person's life differently at different times and under different circumstances. Because we all play multiple roles throughout our lives – mother, daughter, artist, activist, caregiver, prankster – the memories of who someone was change with the role remembered and the relationship that role facilitated for the one remembering. Because the sites of memory, personal and temporal though they may be, are erected in public space, and because the objects left at the site are open to public surveillance, what is private space for personal remembering is also public space that generates cultural memory.

Our memory work seeks obviation of pain, yet painful memories may, in Dominick LaCapra's terms, become necessary in order to avoid the 'covering over of wounds and creating the impression that nothing really disruptive has occurred' because in doing so 'one forecloses the possibility of mourning, renders impossible a critical engagement with the past, and impedes recognition of problems (including the return of the repressed)' (1994, 23). Working through the experience allows healing to begin. Exorcizing the ghosts of the past, LaCapra argues, necessitates distinguishing between acting out and working through trauma. With post-traumatic acting out 'one is haunted or possessed by the past and performatively caught up in the compulsive repetition of traumatic scenes – scenes in which the past returns and the future is blocked' (2001, 21). In trying to cope with the traumatic the individual seeks understanding of, and hence closure to, the unexpected death. Focusing on the place and moment of death is an act of recuperation, but working through trauma, as LaCapra notes, may necessitate forgetting as much as remembering. Just reliving the loss may not be therapeutic. One of our friends talked about his impulse to establish a memorial after the death of his brother in a traffic accident, but explained that his father refused to consider a vernacular memorial. To create a sacred space to make pilgrimages to the place of death, from his perspective was to reduce his son to nothing more than the moment of his death; it meant dwelling on death rather than remembering who his son was in life. For the father, the memorial would lock his son in death, but for the surviving son it was a way to begin the process of healing. Whether the father could not cope with reliving painful memories or had already come to terms with memories in ways his surviving son had not is unclear, but the incident reminds us that, as is the case with official memorials, vernacular memorials are not uncontested.

Simply focusing on death may result in what LaCapra terms acting out – trapping the mourner in a liminal state. The act of constructing or visiting a roadside shrine seeks to resolve liminality and move the visitor to a reaggregated state. In this sense, visiting the shrine is an act of pilgrimage. Reader and Walter (1993) remind us that pilgrimage in a secular sense is less about a physical journey and more a metaphorical glance at the person's life.

In this case, it is conducted through objects that reflect the passage of time and the many facets of how the visitor to a memorial site remembers the victim. Pilgrimage entails 'the idea of quest, of seeking something that lies outside of the patterns of everyday life ... that will enhance or affirm his/her being and existence on one or more levels, that may make him/her whole, more complete' (9–10).

The presence of pilgrims at a shrine creates what Victor Turner calls *communitas* – the temporary sense of identification between individuals who otherwise would not interact (1977, 96). There is an etiquette when strangers converge on the space at the same time. New arrivals wait until those already present move on. When people know one another there is an inclination to tell stories about the dead person, and discuss whether the death is resolved and if the actions taken to 'prepare' the site for public visitation are adequate. *Communitas* may give temporary respite from the isolation that the liminal state of grieving has created, even though the sense of pilgrimage remains as an individual act (Reader and Walter 1993, 21). Roadside shrines offer a place for memory work precisely because they are heterotopian spaces within which to negotiate loss. The space allows performative possibility. As Kennerly notes: 'Roadside shrines are constructed in moments of performance, leave traces that bear witness to those past performances, and invite future performances' (2002, 233).

Objects of memory: Offerings at roadside shrines

The offerings brought to roadside shrines, like those left at public memorials, are entanglements of memory, representation, and negotiation of the pain of loss. They are ways of telling stories about the person who has died and their place in the lives of those who bring the offerings or observe the shrine. They give a physicality to the emotions of grieving; something to touch and see in substitution for the absence of life. These objects are common items that have importance to either the pilgrim or the person who has died. It is important to note, however, the polysemic nature of offerings; meanings vary with the observer and the context. Sarah Henry, interviewed on a PBS film entitled *Objects and Memory*, says it well: 'I believe that objects are the eyewitness of the past, and they are more than that, they are emissaries of the past' (*Objects and Memory* 2008). Objects are a vehicle for making tangible what is intangible and absent. In bringing offerings to the site of tragedy, the pilgrim acquires agency as a concrete step toward coming to terms with trauma. Nonetheless, patterns in offerings at roadside shrines warrant some attention.

The most extensive investigation of vernacular offerings has focused on the Vietnam Veterans Memorial in Washington, DC and its collection of toys, photographs, favourite objects, personal tokens, and symbolic reminders of a life lost. Sturken sees the ritual of leaving these offerings at the Wall as 'an act of catharsis, a release of long-held objects to memory ... talismans of redemption, guilt, loss and anger' (1997, 78). Many of the same kinds of objects are left at roadside memorials. We have identified three broad categories of offerings: firstly, domestic objects, some of which are metonymic personal objects; secondly, ceremonial offerings; and thirdly, objects that we term trauma objects.

Common domestic items – toys, photographs and personal objects – are found at roadside shrines. Many of the shrines we visited included stuffed teddy bears, lambs, monkeys, and smiley faces. Whether brought by children or seen as a nostalgic comfort object, these toys, more commonly seen in a domestic context, are visible even to passersby. About 20% of the memorials include animal representations; in some cases a statue of the victim's pet or a metal ornament of a favourite animal.

The domestic is also reflected in photographs, present in a quarter of the sites we visited. These images define the role and relationship of the victim and the person contributing to the memorial. They include group shots, a snapshot with the family pet, graduation poses, formal career pictures and portraits of the victim. Ludmila da Silva Catela explains the function of the photograph in commemoration:

> the use of photographs to remember an absence re-creates, symbolizes, recuperates a presence that establishes links between life and death, the explicable and inexplicable. Photographs 'vivify.' Like a metonymy, they contain part of the referent to totalize a system of meanings ... By situating the dead and creating a material residue that links them to the living, photography becomes an especially potent representational medium for processing grief. (Quoted in Tandeciarz 2006, 137–8)

The photographs testify to the victim's having-been-there and in this sense they are heterotopian objects collapsing a life fully lived with that person's death. Photographs offer the possibility of triggering memory and are thereby central to the act of mourning and subsequent recovery.

Personal items adorned about 20% of the sites we visited. These include necklaces, glasses, hats, other items of clothing, and awards the person received while living. At times these items are metonyms of the victim – in one case the sheriff's badge, in another a motorcycle. Equally personal are letters written to the deceased, as well as expressive of the loss that the contributor feels. 'To my brother. We miss you always ... you will be in our hearts forever' or 'We love you Kelly! Missing you everyday my friend. Not a day goes by that you are not in our thoughts! Take care of all our everyday heroes!' or 'You are alive in your little girl's [*sic*] faces.' These messages express loss, ask the dead person to watch out for those left alive, and share current events, accomplishments, and concerns with the deceased in an effort to normalize an unordered existence. They are epistolary moments of connection between the living and the deceased and are not intended for other visitors to the site (see Figure 2).

A further domestic gesture uses landscaping materials to ground these spaces. A number of memorials use rocks to anchor the space and thereby give the site constructed a natural substance. Only occasionally are the rocks needed to support a cross. That task is performed at one site by three layers of cement blocks that encircle the cross. On the side of the circle facing the road several dozen 1–2 inch thick pieces of slate form a two-foot wide apron. Decorative bark dust is spread around the remaining two-thirds of the apron (see Figure 3).

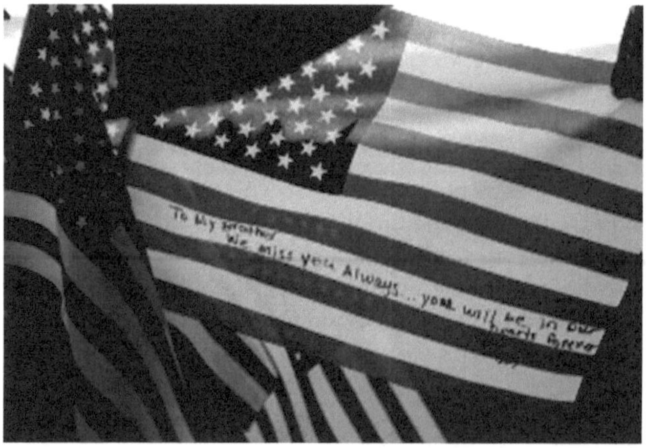

Figure 2. Close-up of Figure 3; Highway 99E south of Woodburn, Oregon.

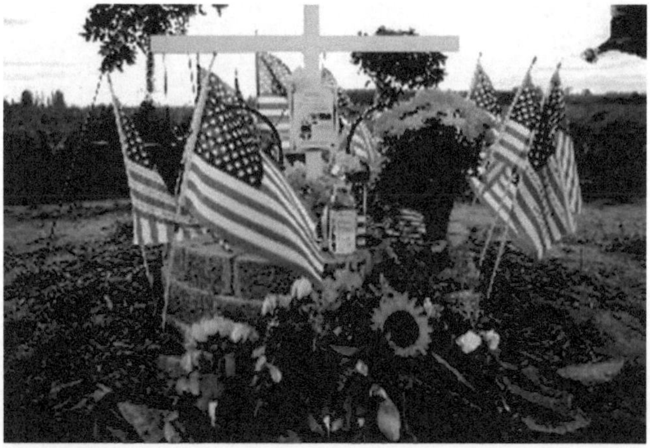

Figure 3. Located on Highway 99E south of Woodburn, Oregon.

When we visited the shrine on the first anniversary of the victim's death we overheard the uncle telling another family member that he had 'cleaned the site' in preparation for the anniversary. A spontaneous shrine filled with common items, the family member nonetheless thought it important to landscape the memorial. At another shrine south-west of Woodburn, Oregon, rocks have then been brought to the cleared site and placed in a loose circle around a white cross. Rather than support the cross, the rocks seem designed to give definition to the space, to mark the sacred from the more profane segments of the memorial site. In one of the newest memorials we have witnessed constant improvements including the addition of several large fieldstones 6–8 inches in diameter that have been added on either side of the central cross area. They serve no function other than to demark the space, to stamp an individual's hand in creating the place (see Figure 1).

In addition to personalized domestic objects, roadside shrines display ceremonial religious objects: crosses, votive candles, flowers and wreaths. Eighty per cent of the shrines we studied include crosses, usually white, either wooden or metal. Bare wooden crosses are also common. Frequently the crosses have identification inscribed on them – the name of the deceased, the date of their death, sometimes the date of their birth – and occasionally a message about the loss felt by the person constructing the cross. One site has eight crosses nailed to a wooden telephone pole, many with messages written on them. Most of the crosses are decorated with artificial flowers and wreaths, especially Christmas wreaths. Relatively few sites have candles but where candles are present they are a prominent part of the display. In one vernacular response to a young Irish man's death by a police shooting there were even extra candles available for visitors to the site. In addition, weeks after the memorial was dismantled, a thick layer of wax covered the road and the sidewalks. Flowers traditionally adorn altars and are used as a symbol of religious celebration. Over 90% of our shrines included flowers and plants. New flowers are added to the shrines on special occasions. These ceremonial offerings set the site apart from the profane space of the roadside and establish a religious ritual identification. In offering ritual space for remembering, they prepare the pilgrim for commemorating.

Trauma objects, our third category, are the most unsettling contribution to the shrine. They are remnants of the accident that vividly bring the force of the trauma to the present.

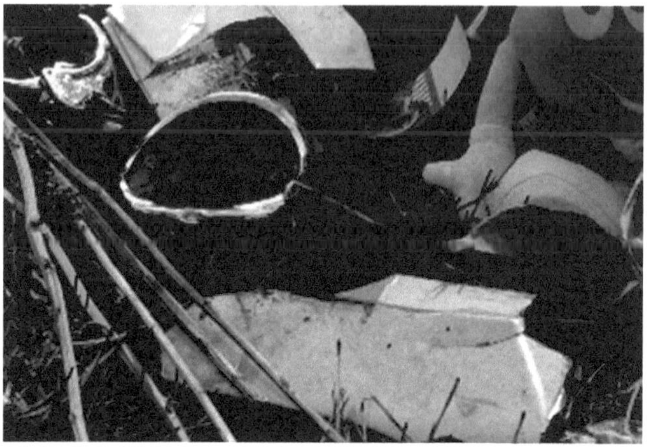

Figure 4. Close-up of Figure 1; Wallace Road, north-west of Salem, Oregon.

Several of the roadside memorials we studied include the moulding strip, windshield wipers, vehicle logo or other mangled car and motorcycle parts. These are the last tangible remains of the vehicle. Several sites also include broken glass from the automobile, even when the memorial site had obviously been cleaned. At times the glass and mangled vehicle parts have been moved onto the pile of offerings (see Figure 4).

In one shrine these material remains are tucked into the spaces within cinder blocks that surround the wooden cross. Over time these leftover remnants of the accident are relocated in the space amidst other offerings. Always prominent, however, is the Harley nameplate at the site of a motorcycle accident. In a similar move to retain the verisimilitude of the crash, the remains of mile markers or fence posts that were twisted at impact are left in place. The remnants of the violence reinforce the heterotopian nature of the place, perpetually evoking the trauma of loss at a site constructed for healing.

Whether in a productive or unproductive way, memory work becomes more pronounced on birthdays and anniversaries, and is marked by increased presence at the shrine and additional offerings. At one site the first anniversary of the accident saw the replacement of a temporary wooden cross with a permanent metal cross, extensive cleaning (grass was cut back all around the memorial and the ground was swept), and the addition of items to represent the young man. A memorial webpage announced the anniversary and invited participation in the remembrance. Because the man who died was a sheriff and on duty, and because the driver of the car that hit him fled the scene and remains at large, the trauma resists closure for family and close friends. In a true heterotopic response, at this particular shrine there are many more personal objects, especially metonymic representations.

Conclusion

Roadside shrines in Oregon exhibit several commonalities despite their variability. They are vernacular rather than sanctioned spaces for memorializing. As such they are highly personalized sites that, while sharing some common characteristics, address the needs of those individuals who construct and add to the shrine. While they are in place, vernacular shrines become sacred space – a place set apart that draws 'attention to the previously ordinary place where some violent event occurred' (Grider 2006, 248). They are temporary because they are often on public or private property not owned by the family of the victim. Furthermore, unlike official memorials, they are made of less durable materials. Because there is no guaranteed maintenance of the site, vernacular shrines depend on those who erected the memorial or on neighbours to the site to maintain them. Over half of the memorials we studied evidence little upkeep. They are heterotopian spaces filled with spatial and temporal ambiguities, but also with the potential stories necessary to the healing process. Finally, they are adorned with transposed domestic, ceremonial, and trauma objects, the meaning of which depends on the visitor and context. They are sites of memory work, of efforts to overcome trauma, but they remain heterotopian spaces of both presence and absence, of necessary forgetting and equally necessary remembering.

Are the roadside shrines restorative? Do they enable those who construct them to find space for negotiating their grief, for coming to terms with the loss they have suffered, and to find, in making the place public, a sense of comfort? Does the offering of objects and the act of constructing a site for grieving position the sufferer to overcome the trauma, or does the loss merely continue to haunt the traumatized visitor? Although answers to these questions are personal, the symbolic act of roadside commemoration holds the potential for trauma work. Visual symbols – the shrine and its offerings – become iconic of the trauma, a placeholder from which to resolve its hauntings. Zelizer and Allan's research on the circulation in the media of images of 9/11 argues that objects bear witness to the events and 'bring individuals together on their way to collective recovery' by moving them 'from the personal act of "seeing" to the adoption of a public stance by which they become part of a collective working through trauma together' (2003, 52). Applying this logic to roadside shrines would suggest that in moving the memorial to public space, in confronting objects contributed by various pilgrims to the site, like the American public's collective participation in the 9/11 trauma through the images, individuals may perceive a collective working through of the trauma they live.

Roadside shrines are also symbolic spaces when adorned with ceremonial, domestic, and personal artefacts that sacralize the place/space. They offer a temporary space for memory work, for remembering and telling stories that work through the trauma and ultimately lead to healing. By their very nature as sites of death, these places become sacred spaces that tell stories to make some sense of inexplicable loss. These commemorative narratives, in James Young's terms, negotiate the chaotic and traumatic event of the past and the desire for an ordered and peaceful future. There is a nostalgic impulse in acts of pilgrimage that these roadside shrines encourage. They allow the individual an opportunity of holding 'on to the past, to what appears to have been lost to the present, and of reconstituting the past in an idealized and romanticized way' (Reader and Walker 1993, 230–1). Roadside shrines hold out the possibility of an at least bearable future.

References

Burke, Kenneth. 1968. *Counter-statement*. Berkeley: University of California Press.

Caruth, Cathy. 1995. *Trauma: Explorations in memory*. Baltimore: Johns Hopkins University Press.

Doss, Erika. 2002. Death, art and memory in the public sphere: The visual and material culture of grief in contemporary America. *Mortality* 7, no. 1: 63–82.

Durbin, Jeffrey. 2003. Expressions of mass grief and mourning: The material culture of makeshift memorials. *Material Culture* 35, no. 1: 23–43.

Everett, Holly J. 2002. *Roadside crosses in contemporary memorial culture*. Denton: University of North Texas Press.

Farrell, Kirby. 1998. *Post-traumatic culture*. Baltimore: Johns Hopkins University Press.

Foucault, Michel. 1998. Different spaces. In *Aesthetics, method, and epistemology*, vol. 2, ed. James D. Faubion, trans. Robert Hurley, 175–85. New York: New Press.

Grider, Sylvia. 2006. Spontaneous shrines and public memorialization. In *Death and religion in a changing world*, ed. Kathleen Garces-Foley, 246–64. Armonk, NY: M.E. Sharp.

Henzel, Cynthia. 1995. *Cruces* in the roadside landscape of Northeastern Mexico. *Journal of Cultural Geography* 11, no. 2: 93–106.

Kennerly, Rebecca M. 2002. Getting messy: In the field and at the crossroads with roadside shrines. *Text and Performance Quarterly* 22: 229–60.

LaCapra, Dominick. 1994. *Representing the Holocaust: History, theory, trauma*. Ithaca, NY: Cornell University Press.

———. 2001. *Writing history, writing trauma*. Baltimore: Johns Hopkins University Press.

Nora, Pierre. 1989. Between memory and history: Les lieux de memoire. *Representations* 26 (Spring): 7–25.

Objects and Memory. Produced by Jonathan Fein. Directed by Brian Danitz. Washington, DC: PBS, 2008.

Reader, Ian, and Tony Walter, eds. 1993. *Pilgrimage in popular culture*. London: Macmillan.

Sturken, Marita. 1997. *Tangled memories: The Vietnam War, the AIDS epidemic, and the politics of remembering*. Berkeley: University of California Press.

Tandeciarz, Silvia R. 2006. Mnemonic hauntings: Photography as art of the missing. *Social Justice* 33, no. 2: 135–52.

Tumarkin, Maria. 2005. *Traumascapes: The power and fate of places transformed by tragedy*. Melbourne: University of Melbourne Press.

Turner, Victor. 1977. *The ritual process: Structure and anti-structure*. Ithaca, NY: Cornell University Press.

Wright, Elizabethada A. 2005. Rhetorical spaces in memorial places: The cemetery as a rhetorical memory place/space. *Rhetoric Society Quarterly* 35, no. 4: 51–81.

Young, James E. 1993. *The texture of memory*. New Haven: Yale University Press.

Zelizer, Barbie, and Stuart Allan. 2003. *Journalism after September 11*. New York: Routledge.

Trauma, bodies, and performance art: Towards an embodied ethics of seeing

Sophie Anne Oliver

School of Psycho-Social Studies and School of Law, Birkbeck College, University of London, UK

The question of how to be an ethical witness to the suffering of distant others is one that has long been a preoccupation of trauma studies scholars. This paper addresses the problem of (un)ethical spectatorship of the traumatized body by engaging with the theory and practice of contemporary performance art. Rejecting the fantasy of the ideal moral witness, the author turns to models of embodied spectatorship suggested by performance-body art to propose ways of seeing that acknowledge and accept the necessary ambivalence of the distant spectatorship of suffering, while at the same time promoting a sense of 'response-ability' and self-reflection.

Introduction

In *The Town Beyond the Wall*, Holocaust survivor Elie Wiesel is cutting in his condemnation of those who, as bystanders to Nazi atrocities, were 'permanently and merely spectators' and, who, in Wiesel's words, 'observed us [the victims], without emotion, while we became objects' (1982, 148). Decades later, the proliferation of visual and other representations of atrocity and human suffering has forced us all to question our role as spectators to the other's pain. This article explores the possibility of imagining ethical ways of seeing the suffering of others, working from a focus upon the traumatized body, by which I mean to refer both to the *traumatized bodies* of atrocity victims that we see represented in visual and other media and, more abstractly, to the corporeal as the conceptual site upon which trauma and its discourses are negotiated. From voyeurism and the 'eroticisation of atrocity' (Jacobs 2008) to the objectification and appropriation of the other's experience, viewing the traumatized bodies of atrocity is an exercise strewn with pitfalls, and yet it is one to which we are all regularly exposed not only through news and media coverage of war and genocide but also in humanitarian campaigns, memorial projects and in artistic representations of suffering and traumatic memory. The question then becomes: how might we be responsive and, to use Kelly Oliver's term, *response-able* to the traumatized body (Oliver 2001)? How are we to move from voyeuristic spectating of the traumatized body as object, to an ethical witnessing of that body as part of the other's, and our own, humanity? In response to such questions, this paper draws on a field of study so far largely unexplored within trauma studies, that of performance art theory.

The scant attention paid to performance art by trauma scholars is surprising when we consider that not only are many contemporary performance artists directly addressing through their work questions of personal and/or collective trauma but also that the very foundations of performance art speak to, of and from the dynamics of power, oppression and the traumatized body. Since the early 'Happenings' and feminist body-art of the 1960s and 1970s, performance art has achieved historical status as negotiator of a new relationship between art and politics (Wark 2006); its repeated engagement with the body as a mode of experience as well as a means of expression has forced audiences both within and outside of the art world to pay attention to embodiment as a cultural and political force. From its earliest manifestations, performance art has sought to redefine discourses of the traumatized body in ways that I suggest may provide the first step towards a model for ethical spectatorship.

The central proposition of this paper is that trauma theorists, in particular those concerned with the visual representation of trauma, would find it useful to consider some of the theoretical insights about experience, embodiment and spectatorship developed in the field of performance art. By its very form and nature performance art suggests the *possibility* of an apparently unique mode of spectatorship that it is argued can and should be transposed onto other contexts in which we are asked to see the suffering of others. What is potentially 'ethical' about this way of seeing is not only its call for a sense of response-ability towards the corporeal subject being viewed (that is, a sense of 'infinite encounter with otherness' as conditional to our own subjectivity [Oliver 2001]), but also, and crucially, the demand for the spectator's own self-conscious relation to the (re)presentation, and the acknowledgement of his or her own embodiment as a performative presence in the moment of witnessing the other's trauma, even in cases of distant or mediated viewing. In this sense, then, performance art may have more to tell us about the *spectating* body of the viewer than about the spectated body of the viewed. Indeed, it is important to note that this essay seeks only to bring into dialogue the theories of *spectatorship* developed within trauma and performance studies; it does not seek to suggest a slippage between the figure of the victim of trauma and the performance artist engaged in self-inflicted pain or mutilation.

The first section of the article provides a brief overview of the ways in which the (not unproblematic) notion of 'unethical spectatorship' has commonly been framed, and explores the proposition that the spectatorship of traumatized bodies is particularly problematic in its potential to induce objectifying and voyeuristic ways of seeing suffering. From here, it is suggested that the corporeal politics of feminist performance art may provide a first indication of how the practice and its theory might serve as a model for an ethics of seeing the traumatized body. The concept of 'ethics' suggested lies not in the absence of feelings of disgust, guilt or voyeuristic pleasure: these are all accepted as genuine responses to the spectacle of trauma. In this sense, performance art proposes a departure from the very concept of unethical spectatorship as it is often conceived in trauma studies. The second section focuses more conceptually on the ontology of performance, which, through its delicate negotiation of presence and absence, and its necessarily dialogic nature, suggests an alternative understanding of 'ethical' spectatorship that, conceptually at least, is fully amenable to trauma theory. In the final section I develop more fully this model of embodied ethical seeing through a discussion of Jill Bennett's theory of sense memory, which, thought in relation to spectator experiences of performance art, brings the performative act of *seeing* into focus, thus suggesting more concretely the possibility of an embodied ethics of spectatorship.

Unethical spectatorship and the traumatized body

The spectator, Wiesel writes, 'has nothing of the human in him: he is a stone in the street, the cadaver of an animal, a dead pile of wood' (1982, 164). Passive, unmoved and unmoving, the figure of the 'unethical spectator' is in the first instance accused of moral indifference; that is, of *turning away*, of pretending not to see and remaining silent in the face of injustice. Elsewhere in Wiesel's account, the spectator of suffering is guilty not only of apathy but also of displaying a morbid fascination with the object of his gaze. Describing an episode in which a group of German workers threw scraps of bread into a freezing, open train carriage of deportees, Wiesel notes how the onlookers appeared enthralled by the sight of these unfortunates as they scrambled and fought for the crumbs turned to gold by hunger. As Wiesel describes it, the fascination with which the German workers watch the deportees is morally and ethically suspect: these bystanders behave as though they were spectators at a freak show, a circus, throwing scraps to the animals at the zoo (Wiesel and Mainac 1958, 156–7).

The image of spectators at a zoo looking on in disengaged interest at the strange animals held captive to their gaze resonates with many of the criticisms voiced today in relation to the visual representation of atrocity. As images of atrocity and traumatized bodies proliferate, it is argued, we, the receivers of these visual representations, become somehow 'immune' to their effect, seeing them simply as *spectacle*, a form of 'infotainment' – the enjoyment of which marks our complicity in the commodification of experience, by which we become merely consumers or voyeurs of suffering (see Kleinman, Das, and Lock 1997, 1–24). Both Lyndsey French and Janet Jacobs have exposed the risks of such commercial or cultural appropriations of suffering for the spectators of photographic exhibitions displaying images of victims and their bodies (French 2002; Jacobs 2008). For French, as for Jacobs, the dangers of unethical spectatorship lie not only in the act of looking away but also, and perhaps even more so, in the act of *looking on*. It is the way we see victims of atrocity and their bodies that presents the greatest danger for the spectator. In her commentary on a MOMA exhibition of genocide photographs drawn from the Tuol Sleng archive in Cambodia, French suggested that by presenting images of victims in ways that remove them from the specific context of their suffering, such exhibitions reiterate a sense of the victims' otherness in the eyes of the viewer (2002, 142). This observation is particularly relevant for thinking about visual representations of traumatized bodies, which are frequently represented as anonymous icons of atrocity, while at the same time provoking an array of visceral, distancing responses that might range from fear and disgust to, in some cases, enjoyment. On the photographic representation of female prisoners of Auschwitz, Jacobs expresses a concern that the images – often of semi-naked, starving women – may encourage 'a sexualized reading of the visual text, an effect of atrocity remembrance that, according to Susan Sontag, may "turn an event or person into something that can be possessed"' (Jacobs 2008, 220, citing Sontag 2003). As female concentration camp survivor Karein Goertz notes: 'there is, after all, such a thing as concentration camp pornography. The idea of having absolute power over others arouses feelings of pleasure' (2001, 179). The contemplation of the spectacle, that is, of the visual exhibition of the traumatized body, Jacobs suggests, places the spectator in an always already compromised position. In French's words, when we stand before such images of suffering we occupy a position of power in relation to the absolute powerlessness of the victims; held by their gaze, 'we stare back at them from the place of the executioner' (2002, 135). To suggest that, as viewers of images of atrocity, we can be said to see from the position of the executioner implies that the spectator is at risk of becoming complicit in the very logic of the degrading, marginalizing, dehumanizing effect of atrocity upon the body. As Elaine Scarry's now landmark study *The Body in Pain* (1985) demonstrates so strikingly, the processes of oppression, desubjectification and dehumanization at work in acts of atrocity such as torture are often, if not always, enacted upon the body, both physically and symbolically. Seeing the traumatized body as *other* or as object, as merely a spectacle to be seen, but not, in Susan Sontag's words, as 'someone (like us) who also sees' (2003, 65) becomes in itself a reiteration of wrongs already committed, continuing in the symbolic rejection of the victim as a subject.

To look upon the spectacle of the other's suffering, particularly when that spectacle is corporeal – and as James Elkins notes, the spectacle is nearly always in some way corporeal (1999, 1) – may give rise to a number of responses in the spectator; from disgust and the desire to look away, to pity, or voyeurism, or even a repetition of dehumanizing perception. Each is problematic in its own way. And yet to talk of an 'unethical spectator' is, I argue, unhelpful because it too easily dismisses certain spectatorial responses as unacceptable, rather than seeking to develop a theory of witnessing that acknowledges and works from the discomfort of seeing. The model of spectatorship suggested by performance art takes as its very foundation the discomfort of the viewer, and in so doing it achieves a clear political goal. Jayne Wark (2006) points to the feminist body art of the 1960s and 1970s as key in resisting dominant oppressive discourses of the feminine body as abject, unstable, and inferior. In acts of mimetic defiance, feminist performance artists such as Carolee Schneemann and Shikego Kubota reclaimed the abjected female body in ways that sought to expose and undermine hegemonic discourses of femininity as mysterious and threatening on the one hand, and passive and powerless on the other. *Interior Scroll* (1975) by Schneemann is iconic in this regard (see Figure 1). Like Kubota's *Vagina Painting* (1965), in which the artist, having attached a paint brush dripping with thick blood-red paint to her underwear, squatted over a large piece of paper which she proceeded to 'paint' as though in menstrual blood, *Interior Scroll* reclaimed the female anatomy, asserting the body's *inside* – usually read as 'a powerful sign of death' (Elkins 1999, 109) – as a source of knowledge, creativity and power (symbolized by the written scroll that the artist appears to be pulling out of her vagina). In another piece, entitled *Meat Joy* (1964), Schneemann brought together a group of partially nude men and women in an ecstatic performance of materiality, their bodies writhing joyously amongst raw fish and meat. Schneemann described this performance as an 'erotic rite', designed as 'a celebration of flesh as material' (www.caroleeschneemann.com). These and countless other performances have been seen to enact a re-appropriation of the objectified and marginalized female body, thereby providing a space for the female subject as both embodied and active, seeing as well as seen. Such a political *coup de force* was possible precisely because the artists were able to anticipate and 'work with' the disgust, anxiety, or voyeuristic pleasure of their spectators.

In no way can performance art cure us (nor does it seek to cure us) of our propensity to eroticize or objectify the people whose bodies we observe. Viewers of performance art are not inherently more 'ethical' than viewers of other forms of visual representation of bodily trauma; indeed, much performance or body art only functions *because* of the existence of negative, voyeuristic or turning away responses towards the abject body. What performance art can (but does not always) do, however, is openly problematize these responses. Vanessa Beecroft's highly political performance at the 2007 Venice Biennale, entitled *vb61: Still Death – Darfur – Still Deaf?* (see Figure 2), is a piece that explicitly brings performance art into dialogue with trauma discourse. In addition to the political question posed by the piece – why do we, as media spectators, remain deaf and apathetic in the face of so much violence and suffering? – it also poses, as all of Beecroft's work does, a set of more complex questions about the nature of voyeurism and the relationship between the viewer, the models and the context of the work, not to mention the relationship of these to the artist. There is something discomforting in the way in which

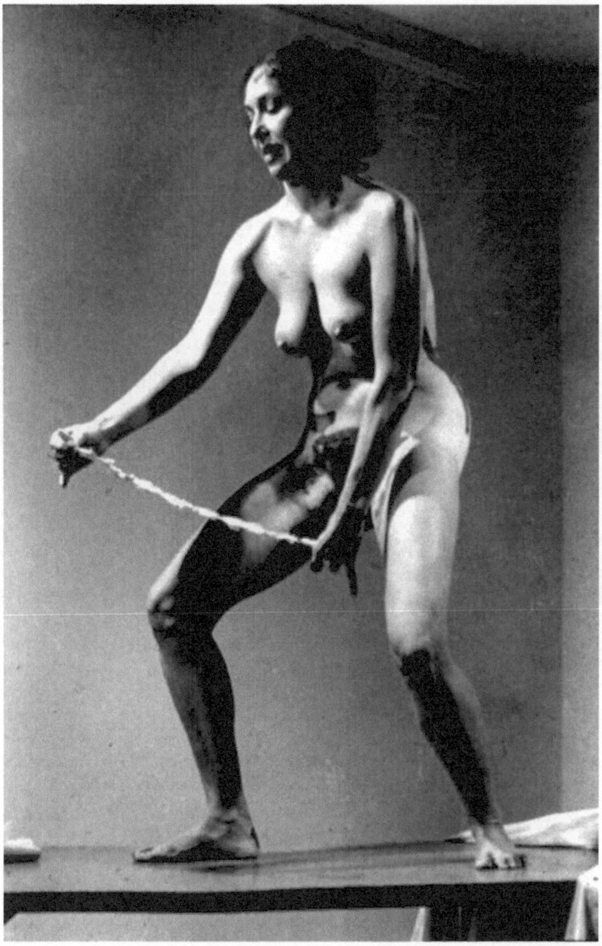

Figure 1. Carolee Schneemann, 'Interior Scroll' (1975). Performance photograph. (Photo: Anthony McCall.)

viewers of this performance observe, photograph, speak over or ignore the blood-covered bodies lying naked on the floor of the gallery space. And yet in posing the question of voyeurism Beecroft is at the same time (re)producing the conditions for that response to occur; as such, she offers to share in her spectator's guilt. Neither she nor her audience can hide from their voyeurism; they are in it together. In acknowledging this fact, the performance suggests, they stand more chance of moving on from their negative responses.

So far, performance art has been identified as *politically* useful in that it exposes and resists our dehumanizing perception of the traumatized or abject body, too easily perceived, like the feminine body, as *other*. In the achievement of this political aim, performance art also encourages us to consider more self-consciously the role of spectator as one which is also always complicit in and *with* the representation, forcing us to acknowledge the unavoidable ethical ambivalence of seeing the suffering of others. In this sense, performance art encourages a revised formulation of spectatorial ethics, one that is not based only in the imposition of ideal or 'appropriate' responses. The following section

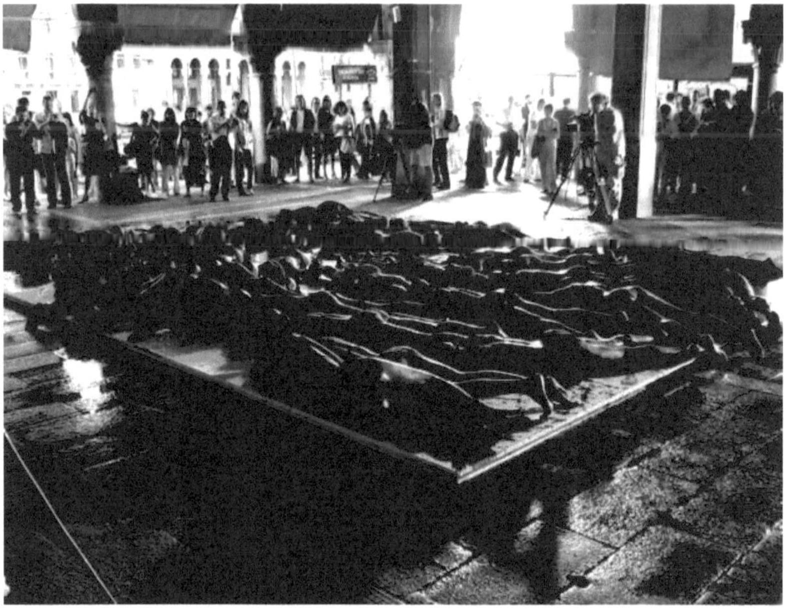

Figure 2. Vanessa Beecroft, 'vb61' (2007). Performance photograph. Image courtesy of Bill Thompson.

explores this theme further, beginning with an analysis of the ontology of performance, which, it is argued, speaks to trauma discourse in ways that merit more attention than they have hitherto received in trauma scholarship.

The ontology of performance: Embodying the spectator

Trauma and performance have long been linked conceptually, from the great Greek tragedies to Freud and Breuer's clinical studies of hysterics. And yet, even if we agree that it is with Freud that the theory of trauma takes flight, two important aspects of his early clinical encounters remain overlooked, namely the significance in the *Hysteria* studies of the patient's *body* and its symptoms as signifiers of trauma, and, even more disregarded, the equally corporeal role of the doctors as interlocutors, or *embodied* witnesses of their patients' suffering. As Peggy Phelan points out in *Mourning Sex*, the *Hysteria* studies painted a picture of the body as performative – part, in these early case histories, of a physical as well as psychical connection or interaction between patient and doctor:

> The fingers of Freud and Breuer press and prod the somatic utterances of their patient's hysterical bodies [...] apply mental and/or physical pressure to the indecipherable bodily signifier, the symptom, until it joins in the conversational. (Phelan 1997, 51)

In these early clinical studies we note, following Phelan, a healing interrelation of trauma, body and performance in which the body of the 'spectator' – in this case the therapist – shares centre stage with that of the spectated. An analysis of Phelan's remarks on the 'ontology of performance' will demonstrate the enduring significance of this interrelation within the theory and practice of performance art, and further suggest how these might usefully influence trauma theories of spectatorship.

For Phelan, the ontology of performance is such that it can never be adequately preserved, described, or documented; in this sense, it may be linked to trauma through a parallel dance of presence and absence:

> Performance's only life is in the present. Performance cannot be saved, recorded, documented, or otherwise participate in the circulation of representations *of* representations: once it does so, it becomes something other than performance [...] Performance's being [...] becomes itself through disappearance. (1993, 146)

Like trauma, performance is unrepresentable, uncontainable. The comparison is at once crude and potentially fertile; existing only in the moment of its happening, performance is always an enactment of loss, of the impossibility of retrieving the past. Trauma theory, too, speaks of impossibilities, of the inassimilable past that forever haunts the present. It is hardly surprising, then, that so many performance artists address the subject of trauma in their work, as though the performance might provide a 'working through' of traumatic experience. The inevitable loss or 'disappearance of the object' in performance, Phelan suggests, 'rehearses and repeats the disappearance of the subject who longs to be remembered' (1993, 147). It is at the same time a political and ethical moment – political because it acts out a moment of rupture, ethical because it calls upon its spectators to join in the rehearsal of loss: 'performance calls witnesses to the singularity of the individual's death and asks the spectator to do the impossible – to share that death by rehearsing for it' (152). In its call to the audience, the performance proposes an alternative *way of seeing* the other that is ethical in a radical, perhaps Levinasian, sense. The performance does not exist without its audience, thus for performance, as for Levinas, ethics precedes ontology. For Phelan, performance art is ethical in that it offers a means of making visible that which is invisible or unmarked in traditional representation; it proposes, Phelan suggests, a model for 'another representational economy, one in which the reproduction of the Other as the same is not assured' (3).

The mode of seeing suggested by performance art is also, as we shall see, thoroughly embodied, adding the last link to the chain suggested by Phelan's reading of Freud. The spectator – situated, a body in space – encounters the other in what performance artist and scholar Anna Fenemore has described as a 'dialogic' mode of vision, experienced as 'a multiplicity of intersubjective relations and intercorporeal perceptions, both of which are marked by a reversibility of trajectory [...] That which is looked upon also acts upon what does the looking' (2008, 7). In dialogic modes of vision we can no longer talk of the 'passive' spectator, acted upon by the text; the spectator of performance art is one who also *performs* and acts upon the representation. Expanding on her argument, Fenemore draws our attention to a piece by Martin Jay, entitled 'Sartre, Merleau-Ponty and the search for a new ontology of sight'. Jay distinguishes between two opposing modes of vision, one epistemological and one ontological. The former is characterized by spectatorial distance and objectification, and corresponds to a 'staring gaze', which, Jay suggests, is not only aggressive but also 'rigid, ego-logical and exclusionary' (1993, 148). This corresponds to the gaze of the so-called 'unethical spectator' outlined above. The latter ontological mode, on the other hand, is embedded; the viewer is situated within the visual field, not outside it, and 'his relationship to the context in which he is embedded is nurturant, not controlling'. It is an *aletheic* gaze: 'multiple, aware of its context, inclusionary, horizontal and caring' (148). It is this embedded, embodied mode of seeing that Fenemore claims is characteristic of audience experiences of many performance art pieces. In this sense, viewing performance, as an embodied experience of the soon-to-be-lost present, entails something other than an appropriation or objectification of that which is seen; performance mirrors and (re-)enacts the dynamic of loss experienced in trauma and its memory, and in so doing it returns the gaze of the spectator, calling him in, demanding that he, too, perform.

One of the clearest examples of this call to spectatorial performance is evident in the work of Serbian-born artist Marina Abramović, whose performances have repeatedly sought to interrogate the emotional and ethical relationship of the audience to the work and to the performer. Her 1974 performance *Rhythm 0* tested this relationship to its limits. Here, the audience was instructed to act: given the choice of an array of over 70 different objects they were told to use these objects upon Abramović's body as they saw fit. By the end of the six-hour performance, Abramović had been 'stripped, painted, cut, crowned with thorns, and had the muzzle of a loaded gun thrust against her head' (McEvilley 1999, 186). Once again, the possibility that audiences of performance art might *act* unethically was exposed, although somewhat paradoxically. Abramović's piece still suggests a thoroughly ethical mode of spectatorship because, precisely, it engaged her audience in an intersubjective, dialogic way of seeing that emphasized their own performance.

Re-reading the squirm: Sense memory and the empathic body

In *The Lips of Thomas*, originally staged in 1975 but re-performed in 1993 and 2005, Abramović consumed a kilo of honey and drank a litre of wine before engaging in a series of progressively violent acts upon her own body, including self-flagellation and self mutilation, and lying for lengthy intervals upon a block of ice. The performance culminated in the now iconic image of the five-pointed star, which she cut into her stomach with a razor blade. Many were visibly disturbed by her 2005 re-performance, with one spectator exclaiming as Abramović brought the blade to her stomach: 'you don't have to do that again!' (Carlson 2005). The earlier performance of this piece had ended with the artist being physically carried off the ice block by the audience, who were, apparently, unable to take anymore. These performances were so important because, as one commentary posted on the Netherlands Media Art Institute website notes:

> Abramović is not only threatening the integrity of her body and, thus, destabilizing the binary opposition between inside and outside, but is also questioning the distinction between public and performer. In the end, the members of the audience can no longer hide behind their passive status as observers, but are forced to take the decision to perform an action of their own. (Netherlands Media Art Institute)

The performance of the artist gives way, finally, to that of the audience. Horror in this case invokes the action of the spectator, whose intervention is born also of disgust, guilt and ambivalence. This ability of performance art to accommodate spectatorial ambivalence is key to the contribution it may be able to make to developing a model of ethical spectatorship of the traumatized body. Art historian Jill Bennett draws attention to the potential creativity of spectatorial ambivalence, which she understands as part of the viewer's embodied response to the visual (re)presentation of trauma. Considering spectators' reactions to Dennis Del Favero and Justin Kramer's photomedia installations on sexual child abuse, and to the self-mutilating performances of Abramović described above, Bennett describes the importance of 'the squirm' – the physical manifestation of the viewer's disgust and unease at the sight of the mutilated or suffering flesh of the other/performer's body. A visceral response that alerts us to Kristeva's abject, the squirm, Bennett suggests, nonetheless signals an engagement with the artwork that is itself an embodied performance:

> Although the squirm is a recoil, a moment of regrouping the self, it is also the condition of continued participation, the sensation that works with and against the deeper level response, which on its own is 'unbearable'. The squirm lets us feel the image, but also maintain tension between self and image. It is a part of a loop in which the image incites mimetic contagion acted out in the body of the spectator, which must continue to separate itself from the body of the other. (Bennett 2005, 37)

By this description, the visceral response-performance of the spectator to the traumatized body echoes the structure of the empathic response that is apparently so key to ethical concern and altruism; in this case, it is an empathy in and of the body that, as in the psychological definition of the term, suggests the capacity to put oneself in the place of the other while always returning to the self.

In his article 'Feeling Performance, Remembering Trauma', Patrick Duggan gives an account of his attendance at Kira O'Reilly's 2007 performance of self-mutilation in *Untitled (Syncope)*. He refers to a similar spectatorial response to that described by Bennett, which he calls 'kinaesthetic empathy' – the process by which 'an embodied and experiential experience of performance can give the effect of the trauma's presence' (Duggan 2007, 56). This is not a claim to vicarious trauma; empathy here should be understood as a return to self through the lived encounter with the memory of the other's trauma (individual or collective), *not* as an appropriation or ingestion of the performer/other's suffering. Duggan describes his experience as one of contradictions, inducing both excitement and guilt, suggesting both proximity and distance:

> The experience of watching someone willingly slice into their flesh connected on a bodily level in the anticipation of pain I expected to feel, a sensation that was undeniably shared by others in the audience as they variously winced, gasped, tensed muscles, or looked away holding hands to mouths. I felt strangely culpable, as though I should have stopped her. I became, as Hand and Wilson put it in their examination of the theatre of Grand-Guignol, a 'willing witness.' (53–4)

Duggan's 'gut' reactions to the spectacle of pain before him, of which he felt both uncomfortably a part and guiltily separate, indicate not only a corporal or kinaesthetic empathy towards O'Reilly in her physical suffering but also give rise to a deeper, individual sense of traumatic memory:

> The connection I felt to Kira O'Reilly's body kept drawing me to make associations in my memory, it put me in a space where I began to reconnect with past moments of traumatic experience – my first memory of pain, the image of watching a friend's forehead split open on a curb, and the sickening experience of guilt and helplessness when a loved one tried to commit suicide. I did not want to remember. The performance placed me in a position of remembering and re-experiencing my own personal traumas. (56)

In psychoanalytic terms, this visceral reaction of the body of the spectator may constitute a repetition not of the other's trauma but of the spectating subject's own early mourning process – their sense of, as Phelan puts it, an 'evisceration at birth' that in no way corresponds to the spectated trauma but nonetheless provides a means of comprehending or 'feeling' that trauma.

Jill Bennett also relates the notion of embodied spectatorship to a theory of traumatic memory. Drawing on Holocaust survivor and poet Charlotte Delbo's formulation, she proposes that we think embodied spectatorship in terms of 'sense memory', a mode of remembering that registers 'the physical imprint' of trauma rather than its facts. For Delbo, sense memory provides something that ordinary or 'common' memory cannot; the aspects of traumatic experience that elude historical memory are, she claims, registered in the experience of sense memory in and of the body, producing an alternative mode of knowledge which breaks from the epistemic in a similar way to the aletheic gaze to which Martin Jay refers. As Bennett writes:

> Sense memory operates through the body to produce a kind of 'seeing truth' rather than a 'thinking truth', registering the pain of memory as it is directly experienced, and communicating a level of bodily affect. (Bennet 2005, 29)

While Delbo's account focuses on the experience of sense memory for survivors of trauma, Bennett considers the address made by art to the *spectator's* bodily memory, conceiving of art as 'registering and producing affect' in the spectator as well as the artist (Bennett 2005, 32). The reader's metaphorical gaze is thus turned towards the spectator; it is she who experiences, remembers, performs her own bodily sense as she views the fragmented and pained body or bodies exhibited before her. In acknowledging this embodied aspect of vision, the spectator is also made aware of her own ambivalent position as viewer of the visual representation of suffering. As Bennett notes:

> Sense memory doesn't just present the horrific scene, the graphic spectacle of violence, but the physical imprint of the ordeal of violence: a (compromised and compromising) position to see *from*. (34)

According to Bennett, 'bodily response precedes the inscription of narrative, of moral emotion or empathy' (32). By this view, the corporeal (inter)actions of the spectator – however problematic – form a necessary stage in establishing the conditions for actual ethical engagement. Through the present, embodied experience of viewing the traumatized body the spectator comes him or herself to *perform*, a way of seeing which is by no means liberated of the ambivalence or complicity of so-called 'unethical spectatorship' but that is nonetheless ethical in a more fundamental sense and, by allowing for the self-conscious acknowledgement of one's own guilt or discomfort, may create a space for ethical action in the more common sense to emerge.

Conclusion

This aim of this article has been to explore and demonstrate the ways in which the practice and theory of performance art might prove useful to trauma studies, in particular in relation to those issues associated with the (un)ethical spectatorship of the traumatized body. At the very least, the examples discussed have established that this mode of enquiry is worth pursuing. The theory of spectatorship proposed by performance art is useful for thinking about the ways in which we see traumatized bodies of atrocity through other forms of visual representation in three core ways. Firstly, it reinterprets the notion of 'ethical spectatorship' to focus not on the absence of negative responses but on the performative act of seeing, which is understood as dialogic and intersubjective, and thus as responsive and response-able to the other of representation. Secondly, performance art rejects the distinction between active artist and passive spectator and forces us as viewers to acknowledge our own role in the performance of representation; by becoming conscious of the presence of our own bodies in the act of spectatorship we may be better equipped to resist the temptation to turn away from the traumatized body of the victim; instead, we are called upon to accept this body, along with our own, as part of what it is to be human. Thirdly, performance art challenges us to view the traumatized body in new terms, opposing our preconceptions of the body as object, alien, other and asserting the significance of the corporeal as a site of resistance and expression in the face of trauma.

Performance art offers an ontological and structural model through which the concept of embodied ethical spectatorship might begin to be imagined; our ambivalence as spectators of suffering is accepted as part of the embodied vision that allows us, in the end, to bear witness in a fundamental ethical sense. If there is reluctance among trauma studies scholars to engage with performance art, it may be less a criticism of the mode of (re)presentation at work in the genre and more a reflection of our unease and unwillingness to face our own ambivalent performance as spectators and commentators of the other's suffering. The model of embodied witnessing proposed in this reading of performance art practice and theory does not overcome the challenge of ethical (in)action. It offers no fixed or *fixing* solutions for trauma theory; what it may do, however, is provide alternative ways of framing the problems.

Acknowledgement

This paper was written as part of a PhD funded by an Arts and Humanities Research Council Grant.

References

Bennett, Jill. 2005. *Empathic vision: Affect, trauma, and contemporary art, cultural memory in the present*. Stanford: Stanford University Press.

Carlson, Marla. 2005. Marina Abramovic repeats: Pain, art and theater. *Hunter on-line theater review*. http://www.hotreview.org/articles/marinaabram.htm

Duggan, Patrick. 2007. Feeling Performance, Remembering Trauma. *Platform* 2, no. 2: 44–58.

Elkins, James. 1999. *Pictures of the body: Pain and metamorphosis*. Stanford: Stanford University Press.

Fenemore, Anna. 2008. The pleasure of objectification: A spectator's guide. *Performance Research* 12, no. 4: 4–13.

French, Lindsay. 2002. Exhibiting terror. In *Truth claims: Representation and human rights*, ed. Mark Bradley and Patrice Petro, 131–56. London: Rutgers University Press.

Goertz, Karein. 2001. Body, trauma and the rituals of memory: Charlotte Delbo and Ruth Klüger. In *Shaping losses: Cultural memory and the Holocaust*, ed. Julia Epstein and Lori Hope Lefkowitz, 161–85. Illinois: University of Illinois Press.

Jacobs, Janet. 2008. Gender and collective memory: Women and representation at Auschwitz. *Memory Studies* 1, no. 2: 211–25.

Jay, Martin. 1993. Sartre, Merleau-Ponty and the search for a new ontology of sight. In *Modernity and the hegemony of vision*, ed. D.M. Levin, 143–85. Berkeley: University of California Press.

Kleinman, Arthur, Veena Das, and Margaret M. Lock. 1997. *Social suffering*. Berkeley: University of California Press.

McEvilley, Thomas. 1999. *Sculpture in the age of doubt (aesthetics today)*. New York: Allworth.

Netherlands Media Art Institute. 2009. *Catalogue: Marina Abramovic work – biography Thomas Lips (1975)*. Netherlands Media Art Institute. http://catalogue.montevideo.nl/

Oliver, Kelly. 2001. *Witnessing: Beyond recognition*. Minneapolis: University of Minnesota Press.

Phelan, Peggy. 1993. *Unmarked: Politics of performance*. London: Routledge.

———. 1997. *Mourning sex: Performing public memories*. London: Routledge.

Scarry, Elaine. 1985. *The body in pain: The making and unmaking of the world*. Oxford: Oxford University Press.

Schneemann, Carolee Website. http://www.carolee.schneemann.com/meatjoy.html

Sontag, Susan. 2003. *Regarding the pain of others*. London: Penguin.

Wark, Jayne. 2006. *Radical gestures: Feminism and performance art in North America*. Montreal: McGill-Queen's University Press.

Wiesel, Elie. 1982. *The town beyond the wall*. New York: Schocken.

Wiesel, Elie, and F. Mainac. 1958. *Nuit*. Paris: Editions de Minuit.

Poetic witnessing in the archive: The database narrative of *Life after Wartime*

David Carlin

School of Media and Communication, RMIT University, Melbourne, Australia

In this paper I analyse the textual strategies employed in Ross Gibson and Kate Richards's interactive database narrative project *Life after Wartime* (2002), which I argue generates a form of narrative that embodies a 'poetics of haunting'. Shifting juxtapositions of image and text, archive and fiction within *Life after Wartime* serve to foreground the ambiguities within testimony and to set in motion the connections we make with the past. I explore whether *Life after Wartime* may be productively viewed as a distinctive new media model of a 'trauma text', one eschewing notions of narrative or therapeutic closure, in which complex interconnections between memory, history and fantasy are played out.

Introduction

In this paper I will examine an interactive media project, Ross Gibson and Kate Richards's *Life after Wartime*, that I believe suggests some interesting and productive ways in which experimental forms of narrative can be engaged to evoke the complex reality of traumatic events. This is neither trauma as direct testimony nor trauma as confessional or curative discourse. Rather, in encountering this work as a viewer/player, one enters a hybrid work in which elements of direct historical reference to traumatic events are played out in a kind of meditative interior dialogue with other textual elements that are allusive and poetic.

Life after Wartime is based around a 'found' archive of police photos of crime scenes, taken in Sydney between 1945 and 1960. These photos, we are told by Gibson in the CD-ROM credit notes (Gibson and Richards 2002), are now kept in a Sydney museum but over the past 40 years have suffered the effects of natural disasters (floods) and neglect, such that they have become unmoored from much of the original documentation that anchored them to particular cases, characters and events. Gibson and Richards have grasped this lack of concrete documentary reference within the archive as an opportunity to pursue the more allusive, affective and poetic connections the photographs may prompt us to make with the past

The project takes a number of forms, including an interactive CD-ROM and several non-site-specific museum installations.[1] I am discussing here only the single-screen (CD-ROM) version. This is an experience somewhat like an interactive slideshow, although such a description does not do justice to its intriguing complexities. In playing, I soon learn I can switch between two recurring 'scenes', both of which consist of ambiguously circulating media fragments. In one there are the crime scene photos writ small, several at once, continuously appearing and disappearing out of the darkness in different sections of the screen, in a succession long enough to seem endless. In the other scene, transit to which

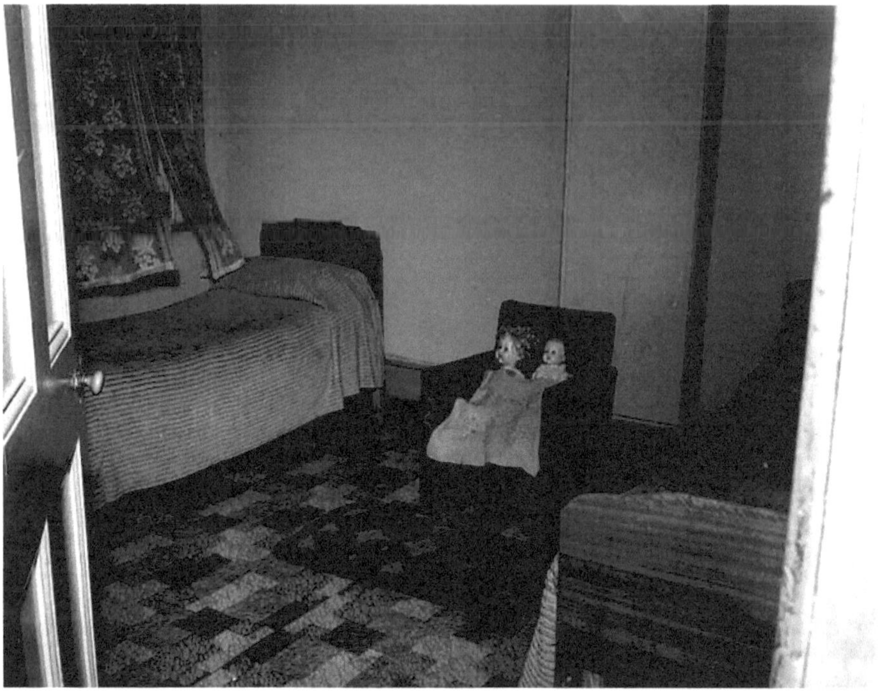

Figure 1. 'Assault. Marrickville. 1954', NSW Police archive (courtesy Ross Gibson).

is each time prefaced by a three-line text of enigmatic poetic observation relating obliquely to the photos, it is words that circulate, crazily, like blowflies. If I try to catch one of the fly/words with my cursor, it will stop for me in midair, whilst the others continue about their way. My previous media literacy in this form of interactivity encourages me to click my mouse on the word; sure enough it leads me elsewhere, to a new scene: a little elaboration through words and photos of the character or location in which I had expressed an interest. The fly/words themselves are allusive, suggestive of drama and narrative: for example, 'courtesan', 'fiend', and 'child'. But the scenes they lead me to always provoke questions more than provide answers – there are, each time, three photos, linked variously to 'fact', 'rumours' or 'glimpses'. When I click on a photo stamped 'fact' or 'rumours', a further short text will appear, which I may choose to evaluate, or attempt to make sense of, in the context of its apparent truth-category.

When I feel I have comprehended the nature of the game in the buzzing word/fly scene, I return to the dissolving photo scene, to discover its grammar of interactivity and its surprises. There, too, I find a relatively restricted succession of formal possibilities, within which the separate elements nevertheless circulate in complex flows of relationships. There are words and sentences that function as ambiguous captions to particular photos, but the same photos may later reappear with new captions attached, captions that do not relate in any direct way with their predecessors.

A haunting machine

Gibson and Richards attempt to construct, with *Life after Wartime*, what I describe as a 'haunting machine'. Theirs is a computer game experience of a singular kind, in which the game is to reflect upon and interact with mediated traces of the recent historical past, traces

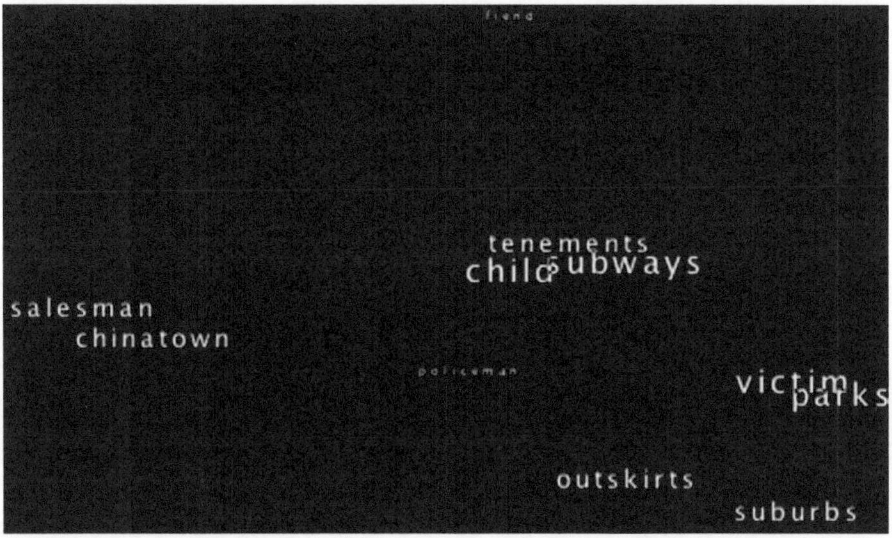

Figure 2. The 'fly/words' of *Life after Wartime*, screenshot (Gibson and Richards). Use of screenshot image authorised by Ross Gibson.

which are by their nature implicitly replete with stories, horrors, violence, tragedy and emotion, of which we receive tantalizing clues but no more. These are fragments of narrative designed to engage our fantasies to fill in the gaps. The design of the interactive interface reflects this purpose: I see pulsing, fleeting visions that circulate ceaselessly, as if teasing my gaze, until I see one I can't resist and grab it with a mouse-click to make it divulge itself in greater resolution as well as the intrigue of its caption. Characters and locations begin to appear, allusively sketched through text and photo. Later they will solidify further, with interconnections suggested between them. So the 'mulatto child' is the son of the 19-year-old 'waitress'? Who is an acquaintance of the 'courtesan'? But the machine, and its makers, are witty enough to play tricks on me, as I navigate their dark labyrinth of ghosts: I return to a place I have been to earlier and things are no longer the same – 'facts' have disappeared, the 'waitress' is no longer to be found. Just as I had become interested in her, and her story, she has vanished – withheld, inaccessible within the database/archive.

The texts, written by Gibson, that accompany the photos, encourage a restless movement between fiction and history, fantasy and memory. The power of the photos lies in their status as genuine historical documents of the archive: indexical signs denoting specific locations and, sometimes, events. A woman's body lies prone in a grassy field; two elderly people lie together dead on a kitchen floor, their heads resting in the gas oven. But the photos prompt many narrative questions for the viewer: who are these people? What led them to this death? Who else was involved? The accompanying captions, which in conventional documentary reportage would provide anchoring facts, instead invite more speculation, reverie, imaginings.

The story *Life after Wartime* tells us is that the past cannot be locked down into a succession of 'key facts'.[2] The archive can only present a necessarily contestable and inconclusive series of 'facts, rumours, glimpses'. Always there will be gaps or ambiguities in the historical evidence of the archive, be it photographs or written testimony. Into these

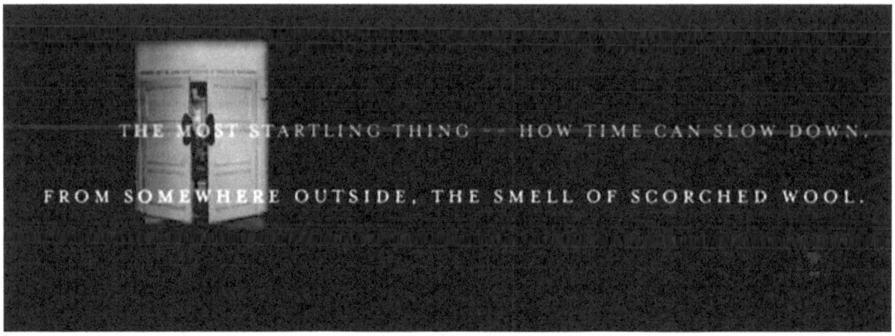

Figure 3. From the opening sequence of *Life after Wartime*, screenshot (Gibson and Richards). Use of screenshot image authorised by Ross Gibson.

gaps flows the unconscious desire of the viewer/reader/receiver, creating links, constructing stories, reconnecting snippets of their own memories and dreams.

Some of the photographs in the series offer no direct hint of a narrative: a set of stairs leading down to an underpass; a busy daytime street; a suburban driveway gate in close-up. If we are to take them as crime scene photos, the nature of the crime can only be imagined. Here again, the design of the interactive artwork playfully engages the player's desire: time and again I reject, for example, the banal image of the gate when it appears, disinterested in clicking on it. I do not want to discover more about this gate. However, apparently, the more I deny it, the more insistently it returns to haunt me, returning regularly to the screen until my curiosity is piqued and I succumb to the hope of its potential story: I click.

And yet, even with this story of the gate-photo, I must confess to an uncertainty. The causal mechanisms and internal logic of the game are sufficiently obscured for me to doubt my own memory of my experience of it. Did I simply imagine that the gate-photo returned more frequently than others that had been clicked because I had refused to click on it? If I returned to the game and played again, would the same thing happen? This sense of ambiguity, of a mirage-like complex system of shifting and slipping connections, is surely at the heart of Gibson and Richards's project.

The trauma of the archive

To turn now to the nature of the archive that Gibson and Richards have appropriated and opened up to our inspection in the very particular way described above. As we have heard, the archive itself has suffered a traumatic, turbulent existence, undergoing an almost biblical[3] journey of survival through floods and neglect – and with the loss of its accompanying files it is as if the photo-archive has experienced an amnesia: forgotten itself. One could observe that this is a risk faced by all images or collections thereof, and indeed by all cultural artefacts that become divorced from markers of their original reference. But it is especially ironic in a case such as this, where the intention behind the original taking of the photographs was to provide legal documentary evidence of specific real-world crimes. And certainly, the violence experienced by this archive and what we might personify as its attendant 'loss of memory' is apt, given the nature of the images it contains. By their nature as police crime scene shots these are visual evidence of the dangerous edges of modern society, where normative standards of behaviour slip into deviance and transgression. They represent the repressed violence and moral taboos of our culture; that which is officially denied but at the same time fascinating, as evidenced by the continuing popularity of crime fiction and crime investigation programmes on television. The photographs return to haunt us, insistent, appearing repeatedly out of the darkness of the interface, stubbornly refusing, as is the way with all photographs, to reveal on their surfaces any more or less than the fixed patterns of light and shade engraved there, and yet in concert generating proliferating cascades of allusion and speculation.

The final poetic message on the CD-ROM states: 'Your bosses all say the case is now closed. But you go home every night and sit with the dead' (Gibson and Richards 2002). This makes explicit what is omnipresent if elsewhere less tangible: that we are called upon to identify not only with the victims, the perpetrators, the witnesses to these crimes, but, even more so, with the police themselves, the detectives and the crime scene photographers whose job it is to collect this catalogue of horrors and mysteries. Although 'the case' may now be closed, the official narrative completed, the traumatic memory embodied in the photograph(s) lingers.

Narrative and the poetics of the database

Gibson and Richards, in *Life after Wartime*, employ the opportunities that new media afford to tell their multiplicitous story of a city and its past. In lieu of traditional narrative, they harness what might be called a poetics of the database to create their 'haunting machine'.

Lev Manovich (2000) notes that narrative and database have had a long and intertwined history in Western thought, the first being the tradition of Homer and Chaucer and the second the impulse towards encyclopaedias and dictionaries. He argues that narrative and database are, fundamentally, 'natural enemies' in the way they make sense of the world, since 'the database represents the world as a list of items, and it refuses to order this list. In contrast, a narrative creates a cause-and-effect trajectory of seemingly unordered items (events)' (225).[4]

While some cultural forms such as the novel and cinema privilege narrative, others such as photography lend themselves more to the logic of the database. Manovich argues that in new media the database is the dominant term of the pair, since all new media works, whether narrative or not, have an underlying database structure.

Marsha Kinder (2003), who posits a more fluid interrelationship between the two terms, has challenged Manovich's binary opposition between narrative and database.[5] Kinder introduces the notion of the 'database narrative' as a combinatory mode with long-standing roots in novels (since Sterne's Tristram Shandy) and cinema (since Bunuel):

> By database narratives, I am referring to narratives whose structure exposes or thematizes the dual processes of selection and combination that lie at the heart of all stories and that are crucial to language: the selection of particular data (characters, objects, settings, sounds, events) from a series of databases or paradigms, which are then combined to generate specific tales. Such narratives reveal the possibility of making other combinations, which would create alternative stories, and they encourage us to question the choice of categories and of what is included and omitted. (Kinder 2003, 113)

Gibson and Richards's project can be approached in the light of the theoretical debate between Manovich and Kinder. The originating database is, of course, the archive of police photos; this has been set into play with a parallel database of fictionalized textual fragments, one set of which links to specific photos (but in a plural, not a one-to-one correspondence) as 'captions', another set of which appears as haiku-like poems, a further set appears as the single circulating ('buzzing') words. Within the project's software codes, then, lie lists of texts, linguistic and photographic. Manovich tells us that 'in general, creating a work in new media can be understood as the construction of an interface to a database' (2000, 226). Here we have a strictly delimited linked pattern of interfaces to the database, basically following a binary structure within which we have no choice but to cycle back and forth between the two interfaces. This 'database logic' departs from the conventional narrative logic of cinema and the novel in so far as the player's movement through the work is defined less by syntagmatic shifts (what will happen next? Where will we go next?) than by paradigmatic shifts (when we return to where we have been, what will be different this time?). In *Life after Wartime* a rhythmic repetitive movement of images and text dominates, but with new information continually surfacing alongside the old. Eisensteinian notions of the clash of meanings created with temporal montage are displaced by what Manovich calls 'spatial montage' (325), in which 'the logic of replacement, characteristic of cinema, gives way to the logic of addition and coexistence'.

This is certainly not an absolute disavowal of narrative; this is not a database arrayed for random access, like a library catalogue stacked in alphabetical order or under the sign of Dewey. Gibson and Richards have embedded a number of strategic elements within their computer codes to satisfy the player's desire for narrative within the database.

Firstly, and crucially, there is a beginning and at least the promise of an end. A sense of forward movement is thus created, so the circular movements back and forth between images and texts can be understood as a spiralling path further into the haunting machine, rather than an endless repetition or bouncing between elements. At the beginning there is a cinematic-style opening sequence inducting us into the experience. We may not reach the end in a single sitting, but the sense that we can and should hold onto the progress that we have made is fostered by the option given to 'save' the coded record of our journey so that we can 'reload' it next time and continue on our path from where we left off. Thus, within this non-linear experience of oblique connections and fleeting associations, we are encouraged to retain the anchor of linearity: like colonial explorers traversing unsettling and uncertain seas, we can cling to the promise that progress is being made.

Secondly, as noted above, amidst the repetitions of the interface, and just as we may become frustrated having mapped the available paths open for us to travel through the work, the codes are programmed to throw in a new narrative element. For instance, when I first encounter the 'buzzing words' interface, none will stop to allow me to discover its secrets. Later, when I return, one or two words are available to be explored, but 'policeman' is not one of them. Later still, and now 'policeman' can be selected, whereby a single 'fact' is revealed, relating the name of a police photographer, Walter Keith Machin (opening up the intriguing thought that he may or may not have been behind the lens of some or all of the photographs we are viewing). Later again, when I select 'policeman', a series of further 'facts' pertaining to Walter Keith Machin unfolds with the clicking of my mouse; amongst other things I discover he was an acquaintance of another character I have uncovered in the meantime: 'the courtesan', a woman called Dulcie MacTavish who masqueraded by the name of Vasca de Merenos.

This, then, is a third important narrative element: character. A select number of identifiable characters gradually emerge from the anonymity of the police archive. To begin with we may take them to be isolated disconnected individuals but as we explore further we discover that, as with Walter Machin and Dulcie MacTavish, there is a unified narrative world in which the characters know and relate to each other. We discover that 'x' is 'y's' friend, and 'y' is 'z's' mother. These characters constitute affect-banks in which we can invest our desire, deepening our fantasy engagement with the world of the database.

However, these narrative connections remain tentative and allusive, with many more gaps than connections, many more questions than answers. Any instrumental impetus to 'leap ahead', as it were, back and forth between the interfaces to speed up the unfolding of the narrative, is bound to be disappointed. Few, if any, more details regarding relations between, or the course of events affecting, Walter and Dulcie, for instance, will be forthcoming.

Thus there is an inherent tension within the work, as it becomes clear that a desire for narrative conclusion will be thwarted. Many twentieth-century critics have argued that meaning is constructed retrospectively in narratives (Douglas 1994), that when we read or watch cinema we do so in anticipation of the ending that will complete the meaning of what has gone before. However, as J. Yellowlees Douglas puts it, when discussing language-based interactive narrative forms, something different is at play:

> Where the number of probable and plausible narrative outcomes conventionally progressively dwindles in print narratives the nearer we approach their endings, the more of the narrative we read in interactive narratives the more these seem to multiply. (12)

Douglas is considering text-only hypertext narratives but we can see that, likewise, in the hybrid image-and-text-based realm of *Life after Wartime*, the narrative connections multiply the longer we play.

What we are left with, finally, are the images: the photographs. In the computerized audiovisual archive, these are available to circulate seemingly endlessly, never resting. The events they represent resurface in our vision over and over, enacting Freud's 'compulsion to repeat' like traumatic nightmares, always the same in themselves, in their fixed photographic forms, but re-visioned in the light of their shifting poetic captions.

The police photographs in the archive Gibson and Richards have appropriated have been set adrift from their original instrumental context, as evidentiary tools in police crime investigations. As Gibson points out, this was an effect of time, misfortune and neglect, as the photos became accidentally separated from accompanying documentation that identified the individuals and places depicted or at least the circumstances surrounding the taking of the photograph. But rather than try to rethread the links to the historical past in a literal and direct way through their own detective work, attempting to 'solve the puzzle' of the various images through forensic research, Gibson and Richards have viewed the 'unmooring' of this archive as an opportunity to construct a new relation with the past through what we might call a 'photographic unconscious'.

In doing so, and especially in so far as many of the images they choose to include in their database are scenes of murder, rape and violent assault, it may be argued that they open themselves to the charge of aestheticizing trauma. The specificity of each historical event photographed, with its particular circumstances and consequences, its particular human actors, suffering and injustice, is, to pursue this line, potentially subsumed within an action of poetic generalizing.[6] After all, *Life after Wartime* is an aesthetically beautiful media object, with its elegant fonts, contemplative music and sleek black-dominated visual interfaces. The question at root is whether there are valid political or ethical objections to be raised against the form in which Gibson and Richards have appropriated the archive.

The strategy that Gibson and Richards use, which to my mind has the effect of circumventing such objections, is the self-reflexivity bound up in the structure of the work. The project is prefaced with the story of the 'unmooring' of the archive from its original referents. The focus of the project is not on the traumatic or non-traumatic events depicted but on the materiality of the photos themselves, and not each in isolation but en masse as a collection. As against what LaCapra calls a 'sacralization of the [traumatic] event' (2001, 93), Gibson in his Credits note to the CD-ROM eulogizes the photos themselves, stressing their 'richness, verging on sacredness' (Gibson and Richards 2002). But this is a sacredness rooted in the conventions of popular culture, and with an ironic eye to the over-determined figure of the police officer/detective within that culture. The captions and textual fragments read like an amalgam of Raymond Chandler, Jean Paul Sartre's existentialism and Eastern philosophy:

> 'Walking is just a struggle with falling.'
> 'Clues crawl over every surface in the city.'
> 'This city – what say you could hear its confession?'
> 'You must show no sign of emotion when false answers are given.' (Gibson and Richards 2002)

The texts encourage a dual action – on the one hand identifying (in particular with their frequent use of the second person) with a fictionalized police subjectivity, and at the same time providing an ironic distancing effect.

Closure, trauma and narrative

Gibson and Richards' approach to the 'crime genre' forms a stark contrast with the classic detective stories of the nineteenth century. With the latter comes the claim 'that all action is motivated, causally explained and eventually comprehensible as such to the perceptive observer' (Brooks 1984, 269). Clues mount up inexorably, one thing leads to another, and finally to the conclusion in which all narrative threads are tied up and the preceding chain of events becomes crystal clear in retrospect.

As Brooks points out, an analogy may be drawn between the emplotment of detective novels such as those of Conan Doyle (of which Freud was very fond)[7] and preliminary understandings of the work of psychoanalysis. Freud in his early analytic work (Breuer, Freud, and Brill 1936) 'almost explicitly assumes a Holmesian posture … [searching for] symptomatic clues, reaching back to uncover a moment of trauma, a scene of crime that makes sense of all subsequent events' (Brooks 1984, 270). As Freud's ideas developed, his notion of psychic causality became more complex. For instance, with the Wolf Man case, Freud initially uncovered what he took to be the 'primal scene' that had led to the Wolf Man's neurosis, but later conjectured that it was equally possible that this originary point was in fact a 'primal phantasy', and that his illness reflected the traces of this fantasy rather than of an actual event he had suffered (Brooks 1984, 276–7). Freud ends up leaving these two possible versions of the story superimposed one upon the other; in suspension, as it were, with neither one totally conclusive. The detective novel promises that in the end we will discover the beginning – whodunit! – but Freud is now telling a differently structured story, in which narrative closure 'is always provisional, as-if, a necessary fiction' (Brooks 1984, 281).

However, it can also be argued, as Susannah Radstone (2000) has shown, that much of the recent 'turn to trauma', in various parts of the academy and in wider cultural discourse, has been underwritten with a re-turn to the narrative of the early Freud, to the therapeutic certainties of causation and closure.

The desire for closure in historical narratives is a quest to apply moral meaning to events, to stamp a moral authority across them, to corral them within a certain form of containable and controllable sense-making. Hayden White points out the importance in this endeavour of the 'moralizing ending' (2004, 77). As White goes on to say, the unacknowledged truth behind this type of moralizing history-making is that it is in an important sense based on a fantasy: for 'real events [to] display the coherence, integrity, fullness and closure of an image of life that is and can only be imaginary' (78). It is this fantasy of moral finitude, this desire for closure that we find being playfully subverted in *Life after Wartime*.

'Trauma texts'

In what sense is it possible or useful to think about Gibson and Richards's *Life after Wartime* as a 'trauma text', a work engaged with the concept of trauma?

In recent years, as trauma has become increasingly popular as a trope in the humanities, there have been a number of attempts by scholars to gather together diverse texts in different forms under the umbrella of 'trauma'. Notable monographs have included Janet Walker's *Trauma Cinema* (2005) and Anne Whitehead's *Trauma Fiction* (2004).

Walker looks at various filmic sub-genres, including representations of the Holocaust and documentary investigations of incest and family violence. She proposes a definition of 'trauma cinema' as comprising films in a variety of genres and national cinemas 'dealing with world-shattering events in a non-realist style that figures the traumatic past as meaningful, fragmentary, virtually unspeakable and striated with fantasy constructions' (Walker 2003, 109)

Meanwhile, Whitehead, in *Trauma Fiction*, discusses contemporary novels by prominent writers including Toni Morrison, W.G. Sebald, Pat Barker and Caryl Phillips. She comments that:

> Novelists have frequently found that the impact of trauma can only adequately be represented by mimicking its forms and symptoms, so that temporality and chronology collapse, and narratives are characterized by repetition and indirection. Trauma fiction overlaps with and borrows from both postmodern and postcolonial fiction in its self-conscious deployment of stylistic devices as modes of reflection or critique. (Whitehead 2004, 3)

Whitehead's notion of the 'self-conscious deployment of stylistic devices as modes of reflection or critique' can be seen to align with and elaborate upon Walker's focus on 'a non-realist style'. Both critics highlight textual strategies that depart from traditions of naturalism and realism in order to mirror the radically unsettling effect of trauma upon the psyche.

Fragmentation, as both Walker and Whitehead tell us, echoing Shoshana Felman, is a particularly appropriate narrative strategy to convey stories of trauma. Fragmentation may enable the emergence of a polyphony of voices, which in turn can express the unsettling of psychic identity that is constituent of trauma.

Life after Wartime gathers together images of and allusions to a heterogeneous set of shocking and not-so-shocking events from a cross-section through time of a city (Sydney)'s history, and it sets them into intertextual play with each other. They are figured as a past that haunts us inter-generationally as a time variously within and before living memory; and, crucially, as a time that is itself haunted by the world-shattering historical events that have gone before: here the title itself is of utmost significance as a constant reminder that what we are seeing is 'Life after wartime'.

The computer-based interactive game form, in which Gibson and Richards are experimenting with *Life after Wartime*, presents some exciting new possibilities for engendering an interplay between history, memory and fantasy when considering how we might approach the past and its traumatic traces. The particular elements Gibson and Richards engage to pursue their narrative strategy in *Life after Wartime* are, in many cases, 'new media' elaborations of the stylistic moves outlined by Walker or Whitehead within their own narrative forms. These can be summarized as follows:

(1) The fragment, and in particular the database as a resource of textual fragments, of which the meaning of each remains open.
(2) A finite but shifting and multi-layered system of connections between the fragments.
(3) A dialectical engagement between the two classes of fragment: the photographic text and the written word, as well as with the third textual layer of the soundtrack.
(4) The time-based nature of its presentation, and in particular the recurring motif of the dissolve, whereby the appearance of words and photos is fleeting and rhythmical.
(5) Intrinsically linked with the previous element, interactivity via the mouse-click designed to offer the promise of satisfying the user's moment-by-moment curiosity and fascination: if I click on this word or photo quickly, before it disappears, I can hold onto it a little longer, or see it more clearly or find out more about it.

Fragmentation, as both Walker and Whitehead tell us, has often been seen as an appropriate narrative form to convey stories of trauma. Fragmentation enables the emergence of a polyphony of voices, which in turn is better able to express the unsettling of psychic identity that is constituent of trauma. But we need to be careful to apply nuance to the concept of fragmentation, which may suggest movement from a unified whole towards discontinuous sub-units.

With *Life after Wartime*, for instance, we are not dealing with a singular narrative broken up into fragments. There is no originating fabula, as defined in Mieke Bal's words as 'a series of logically and chronologically related events that are caused or experienced by actors' (1997, 5). We may posit that the actor is the anonymous police photographer and that there is some level of logical relation between the events (the taking of each photograph) in that they all took place within a discrete (albeit heterogeneous) time and place – Sydney and surrounding areas in the late 1940s. Nevertheless there is no 'logical sequence' (214) to the events – we can agree that the events 'happen during a certain period of time' but not that 'they occur in a certain order' (208). Even if dates survive on the backs of the physical photographs in the archive, to indicate when each was taken, these dates are, with presumably few exceptions, arbitrary in so far as the succession of crimes across the city unfolded in a random and unmotivated fashion. We return to the fact that this text has its origins in a database, an unordered list of items.

This is an approach to history that begins with fragments – isolated photographic images that fix a series of moments in time. It brings what was once seen (by the police photographer) and distributed, and then forgotten (by the institution of the police force and the culture more generally), back into public circulation as 'prosthetic memories' (Landsberg 2004).

As with W.G. Sebald's textual labyrinths,[8] the narrative strategy here is of interweaving connections between fragments. Gibson and Richards have constructed a machine for generating narratives, rather than for the opening, unfolding and closure of a specific narrative journey. I would argue that their work constitutes an example of what Manovich calls, when discussing the style in which new media remediates old media forms (Bolter and Grusin 1999), an 'aesthetics of continuity as exemplified by compositing, morphing, and navigable spaces' (Manovich 2000, 285). Whilst discontinuities in terms of abrupt shifts between the different interfaces are programmed into the work, over and above these is continuity, in large part underpinned by the soundtrack, the black graphic background and the rhythmic flow of predictable elements. So we have, in fact, a seemingly paradoxical aesthetic alliance between fragmentation and continuity.

The unsettling effect of this 'aesthetics of continuity' in *Life after Wartime* is generated by the heterogeneous quality of the textual connections within this flow of predictable elements. These connections themselves – typically, for example, between image and accompanying text – are designed to be anything but predictable. The effect is to prompt a state akin to daydreaming, with the invitation to engage a dream logic of condensation and displacement in response to the images. This may remind us of the acute observation of Marsha Kinder as to the fundamentally oneiric quality of interactive database narratives. Kinder writes:

> . . . dreams are the ultimate model of interactive database narrative, for they rely on a dialectic play between the disruptive power of seemingly random images (which deliver a surrealist jolt) and a repressive narrative drive that imposes chains of causality. (2003, 114)

Photography, Marianne Hirsch tells us, acts to 'bring back the past in the form of a ghostly revenant, emphasizing, at the same time, its immutable pastness and irretrievability' (1997, 20). However, the 'ghostly revenants' of *Life after Wartime*, through their repetitive circulation and their changing textual linkages, suggest a past that is mutable in the way we perceive and imagine it. This is an understanding of the past that brings echoes of Freud's idea of *nachträglichkeit*, or afterwardsness (sometimes translated as deferred action), the concept that (traumatic) events may achieve a new significance when viewed retrospectively in the context of a later experience (Laplanche and Pontalis 1974). Instead of the relation between past and present being configured as strictly linear, afterwardsness implies a back and forth motion, a revisiting of the past in which the original memory is overwritten by a new one. In *Life after Wartime* we return to a photograph to find its surface image unchanged, but with a revised caption that encourages us to read the image in a new light: as if we return to the scene of the exact-same memory (crime) only to find the exact-same memory has changed. Such a doubling of the image-as-memory invokes ideas of the uncanny, the strange sense that something is both familiar and unfamiliar.

Conclusion

Trauma texts, such as those literary works surveyed by Whitehead (2004) under the banner of 'trauma fiction' or the cinematic and televisual ones that Walker (2005) gathers together as 'trauma cinema', can be defined as narrative constructions that seek to testify or bear witness to the lived reality of a historical 'trauma'.

How does *Life after Wartime* testify or bear witness? Where does it fit within the context of what Radstone has referred to critically as a 'culture of testimony' (2006)? As I have argued above, its shifting juxtapositions of image and text, archive and fiction serve to foreground the ambiguities within testimony and to problematize the connections we make with the past. There is, certainly, a haunting pathos attached to the photographic images in the police archive, but it is a pathos engendered in the fragility of their fullness of reference: they tell us something but never enough, and we become complicit in making up the difference.

Clare Kahane writes of the way in which fantasy is implicated in our responses to the spectacle of 9/11, and in particular the bombing of the World Trade Center.[9] She follows Žižek in claiming that 'the most deeply unsettling traumas are not those that are entirely unexpected but those that are anticipated in fantasy, those in which one has a libidinal investment' (Kahane 2003, 108).

When we look at the NSW police archive photographs, they are, I would argue, images we have already anticipated in fantasy: pictures of an old couple lying on the floor with their heads near an oven as if asleep, a little girl in a dress face down on some grass – they are shocking yet familiar, confirming our worst nightmares.

Notes

1. Most recently (in 2008), Ross Gibson has published an experimental book of fiction incorporating a selection of the police archive photographs, entitled *The Summer Exercises.*
2. In Australia's recent past, the 'key facts' view of history has been a politically charged issue, with former Prime Minister John Howard pushing, against the advice of experts in the field, for high school students to learn Australian history via a list of 70 'key dates' (Hirst 2008).
3. Although here, unlike in the Bible, there are no moral judgements made as to the worthiness of what has been lost along the way.
4. Manovich's binary formation immediately invites challenge: for instance, it can be argued that encyclopaedias contain a series of narratives within them, and that other forms, such as the taxonomies of the natural sciences, shape their data into precise orders based on narratives of evolution or connection between species.
5. Kinder is not only a theorist but a practitioner in the field of database narrative, and is the Director of the Labyrinth Project at the University of Southern California, which has produced a number of award-winning 'database documentaries' designed as 'interactive transmedia networks' (Kinder 1997).
6. Dominick LaCapra (2001, 94) cautions against the attractions of a 'negative sublime' in the representation of traumatic events, whereby the unrepresentable excess of trauma assumes a hyperbolic allure.
7. Freud's patient, the Wolf Man, noted in his memoirs Freud's interest in Conan Doyle (Brooks 1984, 270).
8. See Sebald's novels, for example *Austerlitz* (2001).
9. American culture had rehearsed 'airplane-themed' and skyscraper destruction fantasies, up to and including the burning of the twin towers themselves, in various disaster movies over the preceding decades including *Independence Day* (Emmerich, USA, 1996), *Towering Inferno* (Guillermin, USA, 1974) and *Armageddon* (Bay, USA, 1998) (Keane 2006, 90).

References

Bal, M. 1997. *Narratology: Introduction to the theory of narrative.* 2nd ed. Toronto and Buffalo: University of Toronto Press.

Bolter, J.D., and R. Grusin. 1999. *Remediation: Understanding new media.* Cambridge, MA and London: MIT Press.

Breuer, J., S. Freud, and A.A. Brill. 1936. *Studies in hysteria.* New York: Nervous and Mental Disease Pub. Co.

Brooks, P. 1984. *Reading for the plot: Design and intention in narrative.* Oxford: Clarendon.

Douglas, J.Y. 1994. 'How do I stop this thing?' Closure and indeterminacy in interactive narratives. University of Florida. http://web.nwe.ufl.edu/~jdouglas/stop.pdf

Gibson, R., and Historic Houses Trust of New South Wales. 2008. *The summer exercises/Ross Gibson.* Crawley, WA: University of Western Australia Press.

———, and K. Richards. 2002. *Life after wartime*. Sydney. CD-ROM.
Hirsch, M. 1997. *Family frames: Photography, narrative, and postmemory*. Cambridge, MA: Harvard University Press.
Hirst, John. 2008. Australia, the official history. *The Monthly*, February.
Kahane, C. 2003. Uncanny sights: The anticipation of the abomination. In *Trauma at home after 9/11*, ed. J. Greenberg, 107–16. Lincoln and London: University of Nebraska Press.
Keane, Stephen. 2006. *Disaster movies: The cinema of catastrophe*. 2nd ed. New York and London: Wallflower.
Kinder, Marsha. 1997. The Labyrinth Project. University of Southern California; Annenberg Centre for Communications. http://college.usc.edu/labyrinth/laby.html
———. 2003. Honoring the past and creating the future in cyberspace: New technologies and cultural specificity. *The Contemporary Pacific* 15, no. 1: 93–115.
LaCapra, Dominick. 2001. *Writing history, writing trauma*. Baltimore: Johns Hopkins University Press.
Landsberg, A. 2004. *Prosthetic memory: The transformation of American remembrance in the age of mass culture*. New York: Columbia University Press.
Laplanche, Jean, and J.B. Pontalis. 1974. *The language of psycho-analysis*. New York: Norton.
Manovich, Lev. 2000. *The language of new media*. Cambridge, MA: MIT Press.
Radstone, Susannah. 2000. Screening trauma: Forrest Gump, film and memory. In *Memory and methodology*, ed. Susannah Radstone. Oxford: Berg.
———. 2006. Cultures of confession/cultures of testimony. In *Modern confessional writing: New critical essays*, ed. Jo Gill, 166–79. London: Routledge.
Sebald, Winfried Georg. 2001. *Austerlitz*. Munich: Hanser.
Walker, Janet. 2003. The traumatic paradox: Autobiographical documentary and the psychology of memory. In *Contested pasts: The politics of memory*, ed. Katherine Hodgkin and Susannah Radstone, 104–19. London: Routledge.
———. 2005. *Trauma cinema: Documenting incest and the Holocaust*. Berkeley: University of California Press.
White, Hayden. 2004. The value of narrativity in the representation of reality. In *Narrative theory: Critical concepts in literary and cultural studies*, ed. Mieke Bal, Vol. IV, 58–80. London: Routledge.
Whitehead, Anne. 2004. *Trauma fiction*. Edinburgh: Edinburgh University Press.

Bearing witness to the trauma of slavery in Kara Walker's videos: *Testimony*, *Eight Possible Beginnings*, and *I was transported*

Vivien Green Fryd

Department of History of Art, Vanderbilt University, Nashville, USA

This essay shows that Kara Walker creates in her film and video work a repetitive traumatic site that surrounds, involves, and challenges the viewer to witness, acknowledge, and remember the individual and transgenerational trauma of slavery and contemporary racism in the United States, contributing to cultural remembrance and forcing the viewer to bear witness to her topsy-turvy world. Walker represents the 'intergenerational transmission of trauma' as postmemory, which is defined as the relationship of previous generations to powerful, often traumatic, experiences that preceded their births but that were nevertheless transmitted to them so deeply as to seem to constitute memories in their own right, though they can never be fully understood nor re-created. In doing so, she creates art that functions as a ritualized site for a kind of witnessing that becomes visible in her films and videos, a medium that by its own nature performs the act of bearing witness. The paper goes on to show that in her film and video work Walker disrupts conventional US histories and embodies formally and textually trauma's capacity to disrupt, thereby re-enacting or performing the phenomenological structure of trauma. Rather than suggest an opening or release of trauma's repetitive cycles, Walker embodies the hopeless and helpless repetition of trauma among individuals and generations who lack the healing potential often implied in the act of testimony. The viewer is, therefore, unable to imagine trauma as residing solely in the past but rather witnesses it as relentlessly and continuously invading the present in the form of post-traumatic slave syndrome (PTSS), thus failing to enable recovery, healing, or closure.

Kara Walker, the controversial African-American artist who won the MacArthur 'genius' grant in 1997, had a retrospective of her film and video work at the Walker Art Center in Minneapolis that travelled to the Whitney Museum of American Art in New York City and the UCLS Hammer Museum in Los Angeles. The retrospective included three animated works. The first one was *Testimony: Narrative of a Negress Burdened by Good Intentions* (2004), a silent black-and-white work shot in 16 mm film and video and later transferred to DVD.[1] The second work was *Eight Possible Beginnings; Or the Creation of African-America. A Moving Picture by the Young, Self-taught Genius of the South Kara E. Walker* (2005), also a 16 mm black-and-white film and video transferred to a DVD, which includes sound along with text.[2] Thirdly, the retrospective included ... *calling to me from the angry surface of some grey and threatening sea. I was transported* (2007), a five-part, 11-minute video installation with colour and sound.[3] Like her well-known silhouettes, such as *Gone, an Historical Romance of a Civil War as it Occurred between the Dusky Thighs of One Young Negress and Her Heart*

(1994) and *The End of Uncle Tom and the Grand Allegorical Tableau of Eva in Heaven* (1995),[4] these films and videos re-member and re-interpret the trauma of slavery, contributing to a collective remembrance and forcing viewers to bear witness to Walker's world filled with obscene, haunting, humorous, and arresting images.[5] Thus, in her silhouettes and film and video works Walker realizes what the art historian Gwendolyn Dubois Shaw calls the 'discourse of the unspeakable':

> a discourse made up of the horrific accounts of physical, mental, and sexual abuse that were left unspoken by former slaves as they related their narratives and unfathomable bits of detritus that have been left out of familiar histories of American race relations. (2004, 7)

This discourse creates a 'traumatic site' that can be 'rememoried' (7). Her visible taboos significantly show the intersection of race, rape, and representation in troubling ways. This is so not only because she recovers the perversity of slavery in the past and its effect on the present but also because her art ultimately provides unresolved, ambiguous images and messages about racial and gender biases as well as the legacy about slavery and racism in the United States. Walker thus re-writes US history by reconsidering and re-imagining racial politics and relationships from the nineteenth century to the present, while examining the dialectics of pleasure and danger, fulfilment and guilt, desire and fear, race and class.

This essay shows that Walker not only constructs and performs trauma but also re-members and re-interprets both individual and transgenerational traumas of slavery that affect both the enslaved and slave masters. E. Ann Kaplan explains that individual trauma is that experienced directly by a person (2005, 1, 4), while Joy DeGruy Leary terms the 'legacy of trauma' – transgenerational trauma – transmitted 'from generation to generation through the family, community and society' as post-traumatic slave syndrome (PTSS) (2005, 121, 129). In her videos Walker creates a repetitive traumatic site that surrounds, involves, and challenges the viewer to witness, acknowledge, and remember the individual and transgenerational trauma of slavery and contemporary racism in the United States. In this way, she contributes to cultural remembrance by forcing the viewer to bear witness to her topsy-turvy world. Walker represents the 'intergenerational transmission of trauma' as postmemory (Hirsch 2002, 73): the relationship of previous generations to powerful, often traumatic, experiences that preceded their births but that were nevertheless transmitted to them so deeply as to seem to constitute memories in their own right, though they can never be fully understood nor re-created (Hirsch 1997, 22). In doing so, she creates art that functions as a ritualized site for witnessing, which becomes even more visible in her videos, a medium which in itself performs the act of bearing witness. This paper shows that in her videos Walker disrupts conventional American histories and embodies formally and textually trauma's capacity to disrupt, thereby re-enacting or performing the phenomenological structure of trauma. Rather than suggest an opening or release of trauma's repetitive cycles, Walker embodies the hopeless and helpless repetition of trauma among individuals and generations who lack the healing capacity often implied in the act of testimony. She renders what Dominick LaCapra calls the 'aftereffects' of trauma, 'the hauntingly possessive ghosts' that are not fully owned by anyone but affect everyone (LaCapra 2001, xi), in this case not only blacks but also whites.

The 'ghostly presence' of Walker's silhouettes

Walker's film and video works combine silhouettes in the form of puppet animation with text and, in *Eight Possible Beginnings* and *I was transported*, sound. Her signature silhouettes function, I argue, as 'ghostly presences'. In an analysis of 'ghostly matters', the sociologist Avery F. Gordon explains that 'the ghost or the apparition ... is one form by which something lost, or barely visible, or seemingly not there ... makes itself known or apparent to us' (1997, 8). Furthermore, Gordon interprets 'the ghostly haunt' as an instance of giving 'notice that something is missing – that what appears to be invisible or in the shadows is announcing itself' (15).

Gordon's theoretical model is useful in this paper's task of describing Walker's silhouettes, which in fact function as 'ghostly presences' that expose 'hauntings, ghosts and gaps, seething absences, and muted presences' (21). The silhouette form enables Walker to enact the very definition of a ghost as a 'faint shadowy trace'[6] that can never be erased and that marks 'that which is present, but that which is absent, but still detectable in absence', that is, 'an absent presence' (Dever 1998, 117–21). 'Ghosting' is thus 'the simultaneity of revelation and concealment',[7] of something visible and invisible. For Walker, these absent presences are the acts of abuse, sexual and otherwise, experienced by slaves on plantations and encountered by blacks since the Civil War. These are, in fact, acts that were elided from the abolitionist re-writing of slave narratives. Walker's 're-memory of the trauma of slavery' (Shaw 2004, 51) recovers these ghostly apparitions that LaCapra calls 'the hauntingly possessive ghosts' (2001, xi), enabling them to become clearer traces or shadows whose presence on the walls of a gallery or museum haunts the viewer, forcing him or her to acknowledge and remember. The trauma of sexual violence and slavery, as inscribed in Walker's works, exists as blank screens upon which her silhouettes adhere. In this way, they allow the viewer to witness and acknowledge the historical fact of sexual violence against the black body and its effect upon society during slavery and afterwards, thus creating cultural remembrance.

In creating silhouettes, Walker follows a tradition that had flourished in popular American print media during the nineteenth century. She takes images of fine-boned aristocratic gentility – portraits of white middle- and upper-class family ancestors – and replaces them with scatological and macabre images of interracial and intraracial desire, sex, and violence, creating a 'mismatch between decorative elegance and taboo-breaking vulgarity that make the pictures grotesque' (Storr 2007, 69). She is aware of the perception of this medium as 'a benign little craft' (Jenkins 1995, 11), that is, as a feminine, democratic, decorative, middle-class, and Victorian art, which functioned rather like the minstrel shows in which white people rendered themselves black, 'making themselves somewhat invisible, or taking on an alternate identity because of the anonymity' (Walker 2006, n.p.). However, whereas nineteenth-century silhouettes were small-scale, single portraits, Walker creates life-size, sometimes larger than life size, and multi-figured shadowed profiles that make up seemingly sequential narratives. By enlarging the scale of the silhouettes and employing them to create narratives, Walker both works within and explodes the limits of the medium, creating a new type of history painting. This is a genre to which she, as a woman and an African-American, would not have had access in the eighteenth and nineteenth centuries, when only white men could create works within the Grand Manner with heroic action, suffering, and noble themes about white men, with moralizing and didactic content.[8]

Walker's black-paper figures, in contrast to history paintings done in the Grand Manner, are neither heroic nor evil, but, in the words of the artist herself, a 'dot, dot, dot ...' ('Projecting fictions', 4). The ellipsis is significant because it marks, as the art historian Richard Meyer explains, 'secrets and structuring absences' that express 'both ignorance and knowledge' (2002, 26). These secrets and structuring absences become nothing and everything, an absent presence of contradictions inherent in the slave system that whites and blacks have attempted to erase and whose traces Walker re-inscribes in her works in the form of silhouettes. By figuring history through shadows, Walker forces us to notice that racism and violence against the black body have always been present in the United States.

Bearing witness through film and video art

More recently Walker has combined her signature silhouette form with film and video art, a more sophisticated medium. In fact, in moving from cycloramas to cinematic technology, Walker replicates the trajectory of popular nineteenth- and early twentieth-century US historical narratives. Her animations, which combine 'performative and multisensory elements of sound' (Cox 2007, 60) with image and text, evolve from the artist's tendency to combine silhouettes with note cards, a technique that emphasizes the importance of narrative, albeit non-normative, to her work. Black-and-white silhouettes appear in Walker's *Testimony* and *Eight Possible Beginnings*, while vivid hues are visible in *I was transported*, where life-size shadow puppets appear to come to life when manipulated on wooden sticks by the artist. The strings and hands that control the silhouetted puppets are also often visible in *Testimony*, while the artist's assistant appears in *Eight Possible Beginnings* both as the puppet master and as an artist who cuts silhouettes.

Lisa Saltzman explains that video as a medium 'asks that we bear witness to its act of witness' (2006, 130). In this case, each video monitor 'testifies to the act of having seen' (130). Walker thus combines her signature silhouette form – which evokes hauntings, gaps, muted presences – with video, 'a vehicle for testimony, a screen of memory' (130), in order to perform the act of bearing witness to that which had been silenced. The artist, whose presence is always evident on the margins of the videos, also serves as a witness.[9] Video is thus an appropriate medium for Walker's shadow puppets, for it easily conveys fragmentary images and narratives, fantasy, and unspeakable acts. She does so in a format characterized by seemingly unsophisticated paper cuts-outs, flickering light, discontinuous and grainy images, disjunctive narratives, intertitles, and in *Eight Possible Beginnings* and *I was transported*, scratchy sound with songs and dialogue that mimics Walt Disney's 'Song of the South' (1946), the initial basis of Walker's *Eight Possible Beginnings* (Raymond 2007, 356; Knight 2005, E1). The formal collision between low tech (paper cut-outs and still images) and high tech (video, sound, and moving images) contributes to the sense of disruption that also exists in the narrative: a disruption of lived experiences and psychic coherence that is characteristic of trauma.

Working through the narrative

Walker's videos demonstrate the working through of trauma that LaCapra considers a desirable form of remembering trauma. He explains that:

> working through ... means coming to terms with the trauma, including its details, and critically engaging the tendency to act out the past and even to recognize why it may be necessary and even in certain respects desirable or at least compelling. (2001, 144)

He distinguishes between acting out, a repetitive process 'whereby the past ... is repeated as if it were fully enacted, fully literalized', and working through, which:

> involves repetition with a significant difference ... [it] is not [a] linear, teleological, or straightforward developmental ... process ... It requires going back to problems, working them over and perhaps transforming the understanding of them. (148)

Indeed, Walker goes back over the problem of slavery, works it over, and transforms its understanding in a non-linear development.

In *Testimony* a large silhouetted profile of a black boy with a huge eye appears between animated scenes with his lips moving, suggesting that the intertitles correspond to his own testimony of the depicted trauma (his massive eye indicating that he is witness to his own testimony).[10] In the film the boy bears witness to a slave revolt and the uprising of two African-American women: the tawny 'negress', with large lips and ribbons in her braided hair, and the house slave with hoop skirt, straightened hair, and 'whitened' facial features.

The cast of characters from Walker's 'picture file' – those found in her silhouettes, drawings, watercolours, and engravings – reappear in this film animation, especially with the 'negress', a persistent stock image in Walker's repertoire that first appeared in *Gone* and was derived from the character of Lydia Brown in Thomas Dixon Jr's *The Clansman: An Historical Romance of the Ku Klux Klan* (1905) (Reinhardt 2003, 153; Saltz 1996, 82). This bestselling novel focuses on racial conflict during Reconstruction and became the basis for D.W. Griffith's ambitious, costly, and spectacular silent film *Birth of a Nation* (1915). In Dixon's characterization, this 'tawny' mulatta is a 'curious or sinister figure' who 'cast[s] a shadow across the history of a great nation' during its 'most corrupt hour', dragging her white lover into her world of transgressive behaviours (Dixon Jr 1905, 94). For Walker, the generic 'negress' is a catlike woman with 'grotesquely large lips' and 'dirty ribbons' in her hair, who becomes a shadow among 'shadows of artificial things, shadows of stereotypes, shadows of things that maybe there's only a written description of' (Saltz 1996, 82). She is related to the 'nigger wench', described by the artist as a 'young and pretty black girl whose function is to be a receptacle: she's a black hole, a space defined by things sucked into her, a 'nigger cunt', a scent, an ass, a complication' (Shaw 2004, 19). Within this context, the process of creating silhouettes – of cutting a hole from paper – literally represents the resultant image. The 'nigger wench' is certainly a black hole that can be penetrated. But, in Walker's world, she can also become a powerful protector or an aggressive and angry woman who refuses to be a receptacle. For Walker, the 'nigger wench' is always in control; 'even in outlandishly perverse situations',

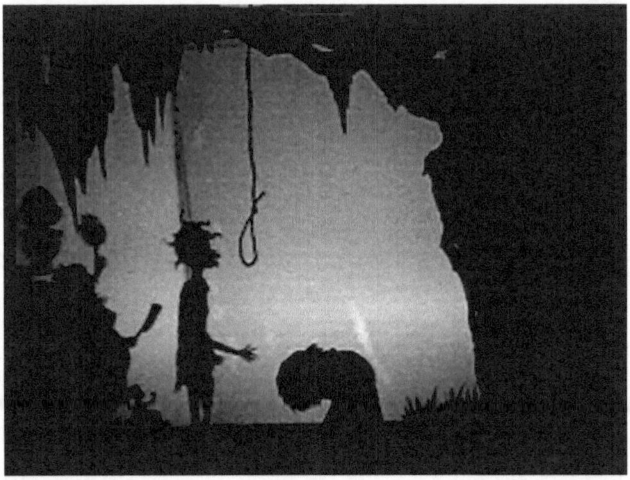

Figure 1. Kara Walker. *Testimony: A Narrative of a Negress Burdened by Good Intentions* 2004. 16 mm film and video. Photo courtesy of Walker Art Center, Minneapolis, MN.

she is a figure 'whose powers overwhelm the "good" and the "just" white people' (Jenkins 1995, 13; Golden 2002, 45).

A sense of uncertainty in terms of which slaves and slave masters alternate in victimizing one another pervades the narrative of *Testimony*. Opening with the text: 'the whites, longing for fulfillment, have sold their bodies to us', the film suggests that the masters have relinquished control to their slaves, and that by appropriating the position of jail keepers, black people police, imprison and ultimately lynch white men. The large-lipped 'negress' similarly takes on a new position by dragging and whipping a pot-bellied white man and then using a broom stick (a domestic tool normally employed by 'mammies' to clean the mansion) as a phallic instrument to sexually violate him. She reappears in another scene in *Testimony* in which she whips another white man, replicating the punishment employed by masters on slaves. Subsequently, three incarcerated white men enslaved by the hoop-skirted house slave escape as 'pisspoor runaways' who were 'due a sound thrashing'. Holding a rifle, the 'negress' and two other black women round up the escaped white men and lynch one of them from a tree, punishing him for his former abuse of slaves. While performing fellatio on the lynched male body, the 'negress' face disintegrates into puddles of watercolour.

This image of fellatio and disintegration arguably signifies the artist's presence as the creator and controller of the staged events – underscoring her visible role as the hand that manipulated the puppets. Alternatively, the paint can be seen to signify semen; and in so far as it covers the 'negress', it marks her as in control – because she is the one responsible for it. However, although she succeeds in gaining agency – castrating and murdering the white man and, as a result, removing his sexual and economic power over black bodies – the presence of the 'negress' is eventually eliminated as she disintegrates behind the puddle of paint. 'The heroine', according to Walker, 'gets it in the end' so that, ultimately, 'no one makes out' (Walker 2007). Thus, *Testimony* suggests that blacks and whites, masters and slaves, experience individual trauma, which implies that even a reversal of order cannot resolve slavery's trauma and its after-effects on future generations.

Through its eight chapters, *Eight Possible Beginnings* narrates the creation of an allegorical land, 'African-America'.[11] It begins with the chapter 'Along the watery road',

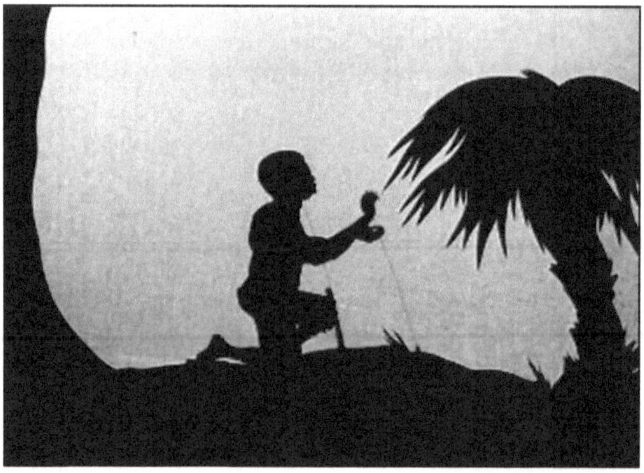

Figure 2. Kara Walker. *Eight Possible Beginnings; Or the Creation of African-America. A Moving Picture by the Young, Self-taught Genius of the South Kara E. Walker.* 2005. 16 mm film and video. Photo courtesy of Sikkema Jenkins & Co., New York.

which refers to a non-specific time during the Middle Passage, while marking the transatlantic slave trade. The animation shows black silhouettes being tossed overboard and drowning in the vast sea while the background sound suggests a storm. This opening scene establishes the individual trauma of the captured Africans as they are transported under horrendous conditions, often resulting in death.

'Motherland', chapter 2, represents the continual trauma experienced by slaves upon arriving in the New World, signified here by the figure of a giant black woman who swallows the captives. In the film they are seen floating down her long, curvy intestinal track, being excreted, and finally morphing into a burly black form with bound hands. The depiction of this process of being swallowed and then 'birthed' (through her anus rather than her birth canal) into enslavement indicates individual traumas.[12]

The following three chapters of *Eight Possible Beginnings* detail abuses that take place in this new 'Motherland' of African-America, indicating both individual and transgenerational trauma. Chapter 3, 'The new world: Enter the king cotton', shows the toil of African slaves forced to grow cotton in a Southern plantation. With a slave field song about picking cotton sung throughout this section, a robust black man, King Cotton, who 'may symbolize the cotton industry, its foundation built on slaves as free labour, its importance in establishing America as a world economical power, and its responsibility in planting seeds of violence and racism in the United States', continuously toils on a cotton field (Raymond and Hooper 2007, 8–9). This reading of the figure of King Cotton is supported by the inclusion of a historical drawing of slaves working at Eli Whitney's cotton gin, which was established in 1793 and not only enabled cotton to become the lead crop in the South but also encouraged the economic expansion of slavery. In the film, while engaged in this labour, King Cotton encounters an older white man with whom he engages in kissing, performing fellatio, and copulating. Caricatures of cotton babies seem to celebrate the men's love making, which at times seems consensual and other times forced. These cartoon-like cotton babies are planted (as seedling children) by the white master into the black man, resulting, visible in a later chapter of the film, in the black man's pregnancy.

'Interlude', the fourth chapter, shows the artist's assistant with headscarf, cutting a silhouette of a white man who models for her (but who also exists as a silhouette). 'We find Bess, a comely negress, taking her master's likeness', claims the intertext, which ends with the praise: 'good job, Bess'. This is clearly an interlude of creativity that also suggests denigration on the part of the slave master who both controls the artist (he presumably commissioned his silhouetted portrait) and denigrates her creativity, casting 'the master–slave relationship ... in artistic terms' (Knight 2005, E1). Ultimately, however, Walker manipulates the entire construction, for it is she who creates the silhouette of the master that serves as a model for her assistant. She both acts out, enacting the past and making it fully literalized, and works through, transforming the understanding of the traumas.

This 'Interlude' disrupts the narrative, which continues in the next chapter. In 'New labors', the film's fifth chapter, a black midwife who is holding a lit candle assists the black man in giving birth, a painful process indicated by his expressions and the text 'rriip', upon the birth of his child. A female slave/midwife delivers the cotton baby, throwing it into a field of cotton where it grows into more cotton. The pregnant man admits that 'Massa knock me up'. Rather than showing the hyper-sexualized black men who threatens white purity and innocence – the prominent stereotype of male black sexuality – Walker constructs the white master as the hyper-sexualized man who cannot control his lust for the male black body, resulting in the pregnancy of the latter and his emasculation. Cox suggests that what this part of the film shows is a male rape scene, exposing in this sense the issue of homosexual rape of slaves by their masters that only recently has been discussed in scholarly literature (2007, 72). Yet the interaction between the figures appears more ambivalent, for they seem to have hypersexualized and frolicking consensual sex, which in itself raises the question: how can a slave who has no control over his body deny his slave master's desires? Whereas Walker seems to indict the white man's insatiable lust after both the black female and the black male body – thus resulting in the abuse and sexual violation of both – she also suggests that the black woman and man may desire the white body, highlighting in consequence complications in sexual relations between those in control and those controlled. As Walker explained about this video: 'There's something about complicity and about abuse and wishes for a kind of wholeness' played out because of the cohabitation of masters and slaves (Cheng 2005, E3). In addition, through the notion of the black man's pregnancy Walker seems to suggest that men as well as women are forced not only into slave labour for production but also for reproduction so that their 'cotton babies' will be born into slavery and constant toil in the fields. The babies' mothers and fathers have experienced individual traumas; they are born into trauma, and their lives are filled with trauma, which will be passed onto and experienced by later generations.

Chapter 6, 'A darky hymn: All I want', depends more on voiceover than imagery: the 'negress' walks in despair, followed by a larger white plantation master who hovers over her as she works in the cotton field. Two voices – that of an older woman and that of a little girl – interweave, acting out personal trauma. Sometimes one repeats what the other says:

> I wonder how long it will last … I can't talk about it … Don't expect too much … I can't talk about it. Everything is good … Very little works out in my life. I understand very little … I wish I weren't so short, people scrutinize me … My momma is calling … I understand very little … Perfection is a godly thing … I wish that I were white. Sometimes I pretend the world is upside down … Maybe all this … will disappear … and I will disappear … I wonder how wishes are made. I bet he wishes the same thing … Next time everything will be all right. I hope and I pray. I wish I could get this thing off me. I can't stand how this feels. I guess this is how it is, go with the flow. I think he is going to hurt me … I wonder what it will feel like. I guess this is what happened to Addy.

This spoken text, accompanied by soulful, mourning humming, combines with the animation to indicate that the black girl – who, while not depicted, is present through her disembodied voice, detached from the body to create a testimony – is forced into slave labour for the Southern economy. The black girl thus exists not only in the realm of production but also within the realm of reproduction, nurturing, and sex. This disembodied voice, however, makes it clear that she feels overwhelmed, scared, lonely, confused, and hopeless. These are characteristic emotions of sexually abused children who are required to be silent about such scarring violations. The girl's voice allows us as viewers and listeners to hear and thus witness her mental mantra, providing access to 'a mechanism that enables a person to quit a place where bad thoughts or events are happening' (Terr 1994, 77–8). Walker accurately conveys, through this moving and repetitious narration, the ways in which a rape and incest victim survives by mentally removing herself from her physical body and its experiences. She furthermore accurately embodies the symptoms of post-traumatic stress disorder (PTSD), the result of an event perceived as threatening to life or bodily integrity and experienced subjectively as helplessness and terror with overwhelming and spinning thoughts. Walker thus creates a narrative of trauma through repetition, another symptom of PTSD, in an attempt to show how sexual violation of the traumatized body results in wounds, disruptions, fear, and a sense of helplessness.

This segment differs from the others because of its refusal to provide humour, ambiguity, or consensual sexual encounters. On the contrary, it makes clear that sexual violation formed an inherent part of the slave system in which the black body existed to be used for labour and sex by the white owner and that the black slave was a human being who experienced traumatic after-effects from rape. It also contains the most sustained spoken narrative that is unrelenting and painful in its continuity and repetitive content. Indeed, the little girl's lament becomes more powerful and unsettling in the absent presence of her impending rape, due to her knowledge and fear that the master is going to hurt 'her the same way that he hurt Addy'.

That the girl is condemned to production and reproduction is made clear in chapter 7, 'Plantin' time', where the formerly pregnant black man continuously waters his cotton ball child with a ladle. After having given birth, his child, a cotton baby, is planted in the field, suggesting that nurturing of his offspring is necessary for the continuation of the Southern economy. The film's visualization of a black man, rather than the little girl, as pregnant and giving birth is not only a humorous construction of the artist's imagination but also a symbol of the suffering of all blacks. His pregnancy powerfully symbolizes the plight of all slaves and their descendants, indicating that everyone is born into sexual and economic slave economy.

Eight Possible Beginnings' final chapter initially appears unrelated to the previous narratives, perhaps suggesting that the rest of the video is part of the story narrated in the Uncle Remus folktales. This is suggested by the title of this eighth chapter: 'The story of br'er Rabbit, br'er Fox and how briar patch county come to be called that', which is derived from both the Uncle Remus tales and Walt Disney's *Song of the South*, which combines animation, live action characters, and songs. The Uncle Remus stories were compiled by Joel Chandler Harris and based on the tales of several black storytellers whom he met in the South during the last years of the nineteenth century. First published in newspapers and magazines and then as a book in 1880 (followed by six more volumes), these tales are recounted in rural black dialect by an elderly former slave, Uncle Remus, to the young grandson of his former master. Created during the Reconstruction era, these animal fables tell of the pursuit by br'er Fox of br'er Rabbit, 'the black slave's alter ego and trickster-hero' (Bickley 2002, 58), and the latter's escape through wit and cunning, echoing the struggle of the slaves and slave owners.

Having revised and retold other canonical texts about the South (notably *Gone with the Wind*, *Uncle Tom's Cabin*, and popular minstrel theatrical productions), Walker reappropriates this well-known children's tale to expose, critique, and reclaim its racist messages. In Walker's retelling, the little boy begs Uncle Remus to tell him 'one of' his "long tales", but the former slave explains that he feels 'mighty worn out today'. The boy then threatens him: 'I'll tell mis Sally if you don't open your mouth', calling him an 'old coon'; 'I own you you dirty prick'. We see the artist place the silhouetted child on Uncle Remus's lap, making it clear that the situation is controlled by the boy and the artist.

Uncle Remus reluctantly acquiesces to the white boy's demands and threats, which Walker exaggerates to indicate that the supposed warm conviviality and audible laughter depends upon the boy's domination, control, and disrespect for the black man. His story, told in black dialect and acted out by the silhouette-puppets, takes place in, as the screen text explains, the 'dead nigger gulch'. In the story, the rabbit and fox lynch three black men, and the fox chases a rabbit, while the theme from the Disney film is sung in an overly sentimental and patronizing manner: 'Oh what a wonderful feeling, what a wonderful day'. Walker thus reappropriates Uncle Remus's voice and that of the white boy, as constructed by Harris, to reconfigure the narrative, making it clear that blacks will no longer remain subservient to white power. This is indicated by the final voiceover – Uncle Remus's proclamation: 'I will be telling no more stories'.

Throughout this scene, the artist's manipulation of the figures is overtly visible, underscoring Walker's role as the narrator of a nineteenth-century folktale that she configures as the tale of white subjugation of black slaves. This last chapter does not continue the history of the founding and settlement of African-America. It instead disrupts the narrative in a manner similar to the earlier interlude. It metaphorically summarizes the plight of blacks in African-America under the control of white slave traders and masters and their subversion of American apartheid's hierarchies. *Eight Possible Beginnings* significantly ends, as in *Testimony*, with the castration and murder of lynched white men, closing with this African-American trickster's moral lessons about escape from submission, the value of cunning, and appropriation of power (Knight 2005, E1). Walker turns Uncle Remus's 'safe' fairy tale onto its ear, realizing the white's greatest fear that the black man will ultimately have power and suggesting that individual and intergenerational traumas existed across the racial lines – both whites and blacks experience such traumas.

I was transported is Walker's most complex cinematic work. It is a video installation that consists of five screens placed on walls. On the larger wall, Walker has three screens: a larger central rectangular panel flanked by two smaller rectangular panels, resembling the format of a Christian triptych, an appropriate format given the video's themes of suffering, entombment, and resurrection. Two smaller screens are placed on the left and right walls, respectively. They are surrounded by an undulating and flickering frame that produces the sense of looking through a picture frame. This is an appropriate metaphor, especially since a series of photographs appears particularly on the left wall. These are nineteenth-century portraits of both blacks and whites, for example, of Abraham Lincoln, as well as silhouettes by Walker, and nineteenth-century colour engravings. These images appear, dissolve, and reappear, looping repeatedly and so quickly that it becomes overwhelming, confusing, and frustrating. Walker does not allow the viewer fully to see these obscure, fragmented, repeated images, suggesting their absent presence throughout history and their traumatic repetition and return with no clear end.

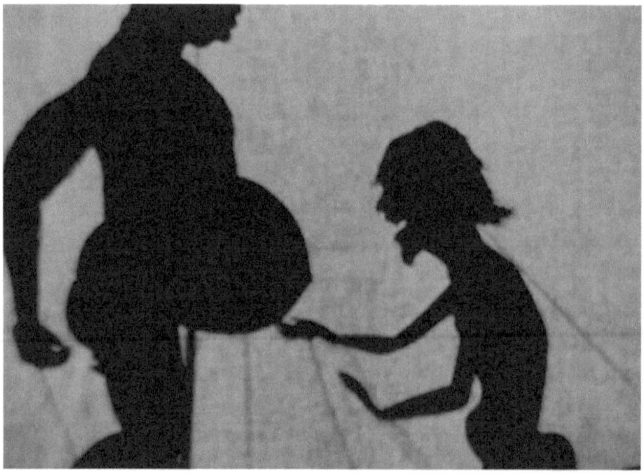

Figure 3. Kara Walker …*calling to me from the angry surface of some grey and threatening sea. I was transported.* Video 5 part installation. 2007. Photo courtesy of Sikkema Jenkins & Co., New York.

The installation's central video screen shows Walker's familiar silhouettes against intense hues in which a narrative emerges, although it is not clear where it begins or ends, suggesting an endless cycle that continually loops and that at times abruptly switches from scene to scene. The setting for this video takes place on a Southern plantation, which is signified by the moss-covered trees and Georgian plantation mansion. Here a slave mother at times nurses her child, who appears too old for such nourishment, while at other times she nurses her white master with whom she engages in sexual acts. Mutilation and murder also take place in this fantastic antebellum world, ending with the entombment of the mother rendered as an outlined body – hollowed out and empty – a field of gaping nothingness.

In this video the artist overwhelms the viewer with a multitude of images and activities that continuously appear and disappear. This functions as an appropriate metaphor for the confused world in which slaves and masters lived. The video images' endless re-looping suggests that the theme of resurrection cannot be a final resolution; instead, murder and entombment continually unfold as a perennial inevitability and haunting repetition.

Performing an act of remembrance

In *Eight Possible Beginnings* Walker works through both personal and transgenerational traumas of slavery first on a slave ship and then on a Southern plantation, the two main foundational institutions of modern slavery (Rediker 2007, 43). She suggests a chronology from the slave ship (which has no specific date) to 1793, when Eli Whitney invited the cotton gin, and to Reconstruction (when the folktales of Uncle Remus were published). In this and her other film and video works, Walker makes the individual and transgenerational trauma knowable and visible, thus suggesting the continuous repetition of dysfunction, sexual trauma, despair, and anger among blacks and whites. Like *Eight Possible Beginnings, Testimony* and *I was transported* similarly work through the individual trauma of slavery on a Southern plantation, implying that these traumas are so ingrained and persuasive that they will be passed onto subsequent generations.

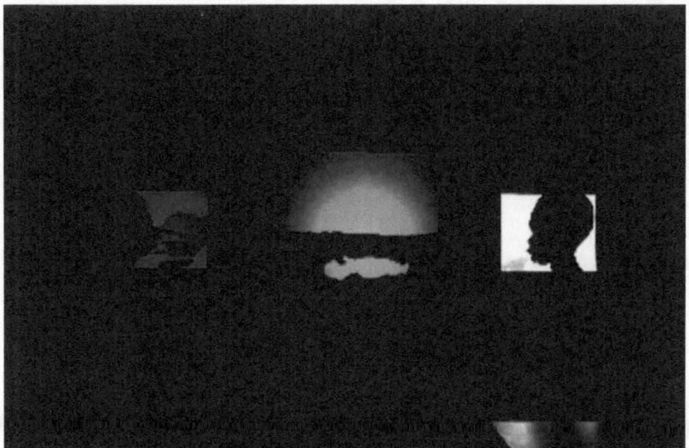

Figure 4. Kara Walker *... calling to me from the angry surface of some grey and threatening sea. I was transported.* Video 5 part installation. 2007. Photo courtesy of Brent Sikkema Gallery, New York City.

As Cathy Caruth explains: 'the striking juxtaposition of the unknowing, injurious repetition and the witness of the crying voice' demands a listener or viewer 'for the belated repetition of trauma' that can only be known after the traumatic event (1996, 204). Walker's ghostly silhouettes of African-Americans and whites deliberately evoke this shame, representing the unspeakable, and thereby signifying an absent presence whose traces are always evident and haunting in US culture. She creates a repetitive traumatic site – 'the belated repetition of trauma' – that surrounds, involves, and challenges the viewer to witness, acknowledge, and remember the trauma of slavery and contemporary racism. It also challenges the viewer to consider how the abuse of power results in contradictory roles that are complex and layered, sometimes resulting in abuse against the white body. Her traumatic narratives have no beginning, no ending, no before, no after, but instead appear timeless and ubiquitous.[13] Her testimony corresponds to the ways in which, according to Shoshana Felman, 'testimony has become a crucial mode of our relation to events of our times' that are:

> composed of bits and pieces of a memory that has been overwhelmed by occurrences that have not settled into understanding or remembrance, acts that cannot be constructed as knowledge nor assimilated into full cognition, events in excess of our frames of reference. (1992, 35)

Since Walker fails to visualize alternative behaviours and conversely repeatedly visualizes the trauma of slavery in her 'bits and pieces' of reconstructed and imagined memory, this unrelenting repetition of horrors as a postmemory is stuck in a closed loop – implying that no resolution exists. The very continuous looping of her videos establishes the repetition compulsion characteristic of PTSD. Rather than suggest that testimony can assist in healing trauma, Walker instead embodies the hopeless, helpless, terrorizing repetition of trauma that becomes transgenerational because of its continuity in the present. Moreover, Walker re-enacts the sensations of trauma through her formal inventions: the non-linearity and disruption of the narrative, the flashbacks, and the fragmentation of narrative and images through the paper cut-outs, rapid splicing, flickering light, and grainy images that create visual disturbances. These formal and textual discontinuities, as noted in this paper, embody the trauma victim's sense of disruption in lived experience and psychic coherence. As viewers, we bear witness to this disruption – as enacted, for example, in the disembodied voice of the sexually abused little girl in *Eight Possible Beginnings* – performing an act of remembrance as a postmemory of the traumatic history of the United States. As a result, the viewer is unable to imagine trauma as residing solely in the past but rather perceives it as relentlessly and continuously invading upon the present as PTSS, disturbing the process of recovery, healing, or closure.

Acknowledgements

I would like to thank the fellows in Trauma Studies at the Robert Penn Warren Center for the Humanities, for the academic year 2008/2009, for assisting me in understanding more clearly trauma theory and its application to Kara Walker's videos.

Notes

1. Hereafter referred to as *Testimony*. 'A genius of the south' has a rich history in African-American literature. The phrase derives from a poem, 'Georgia Dusk', by Jean Toomer that refers to orgies in the Georgia night. It was later engraved by Alice Walker on the grave of Zora Neale Hurston. The line resonates with a long history that associates 'madness' and sexual

promiscuity with the creativity of, in particular, African-American women. In a different essay it would be interesting to explore these histories of 'mad' women in relation to *hauntings* by unspeakable sexual traumas and manifestations of collective postmemory of such works as Toni Morrison's *Beloved* (1987).

2. Hereafter referred to as *Eight Possible Beginnings*.
3. Hereafter referred to as *I was transported*. Walker's 2004 solo exhibition, *Flibbergibbet and Mumbo Jumbo: Kara E. Walker in Two Acts*, at the Fabric Workshop and Museum in Philadelphia, marked her first use of video and performance (Raymond 2007, 369).
4. Hereafter referred to as *Gone* and *The End of Uncle Tom*.
5. My definition of 'collective remembrance' derives from Jay Winter and Emmanuel Sivan who emphasize agency, activity and creativity: it is 'the act of gathering bits and pieces of the past, and joining them together in public' to involve 'a domain beyond that of individual memory' (Winter and Sivan 1999, 6–39; Edkins 2003, 33).
6. *Webster's Seventh New Collegiate Dictionary* (1970, 809).
7. Ibid.
8. Grand Manner refers to the aesthetic style derived from antiquity and codified by eighteenth-century British artists, especially Sir Joshua Reynolds, to describe paintings that embody noble and heroic themes.
9. This is similar to the filmmaker of *Shoah* who, according to Shoshana Felman (1992, 216), also serves as a silent witness.
10. This film is based on research into historic models: Latte Reniger's silhouette film *The Adventures of Prince Achmed* (1926), a colourful, fanciful retelling of *The Arabian Nights*; D.W. Griffith's silent movie about the Ku Klux Klan, 'The birth of a nation' (1915); and the production of the early African-American filmmaker Oscar Micheaux.
11. Walker first exhibited this film in the fall of 2005 at the Roy and Edna Disney CalArts Theater in Los Angeles (Cheng 2005, E3; Cox 2007, 59).
12. This imagery recalls the biblical story of Jonah and the Whale, an allegory of redemption. Jonah, ignoring God's command that he preach to the Ninevites, attempts to hide from God by taking a boat elsewhere. During a storm, the sailors throw Jonah overboard. A whale swallows him, but after three days Jonah issues out unscathed. After emerging from the whale, Jonah sits by a tree, where he wrestles with his anger, knowing he will obey God despite his reluctance. Is the black woman the whale who imprisons the Jonah-like Africans, who must suffer and be obedient to win God's compassion and mercy? God's command that Jonah preach repentance to the gentile Ninevites suggests a parallel with the white/black struggle of the film. That Jonah is associated with the slaves (the oppressed or Other) takes on significance, since it is the oppressed who are called upon to preach repentance.
13. As Dori Laub explains: 'The traumatic event ... has no beginning, no ending, no before, no during and no after' (1992, 69).

References

Bickley, R. Bruce, Jr. 2002. Uncle Remus tales. In *The New Georgia encyclopedia*. http://www.georgiaencyclopedia.org/nge/Article.jsp?id=h-705&pid=s-58

Brasch, Walter M. 2000. *Brer Rabbit, Uncle Remus, and the 'cornfield journalist': A tale of Joel Chandler Harris*. Macon, GA: Mercer University Press.

Caruth, Cathy. 1996. *Unclaimed experience: Trauma, narrative, and history*. Baltimore: Johns Hopkins University Press.

Cheng, Scarlet. 2005. Out of her shadows. *Los Angeles Times*, 19 October, E3.

Cox, Lorraine Morales. 2007. A performative turn: Kara Walker's *Song of the South*. *Women and Performance: A Journal of Feminist Theory* 17, no. 7: 59–87.

Dever, Carolyn. 1998. *Death and the mother from Dickens to Freud: Victorian fiction and anxiety of origins*. Cambridge: Cambridge University Press.
Dixon Jr., Thomas. 1905. *The Clansman: An historical romance of the Ku Klux Klan*. New York: Doubleday.
Edkins, Jenny. 2003. *Trauma and the memory of politics*. Cambridge: Cambridge University Press.
Felman, Shoshana. 1992. Education and crisis, or the vicissitudes of teaching. In Felman and Laub 1992, 1–56.
Felman, Shoshana, and Dori Laub, eds. 1992. *Testimony: Crisis of witnessing in literature, psychoanalysis, and history*. New York: Routledge.
Golden, Thelma. 2002. Thelma Golden/Kara Walker: A dialogue. In *Kara Walker: pictures from another time*, ed. Annette Dixon, 43–9. Ann Arbor: University of Michigan Museum of Art.
Gordon, Avery F. 1997. *Ghostly matters: Haunting and the sociological imagination*. Minneapolis: University of Minnesota Press.
Hirsch, Marianne. 1997. *Family frames: Photography, narrative and postmemory*. Cambridge, MA: Harvard University Press.
———. 2002. Marked by memory: Feminist reflections on trauma and transmission. In *Extremities: Trauma, testimony, and community*, ed. Nancy K. Miller and Jason Tougaw, 71–91. Urbana: University of Illinois Press.
Jenkins, Sidney. 1995. *Look away! Look away! Look away!* Annandale-on-Hudson, NY: Center for Curatorial Studies, Bard College.
Kaplan, E. Ann. 2005. *Trauma culture: The politics of terror and loss in media and literature*. New Brunswick, NJ: Rutgers University Press.
Knight, Christopher. 2005. A South Disney didn't dream of. *Los Angeles Times*, 12 September, E1.
LaCapra, Dominick. 2001. *Writing history, writing trauma*. Baltimore: Johns Hopkins University Press.
Laub, Dori. 1992. Bearing witness or the vicissitudes of listening. In Felman and Laub 1992, 57–74.
Leary, Joy DeGruy. 2005. *Post traumatic slave syndrome: America's legacy of enduring injury and healing*. Milwaukie, OR: Uptone Press.
Meyer, Richard. 2002. *Outlaw representation: Censorship and homosexuality in twentieth-century American art*. Boston: Beacon Press.
Projecting fictions: Insurrection! Our tools were rudimentary, yet we pressed on. In *Art in the twenty-first century*. http://www.pbs.org/art21/artists/walker/clip1.html
Raymond, Yasmil. 2007. Maladies of power: A Kara Walker lexicon. In Vergne 2007, 347–69.
Raymond, Yasmil, and Rachel Hooper. 2007. *Kara Walker: My complement, my enemy, my oppressor, my love*. Gallery Guide. New York: Whitney Museum of American Art.
Rediker, Marcus. 2007. *The slave ship: A human history*. New York: Viking, 2007.
Reinhardt, Mark. 2003. The art of racial profiling. In *Kara Walker: Narratives of a negress*, ed. Ian Berry, Darby English, Vivian Patterson, and Mark Reinhardt, 109–29. Cambridge, MA: MIT Press.
Saltz, Jerry. 1996. Kara Walker: Ill-will and desire. *Flash Art* 29 (November/December): 82–6.
Saltzman, Lisa. 2006. *Making memory matter: Strategies of remembrance in contemporary art*. Chicago: University of Chicago Press.
Shaw, Gwendolyn Dubois. 2004. *Seeing the unspeakable: The art of Kara Walker*. Durham, NC: Duke University Press.
Storr, Robert. 2007. Spooked. In Vergne 2007, 63–74.
Terr, Lenore. 1994. *Unchained memories: True stories of traumatic memories, lost and found*. New York: Basic Books.
Vergne, Philippe, ed. 2007. *Kara Walker: My complement, my enemy, my oppressor, my love*. Minneapolis: Walker Art Center.
Walker, Kara. 1998. Kara Walker's response. *International Review of African American Art* 15, no. 2: 48–9.
———. 2006. Kara Walker. http://www.moma.org/onlineprojects/conversations/trans_kwalker.html
———. 2007. Taped tourguide. *Kara Walker: My complement, my enemy, my oppressor, my love*. New York: Whitney Museum of American Art.

Webster's seventh new collegiate dictionary. 1970. Springfield, MA: G. & C. Merriam.

Winter, Jay, and Emmanuel Sivan. 1999. Setting the framework. In *War and remembrance in the twentieth century*, ed. Jay Winter and Emmanuel Sivan, 6–39. Cambridge: Cambridge University Press.

Young, Kevin. 2007. Triangular trade: Coloring, remarking, and narrative in the writings of Kara Walker. In Vergne 2007, 37–52.

Depiction or erasure? Violence and trauma in contemporary Peruvian film

Iliana Pagán-Teitelbaum

Department of Romance Languages, University of Pennsylvania, Philadelphia, USA

Most of the 70,000 people who died or disappeared during the 1980–2000 civil war in Peru were Indigenous Quechua speakers. It is still proscribed to talk about the violent conflict in this Latin American country on the Pacific, where the high levels of poverty that may have triggered the war continue to affect 40% of the population. In this paper, I discuss the effort of three Peruvian films to respond to the trauma of misery, racism, forced migration, and dirty war experienced by both civilians and soldiers. I analyse how the films *Gregorio* (Grupo Chaski, 1984), *The Lion's Den* (Francisco Lombardi, 1988), and *Days of Santiago* (Josué Méndez, 2004) depict or erase the persons and bodies of the Andean individuals who have suffered violence.

In Seven interpretive essays on Peruvian reality ([1928] 1974), Peruvian intellectual José Carlos Mariátegui asserts that the 'problems' of the Indigenous people in Peru are economic, rooted in the land tenure system of the Peruvian economy (based on the *latifundio* or large landowner system implanted by medieval Spain during colonization). According to Mariátegui, Indigenous people would not escape feudal servitude until they gained control over agricultural lands (50–104). Lacking the political power to achieve land reform, in the 1950s thousands of displaced and landless Indigenous people from the Andes mountain ranges migrated to the coast and settled in slums in the desert outskirts of Lima (Nugent 1992, 31). As Núria Vilanova indicates, 'mass migration is one the most dramatic changes in contemporary Peruvian history, turning the traditionally agrarian people of Peru into urban dwellers struggling for survival in the city' (1999, 15).[1] Coastal people considered themselves 'whiter'[2] and more 'modern' than people from the Andes highlands (Martínez 2008, 1). They rejected the Indigenous highlanders who found it extremely difficult to access housing, education, and work on the coast (Soto et al. 1987, 12).

In 1969, the leftist military regime of Juan Velasco (1968–1975) instituted a Land Reform Law and recognized the Quechua Indigenous language as the second official language of Peru, along with Spanish. Though interrupted by a 1975 right-wing military coup, Velasco's regime generated pressing demands in large sectors of Peruvian society that were beginning to recognize their legal rights as citizens. These sectors would also constitute the core of movements such as Shining Path (Manrique Gálvez 2002, 55). Democratic elections were announced in 1980, but armed political groups such as the Shining Path Communist Party of Peru ('*Sendero Luminoso*' in Spanish)[3] and *Tupac Amaru* Revolutionary Movement (MRTA) had already resorted to armed struggle against the Peruvian state. Francisca da Gama explains that the rise of armed revolutionary groups responded to concrete historical developments in Peru, such as 'political upheaval, government corruption, a weak left, and racism towards the Indigenous population – who continued to live in poverty and be excluded from political decision-making' (2007, 1). Peruvian historian Nelson Manrique Gálvez adds that the devastating violence of the armed conflict in Peru was generated by a 'profoundly excluding and segregationist State, which inherited and adopted a racist and anti-indigenous colonial discourse, that saw Peruvian society as divided in castes, and that considered Whites intrinsically superior, and Indians inferior, for biological reasons' (2002, 57).[4] For Manrique Gálvez, the armed insurrection was a reaction against historical racial discrimination and conservative ideology that blamed the 'Indians' for all of Peru's misfortunes as a nation, and proposed a radical 'solution': the extermination of the aboriginal population (339). In this sense – as in South African *apartheid* (Lincoln 2008, 27) – the 'whiter' Euro-descendent Peruvian minority in power constructed the majority Indigenous population from the Andes and the Amazon as what Robert Jay Lifton calls the 'designated victims': Indigenous people were denied the right to live in their own country and were designated as a group that deserved to be exploited (or eliminated) for the economic and psychological survival of the Peruvian nation (Caruth 1995b, 139). Renowned Peruvian writer Mario Vargas Llosa (a presidential candidate in 1990) provides a relevant example of anti-Indigenous discourse in Peru when he declares that a 'free and decent' modern society can only be achieved in a state in which the 'native population is scarce or nonexistent'. With this objective in mind, Vargas Llosa urges the 'Indians to pay this high price', that is, 'to renounce their culture – their language, their beliefs, their traditions, and customs – and adopt those of their old masters' (1992, 811).

Indeed, most of the Peruvians who were killed or disappeared during the war were Indigenous Quechua-speakers. Since the ethnic composition of the lower ranks of the Peruvian armed forces is mainly of Indigenous descent, Indigenous Peruvians paid the 'high price' of the violence on both sides of the civil war (Manrique Gálvez 2002, 341).[5] A national state of emergency was declared in 1981, but the population of Lima largely ignored the war being waged in the mountains for a decade, until a bomb was placed in an affluent district of the capital in 1992. In November 2000, after two decades of war, an interim government organized new elections and created a Truth and Reconciliation Commission (TRC), which collected 17,000 testimonies from 2001 to 2003. The Peruvian TRC was based mainly on the South African model (1995), with public hearings broadcast on national television, but was also based on prior Latin American models from Argentina (1983), Chile (1990), El Salvador (1992), and Guatemala (1994) (Burneo 2001, 1). The Final Report of the TRC determined that the internal war in Peru led to more than 70,000 deaths and that Peruvian state forces were responsible for the deaths of at least half of the victims (Comisión de la Verdad y Reconciliación 2004, 9). The report also describes the

> feeling of exclusion and indifference experienced by the people and the communities that were the main victims of the internal armed conflict. Many Andeans felt that in the important centres of political and economic power of Peru, people thought that what had happened in Andean towns, houses and families was happening in *another country*. (20)

E. Ann Kaplan points out that it makes a big difference if a catastrophe is perceived as natural, accidental or produced by humans:

> Natural disasters are beyond human control, and accidents happen. But to understand that fellow humans have deliberately brought about one's overwhelming suffering adds to the traumatic effects ... Transmitted from generation to generation, the wound remains open even if split-off from daily consciousness. (2008, 46–7)

To this day, it is still proscribed to talk about the war in Peru, so the social wound or 'collective trauma' (Erikson 1995, 187) of a brutal internal war that damaged social bonds and destroyed trust in individuals, society, and the Peruvian state has not been healed. In a kind of 'sanitized language' that enables the state to assimilate violent deeds into a coherent narrative in order to delay their traumatic effects (Lincoln 2008, 29), the war is denied and is officially referred to as the 'internal armed conflict', 'the violence', or the time of 'terrorism'. An official document of the Peruvian army about its history in the twentieth century makes only brief reference (two sentences) to the 'struggle against subversion' after 1982 in which the soldiers who died are recognized as 'Heroes of Peace' (Ejército del Perú 2009). In similar documents, the Peruvian air force and the Peruvian police force state that they fought against terrorism and narcotrafficking (Fuerza Aérea del Perú 2008; Policía Nacional del Perú 2009),[6] while the Peruvian navy only mentions its participation in two international conflicts with Ecuador in 1981 and 1995 (Marina de Guerra del Perú 2009). In effect, as in the crimes of apartheid, '"nobody" committed them' (Lincoln 2008, 31) and the war does not appear to have happened in the official history of the Peruvian armed forces. Government officials and many intellectuals regularly refer to non-state political militants as 'terrorists'. As in the era of South African apartheid, when political opponents were represented as 'criminals' and the state apparatus as the upholder of 'law and order', in Peru political opponents were posited as terrorists or '"inhuman" enemies of the "legitimate" state' (31).

Even though the wounds of the war must have left personal, collective, and historical scars and residues, little attention has been paid to what Dominick LaCapra terms mourning as a '*social* process or ritual' (2001, 143, 151). Peru seems to lack the sentiment of national tragedy that engulfs civil society in countries of the Southern Cone such as Chile or Argentina, following the consequences of the violent state repression of the 1970s. This is possibly due to the common perception that the Indigenous victims in Peru are as not as deserving of the same human rights as the dominant 'whiter' minority sectors (Manrique Gálvez 2002, 340). As Kaplan puts it:

> The issue of 'national' trauma (and whether such a concept is viable) is complicated: national leaders usually deal with an historical past in which suffering was deliberately imposed on ethnic minorities in political rather than emotional terms. They may be fully aware of what was done, but seek to repress public knowledge so as not to arouse outcry and attribution of blame, to say nothing ... of demands for financial compensation for suffering. (2008, 47)

In February 2009, for example, President Alan García's government was criticized for initially rejecting a $2 million donation from Germany to build a museum for victims of Peru's civil conflict. Peruvian Defence Minister Antero Flores then stated that 'a museum to remember victims of the conflict would be of no use to anybody' (Collyns 2009a). A month later, President García – previously President during the most violent years of the war in 1985–1990 – accepted the German donation, but named Vargas Llosa head of the committee to design the 'memory museum' (Collyns 2009b). *BBC News*'s Lima correspondent, Dan Collyns, points out that

> Mr Garcia's initial refusal to accept the donation brought into focus his own record on human rights dating back to his first presidency in the late 1980s – one of the worst periods in Peru's civil war between state forces and the Shining Path rebels. A government-appointed truth and reconciliation commission found that he was politically but not criminally responsible for several massacres carried out by the military during that period. (2009b)

The persisting structures of domination and violence also contribute to constant 'insidious trauma'. As Laura S. Brown (1995) argues, post-traumatic symptoms can be considered not only 'intergenerational' (as in the case of the children of survivors of the Nazi

Holocaust) but also as an 'insidious trauma' that can 'spread laterally throughout an oppressed social group as well, when membership in that group means a constant lifetime risk of exposure to certain trauma' (107–8).

As the causes and the victims of the civil war continue to be denied, the suffering due to a traumatic history is 'exacerbated by ongoing power relations' (Kaplan 2008, 46). LaCapra reminds us that

> any truly viable reconciliation on a collective level depends not only on such processes as empathy and mourning but also on concrete economic, social, and political reforms in a larger context in which mourning itself has a broader, indeed a political, meaning. (2001, 215)

In Peru, the high levels of poverty and racism that triggered the war still affect a large part of the population. According to national statistics for 2007, nearly 40% of all Peruvians still live in absolute poverty, and most of the poor are Indigenous people (Instituto Nacional de Estadística e Informática 2007, 3). In the national Peruvian media, Indigenous people tend to be erased, caricatured or exoticized. As I have written elsewhere, even though the majority of the Peruvian population is of Indigenous descent, they do not have access to the dominant means of communication (2008, 6). Peruvian television programming is usually produced in Lima, and the owners of television channels 'are all white' (Quiroz 2007, 1). This contributes to the reproduction of Eurocentric patterns in which success, beauty, and desire appear associated with blond hair, light-coloured skin, and a tall stature (as in the discredited advertising campaigns for Gloria milk in Peru).[7] As Kaplan and Ban Wang express it, the 'cultural memory' that could bear witness to the traumatic experience of war is

> subjected to relentless erasure by the transnational media driven by the logic of commodity and consumption. The transnational media, with their soap operas, talk shows, disaster stories, glamorous geography, and historical dramas are erasing traumatic memories of oppression, violence, and injustice in both metropolitan centers and developing countries. (2008, 11)

The question then arises about the possibility of films to break through the 'collective blindness' (Nieto Degregori 2004, 20) and force an audience to 'face the horror' (Salazar Bondy [1964] 2002, 32) in order to remember, gain critical distance, come to terms with, and in a sense help 'work through' (LaCapra 2001, 143) a traumatic past. As Joshua Hirsch states, trauma is 'utterly bound up with the realm of representation' (2008, 98). For Cathy Caruth, art is a privileged place for giving voice to trauma (LaCapra 2001, 190). Janet Walker explores the ability of films to 'externalize, publicize, and historicize traumatic material that would otherwise remain at the level of internal, individual psychology' (2005, xix). Walker defines 'trauma cinema' as a group of films that 'deal with a world-shattering event or events, whether public or personal' through a 'trauma aesthetic' which entails a 'nonrealist mode characterized by disturbance and fragmentation of the films' narrative and stylistic regimes' as well as 'innovative strategies for representing reality obliquely, by looking to mental processes for inspiration, and by incorporating self-reflexive devices to call attention to the friability of the scaffolding for audiovisual historiography' (19). Can a film transform a viewer into some kind of 'witness'?[8] Could a film, as in the case of the enabling of a 'true witness' (Lincoln 2008, 30), allude to the falsity of the narratives that justified violent actions, so that individuals in a society could belatedly experience the traumatic effects of national crimes and thereby be enabled to identify on some level with the victims? In subsequent sections I discuss three Peruvian films that are unusual in that they seriously attempt to portray some of the traumatic historical realities of Peru.

Andean migrants in *Gregorio* (1984)

In 1982, the Grupo Chaski film collective was formed by: Peruvians María Barea, Fernando Barreto, and Fernando Espinoza; Alejandro Legaspi, from Uruguay; and Stefan Kaspar, from Switzerland. 'Chaski' is Quechua for 'messenger' or 'courier' (especially during the Inca era), and 'Grupo' is Spanish for 'group' or 'collective'. The name of the group, in Quechua and Spanish, symbolizes its commitment to communicating important messages to all members of the Peruvian nation. The Chaski collective stated its intention of altering commercial cinematographic practices and making films with and for marginalized communities. The members of the group were conscious of power dynamics in Latin America, and intended to create a space of inclusion for all Peruvians in their films (McClennen 2008, 1).

In their first feature film *Gregorio* (1984), created with the support of Velasco's Film Law, Chaski directors established a bridge between rural and urban cinema.[9] Following the tradition of the Cuzco Cinema Club that produced the first film in Quechua, *Kukuli* [Dove] in 1960, Chaski dared to start their film *Gregorio* in a 'dominated language', the Indigenous language Quechua (Mazzotti 2002, 37–58). According to María Elena García, Quechua had survived as the language of the colonized peoples of the Andes, a condition that placed it 'unequivocally below Spanish'. Furthermore, Quechua was subordinate to Spanish because Spanish had been the language of the new rulers and because Quechua was an oral language (García 2004, 349).

The film *Gregorio* begins in the Peruvian mountain ranges of the Andes, and shows how a poor Quechua-speaking family is forced to migrate to the coastal desert city of Lima. The words spoken in Quechua at the beginning of the film would be heard and understood by the Andean-descendent population, while non-Quechua-speakers had to trust the given translation and read the subtitles in Spanish.

At the beginning of the film, the idealized image of the majestic Andes as a peaceful region of snowy mountain peaks is questioned by consecutive stylized cuts, which are marked by sinister hammering sound effects. With each hammering strike, the beautiful images of nature are replaced by different images of hard physical work, which repeatedly allude to the historical exploitation of Indigenous communities in the Andes. The condition of Indigenous landlessness of Gregorio's family is then discussed in Quechua, with Spanish subtitles. Gregorio's father (Manuel Acosta Ojeda) is warned of the dangers of abandoning the struggle for land and migrating to the city to end up as a 'dish-washer' and 'return crying'. Nevertheless, in the film the lack of access to agricultural land pushes the father to make the long truck journey to the capital, in search of better living conditions. In the 1980s, two-thirds of the Lima population was composed of first- and second-generation migrants. Even though the modern city promised progress and citizenship to all Peruvians, migrants arriving in Lima were not well received. Urban dwellers expected 'civilization to arrive to the countryside' and did not want 'peasants to come looking for it' in the city (Soto et al. 1987, 8–12).

When Gregorio (Marino León de la Torre) and his family arrive in Lima, the father forces them to speak Spanish. The film shows how Quechua-speaking *campesinos* (peasants) are pressured into abandoning their language, because if they speak Quechua in the capital, as Gregorio's father admonishes, 'no one will understand you'. We hear Gregorio's thoughts as he muses (in Spanish) over the loss of his language: 'Here in Lima nobody speaks Quechua.' As Eric Santner points out, the loss of the native language 'stands in, metonymically, for the loss of a formerly intact rural culture as a whole' (1990, 97). Gregorio first loses his Andean community and environment, then his language, and then his father, who dies soon after moving to Lima because of unsafe work conditions, exploitation, and lack of proper housing and access to healthcare when he becomes sick. This death forces his son Gregorio to work as a shoe-shine boy on the streets to help his widowed mother support her three children.

Chaski's film strives to denaturalize urban poverty from the perspective of Gregorio and other working street boys in Lima, who are represented by non-actors and actually talk about their own traumatic experiences of hunger, injustice, and violence in a testimonial style before the camera. The giant close-ups of the boys' delicate, sad faces serve to make visible these unwanted street children, making it impossible to ignore them, forget them, or 'split them off from daily consciousness' (Kaplan 2008, 46). Their testimonies break the realist flow of the film in order to speak directly to the public. We hear about how the boys miss their families, and learn about their efforts to survive on the harsh streets of Lima and in the dangerous, uncomfortable desert slums. Gregorio complains that everything in his straw shack gets constantly full of sand when the wind blows; the community he has settled in with his family lacks all basic services; he cannot attend school; and he fears being assaulted on his way home. The boys' testimonies correct the myth of the city as a place of progress for all.[10] On the contrary, the film demonstrates that privileges are reserved for certain groups and that, despite exploitative hard work, migrant families are unable to escape misery. Given the boys' difficult conditions, their occasional acts of theft are diminished next to society's greater crime of discarding migrant families and their children, who are denied access to citizen rights. In a parallel manner, the film could also suggest that the peasant rejection of the status quo originated from 'real' injustices, as represented in the lives and testimonies of the young children.

Even though *Gregorio* was filmed in 1984, during the deadliest year of the war (by which time more than 5500 Andean *campesinos* had been massacred),[11] the massive rural exodus to the capital caused by people fleeing from violence is not mentioned in the film (CVR 2004, 25). In *Gregorio*, the war is only briefly and discreetly referenced by the inclusion of graffiti in the background, as Gregorio walks alone, defeated by city street life at the end of the film. The graffiti on the wall reads 'Down with the state of emergency' and is signed by 'Red Homeland Revolutionary Movement' (*MR Patria Roja*). Even though the film is otherwise silent about the war, the included graffiti signals that the Chaski filmmakers were aware of the war. While the Chaski collective does not make a film directly about the violent war, it does strive to make visible the indirect violence of the poverty and marginalization that was suffered by Andean farmers and migrants, and that caused the uprising. The film's focus on structural violence could be aimed at provoking a reflection about existing causes of the peasant uprising, even after the efforts to establish 'democracy' in Peru. The film thus provides an alternative narrative that discredits the official state discourse that accused insurgent peasants of being terrorists, evil communists, or drug traffickers without recognizing their demands. The thirst for such an alternative narrative might be one of the reasons for the great box-office success of the *Gregorio* in Lima and in rural regions of Peru, where the film was shown by means of a mobile cinema (Barrow 2005, 44–57).[12]

At the same time as Chaski's film makes visible the traumas of Andean migrant families, some of their casting choices may erase the bodies of the migrants and distance spectators from identifying with actual Andean people outside of the movie screen. As I assert in my essay 'Glamour in the Andes: The representation of indigenous migrant women in Peruvian cinema' (2008, 1), the choice of the 'whiter' Euro-descendent Peruvian actress Vetzy Pérez-Palma for the role of Gregorio's Indigenous mother, Juana, denies Andean women self-representation and replicates dominant Eurocentric codes of beauty. In a similar way, I would add that it is possible that the choice of a 'cute', healthy, light-skinned, fine-featured young boy, Marino León de la Torre, as the film's protagonist might be an effort to approximate the leading role to exotic and Eurocentric notions of beauty.[13] As Rita Barnard states in her essay 'Contesting beauty', beauty is 'always political' and 'standards of beauty function as a peculiarly dense transfer point for relations of power' (2000, 345). Therefore, it is possible to question how the casting choices relate to the 'symbolic politics of visibility' (356), especially when considering that the choice of the beautiful Lima actress Pérez-Palma was approved by the Peruvians and yet disapproved of by the non-Peruvians in the Chaski Group (Legaspi 2008, pers. comm.; Kaspar 2008, pers. comms). The implications of racist casting choices are an extremely sensitive issue in an 'intensely racist' society that denies its racism in official and everyday discourse (Manrique Gálvez 2002, 60). Racism in Peru is unusually complicated because in most cases the discriminating subject cannot easily separate him or herself from the object of discrimination. As Manrique Gálvez points out, Peruvians with

> evident indigenous phenotypical features who insult other Peruvians by using the epithet 'Indian' in a pejorative way can only do so by denying a part of their own – Indian – identity, which means discriminating, hating, and spurning constitutive elements of their own self. Racism, in this case, constitutes a superlative form of alienation, because it implies the impossibility of recognizing one's own face, as reflected by the mirror. (334)

In choosing individuals 'whose deportment, appearance, and style' embody the values and goals of a nation or group (Stoeltje et al., qtd in Barnard 2000, 348), the filmmakers confirm the dominant media requirement that the heroes or heroines on a screen must have a certain light-coloured complexion. This covert ideology then continues to be transmitted to spectators in a country that completely lacks positive representations of Indigenous or Afro-descendent Peruvians in the mainstream media, and in which non-Euro-descendants lack the power to control their own images (Pagán-Teitelbaum 2008, 5). As Ella Shohat and Robert Stam maintain, when the images of marginalized people operate as part of a 'continuum of prejudicial social policy and actual violence against disempowered people' they can place the bodies of those people in danger (2004, 183–4). In the context of a country at war against its marginalized and insurgent Indigenous population, casting choices in a film narrative about Indigenous migrants become even more relevant. As LaCapra argues, 'there is an inverse relation between the degree to which a topic is still intensely invested with emotion and value, and the strictures placed on art' (2001, 187–8). A film about Indigenous peasants made during a traumatic war in which thousands of Indigenous peasants are being killed has an ethical responsibility with regards to the representation of that community. The casting choices in *Gregorio* may therefore 'formally counteract' the film's potential to explore a traumatic historical narrative, and may – like Santner's 'narrative fetishism' – consciously or unconsciously 'expunge the traces of the trauma or loss that called that narrative into being in the first place' (qtd in Hirsch 2008, 106). This 'casting fetishism' that eliminates Indigenous or Indigenous-looking faces from the leading roles of films that purport to be about the elimination of Indigenous rights or lives is a pattern that is, unfortunately, repeated in the two other films that I discuss in this article.

State crimes in *The Lion's Den* (1988)

Four years later and still under the Film Law, the 1988 film *The Lion's Den* [La boca del lobo] by renowned Peruvian filmmaker Francisco Lombardi opens by giving a textual account of 'dirty war' conditions during the period 1978–1983. The opening titles on the screen mention 10,000 dead, and claim that the film is based on 'real events' that occurred in 1983. Lombardi's film makes reference to a massacre in an Andean village and to other violent acts by armed state forces, such as rape, torture, violent interrogations in Spanish of individuals who did not speak Spanish but only Quechua, and the theft and killing of livestock. According to the Peruvian Human Rights Commission, on 13 November 1983, Peruvian police violently invaded a family celebration in the Soccos district of Huamanga, Ayacucho, detaining 36 individuals, including children and old people, raping the women, and lining up everyone to be killed by machine-guns, as portrayed realistically in the film (CVR 2002).[14]

The Lion's Den was made in secrecy, out of fear of censorship by the government of Alan García (President of Peru, 1985–1990 and 2006–present).[15] García was perceived to have an 'ambiguous relationship' with the military, according to Augusto Cabada, one of the screenplay writers of Lombardi's film (Valdez Morgan 2006, 2). After undertaking research in Ayacucho in 1987, the filming took place in the town of Estique, in the mountains of Tacna, far from conflict zones, for two months. To preserve secrecy, the extras acting in the film, who were from the town of Estique, were not told the plot of the film. The secrecy supposedly allowed some collaboration of the army and air forces, which might not have participated had they been aware of the filmmakers' intentions (2).

Together with Chaski's *Gregorio*, Lombardi's *The Lion's Den* is one of the most screened Peruvian films (Valdez Morgan 2006, 3). It screened to 'packed audiences once it was released', and received media acclaim (Gama 2007, 2). Jorge Valdez Morgan remarks that it is unusual and surprising that the film escaped censorship from President García's government and the military, despite its première occurring during the war, and during the period of extreme hyperinflation (2006, 2). I contend that Lombardi's film was not censored because it strategically represents military war crimes as the responsibility of certain lawless and insane individuals such as the unruly Lieutenant Iván Roca (Gustavo Bueno), and not as official state war policy.

In the film, Lt Roca demands the massacre of the Quechua-speaking *campesinos* amidst a failed army career, bouts of alcoholism, and suicidal acts such as risking his life playing Russian roulette with a loaded gun. Gama points out that 'Even his own men refer to him as crazy so that his behaviour is rationalized according to a psychological defect' (2007, 2). This negative military image is neutralized by the positive image of the idealistic soldier, the hero-protagonist Vitín Luna (played by the Euro-descendent middle-class actor Toño Vega) who refuses to take part in the murder of innocent civilians and finally deserts the army. According to Lombardi's film, 'there is a law, one not correctly implemented. The military presence is not the problem, but rather, how the military behaves towards the community' (Gama 2007, 2). Even though the film claims to be about the traumatic war in which thousands of Indigenous people were being killed, the focus is actually diverted to a simplistic Hollywood-type binary opposition between good and evil, which centres on two characters, Luna [moon] and Roca [rock], played by Euro-descendent actors. As Jean Franco suggests, there is an 'inevitable dislocation between stated intent and narrative logic' when films that intend to represent contemporary problems of Indigenous societies give in to 'the demands of narrative structures that belong to the continuing saga of the white man's search for identity' (1999, 183).

Despite taking place in the supposed Andean community of Chuspi, *The Lion's Den* manages to make the Indigenous community anonymous. Andean people who had generally been excluded from Peru's mainstream cinematic tradition are again 'bound by conditions in which intellectual life continues to serve urban cultured elites and set the rules by which the Andean subject can be represented on screen' (Gama 2007, 2).

In the film, the Andean community of Chuspi is viewed as exotic, foreign, and mysteriously 'quiet', from the point of view of the 'good' soldier Luna, who is from Lima, and with whom spectators are encouraged to empathize. Valdez Morgan comments that the Andean peasant community in *The Lion's Den* is almost as absent as Shining Path, not for lack of knowledge, but because the film takes on the perspective of the state armed forces: 'In this way, Quechua-speakers are presented as strange, quiet, distrustful, non-cooperative, and difficult to understand' (2006, 4). The Andean region is portrayed as strange foreign territory, and Andean characters are presented as a collective, with rarely any individual voices or stories. Lombardi's film never portrays any conversations amongst Chuspi inhabitants, for example. Spectators are not given access to the *campesino* point of view with regards to the war, the invasive state military presence, or the actions attributed to Shining Path. Indigenous civilians in the film usually speak briefly (and in Spanish), and only when they are forced to interact with members of the armed forces.

Moreover, the film mystifies the state's political opponents by associating Shining Path's actions with irrational and supernatural forces. In a 2004 interview, Lombardi states that he had the sensation that the Shining Path struggle was seen from the cities as something 'foreign' that was happening 'far away' (qtd in Valdez Morgan 2006, 2). In his film, militants are never seen or even named, leaving only traces of spectacular violence – dead bodies with red painted signs on them, red flags, and red graffiti – as proof of their haunting invisible presence. As historian Steve Stern has observed, the subject of Shining Path is often framed as an exotic and surprising 'enigma', as 'a freakish evil force outside the main contours of Peruvian social and political history – more an invention of evil masterminds and an expression, perhaps, of the peculiarity of a particular regional milieu than a logical culmination or by product of Peruvian history' (1998, 1–2). The soldiers from Lima are the only characters developed with depth, individuality, and a certain degree of complexity. The film emphasizes the feelings of intense fear and disgust felt by the soldiers as they perceive the traces of violence left behind by the invisible militants. Soldiers feel constantly threatened by an impalpable danger that could attack invisibly at any given moment. The violent Shining Path acts are not contextualized and seem to have occurred for no reason: they are inconceivable and impossible to understand. The soldiers' violence, on the other hand, is 'conceivable' under the evident conditions of danger, fear, and stress. All of the soldiers' actions are contextualized so that the causes, if not acceptable, at least become understandable. Even though the film may intend to show and criticize the excessively violent conditions of the state's so-called dirty war, it consciously or unconsciously reproduces the oppressive state narrative in which Andean people appear as a source – and not as victims – of violence (Giroux 2002, 197). Since the film does not analyse the causes of the war, it thereby continues to make invisible the problems of exclusion of the majority of Peruvians from national politics and citizenship. As Peruvian film critic Ricardo Bedoya has pointed out, *The Lion's Den* fails to centrally address the massacre. By focusing on the emotional and psychological turmoil of Luna and Lt Roca, Lombardi manages to depoliticize the film and present a variation of the adventure narrative, a group of paranoid soldiers confronting an invisible enemy in an alien environment (Bedoya, qtd in Gama 2007, 2).

In terms of the politics of visibility and the lead casting choices, a 'whiter' actor, Toño Vega, was unrealistically chosen to represent the 'good' soldier Luna, who resists participation in corrupt and violent state actions, challenges Lt Roca, and risks his career in order to be loyal to his principles. José Tejada, an actor with more Andean features, was chosen to be the 'bad' soldier Gallardo, who rapes a local Indigenous shopkeeper and lies about a supposed attack by villagers who were actually having a wedding celebration;

Gallardo's lie ultimately leads to the massacre and disappearance of all the villagers. Just as in *Gregorio* where the heroic Indigenous mother is played by a 'whiter' actress, in *The Lion's Den* heroic conduct is related to ethnic whiteness. Meanwhile, non-European descendants in Lombardi's film appear connected to immoral and irrational violence (as in the actions alluding to Shining Path) or to the impotent victims of the war. To paraphrase Adam Lowenstein (2008, 147), the overwhelming facts of the destructive state response to the war, the 'controversial political issues of war responsibility', the reality of victim discrimination and censorship by the Peruvian authorities demand 'that representation answer to the traumatic significance of the event'. In limiting the remembering of the traumatic massacre to the point of view of state forces, Lombardi's film fails to dismantle the official state narrative that justifies the genocide of Indigenous people during the war. It is unclear whether the film would relay the 'burden of witnessing genocide' to the public, lending a degree of awareness and empathy to the audience (Hirsch, qtd in Walker 2005, 132). In spite of constituting an effort to reconstruct catastrophic memory, *The Lion's Den* would not qualify as trauma cinema (as defined by Walker) because of its realist mode of representation, its conventional narrative structure, and its lack of self-reflexivity.

The erased veteran in *Days of Santiago* (2004)

The 2004 film *Days of Santiago* (*Días de Santiago* in Spanish) by emerging filmmaker Josué Méndez is an unusual film, created immediately after the so-called 'years of violence' (Bedoya, in *Making of* 2005). Méndez's first feature film considers how Peruvian war veterans who fought in the 1995 Peru–Ecuador border conflict suffer post-traumatic stress disorder (PTSD). For LaCapra, trauma indicates 'a shattering break or cesura in experience which has belated effects' (2001, 186). Caruth states that PTSD is generally described as a delayed response to 'an overwhelming event or events' which may or may not traumatize everyone in the same way: the disorder consists in the '*structure of its experience* or reception: the event is not assimilated or experienced fully at the time, but only belatedly' (1995a, 4). Walker cites the diagnostic criteria for PTSD (as defined in the *Diagnostic and Statistical Manual of Mental Disorders*, DSM-IV) according to which 'traumatic events are "persistently experienced" as "recurrent and intrusive distressing recollections of the event" including dreams, flashback episodes, hallucinations, illusions, and the "feeling of detachment or estrangement from others"' (2008, 128). As Hirsch indicates, in post-traumatic memory, linear chronology collapses (as opposed to narrative memory) and time becomes 'fragmented and uncontrollable. The past becomes either too remote or too immediate. It remains inaccessibly in the past (amnesia), or presents itself uninvited, seizing consciousness (hypermnesia)' (Hirsch 2008, 103).

In *Days of Santiago*, the protagonist Santiago is constantly perturbed by the lasting effects of the war. In a remarkable displacement, Méndez substitutes the most recent and traumatic Peruvian conflict (the two-decade internal war in which the state confronted Shining Path and other political groups) with a brief border conflict known in Peru as the Cenepa conflict, which lasted a couple of months in 1995, in the Cenepa River region of the Amazonian Peru–Ecuador border. Even though Santiago is supposed to have fought in the Cenepa conflict, the Peruvian audience would recognize that Santiago actually represents a veteran who fought in the internal war because he mentions the fear of fighting against the '*terrucos*'. '*Terruco*' is a derogatory term used in the military to refer to anyone deemed to be associated with Shining Path, that derives from the word 'terrorist', but also sounds like '*tierra*' or land in Spanish, with the added negative suffix '*-uco*'.

The displacement could be seen as a cultural sign of a traumatized nation that has still not come to terms with its past, or as a strategy to avoid censorship by the powerful military that prefers not to officially acknowledge its violent participation in the internal war.

Days of Santiago carefully examines the lack of opportunities for soldiers' reinsertion into a 'peaceful' society, and denounces the violence of the invisibility and anonymity with which war heroes (who supposedly fought for their homeland) return to civil society in Peru. When Santiago returns to Lima, the difficulties of returning to civilian life reveal that even though he risked his life for the safety and well-being of his nation, his nation does not care about him. Santiago cannot find employment, his pension is insufficient to sustain his family, he cannot obtain credit to buy a refrigerator even though he proudly shows his military documents to prove that he is a veteran with a pension, and he does not have access to educational benefits. In a similar situation, some of Santiago's unemployed veteran colleagues get caught trying to rob a bank, while a veteran friend who is disabled hangs himself. Santiago grows increasingly unstable, sleeping in full military gear, performing ritualistic military practices on the beach, and violently overreacting to human proximity. Kai Erikson explains that

> Traumatized people often scan the surrounding world anxiously for signs of danger, breaking into explosive rages and reacting with a start to ordinary sights and sounds, but at the same time, all that nervous activity takes place against a numbed gray background of depression, feelings of helplessness, and a general closing off of the spirit, as the mind tries to insulate itself from further harm. Above all, trauma involves a continual reliving of some wounding experience in daydreams and nightmares, flashbacks and hallucinations, and in compulsive seeking out of similar circumstances. (1995, 184)

In the film, Santiago constantly scans the streets of Lima for danger. He prepares safety strategies and never uses the same route twice, even when he starts working part-time as a taxi driver. He explodes in rage when he perceives people to be acting 'wrongly'. These rages are sometimes expressed through actual fights with his family, but also through 'imaginary' scenes that Santiago acts out realistically, before it is revealed to the public that he is actually immobilized by his rage, and that everything seen on the screen represents images that occurred only in Santiago's mind. This entrance into Santiago's psyche is magnified by the contrasting use of black and white effects within the colour film. The 'numbed gray background' of depression and helplessness is exteriorized as a disturbance in the colours that Santiago (and the film viewers) can see. In this way the film makes visible some of the PTSD symptoms suffered by veterans.

The film focuses on what LaCapra calls 'the problem of perpetrator trauma' (2001, 120). As in the context of the Vietnam veterans, the Peruvian war circumstances enabled soldiers

> to perform actions that would otherwise be abhorrent to them. The result is a 'psychic numbing' that acts as a delay mechanism, displacing the traumatic effects of war crimes and allowing soldiers to continue performing apparently without psychic damage. It is only once these veterans return to 'normal' society and are confronted with the 'traditional world of justice' that they belatedly recognize the horror of what they have done and thus undergo traumatic responses. For these men, the restoration of 'normality' constitutes a trauma, since it reveals the hollowness of the narratives that have sustained them thus far. (Lincoln 2008, 29)

Santiago's return to society serves to dismantle narratives kept alive during the war to justify violence. Peru does not seem to have become a safer or better place for Santiago after sacrificing his youth fighting against 'terrorism' in the compulsory military. Upon his return to Lima, Santiago's veteran status is meaningless and nobody seems to be aware of the recent war. Santiago feels estranged when, instead of being received as a hero, he joins the ranks of millions of oppressed Peruvians (many of whom had tried to fight for social change, which he possibly contributed to suppressing).

Méndez based *Days of Santiago* on extensive interviews with a real veteran who was a friend of the family, named only as 'Santiago'. The fiction film was based on the experiences of the veteran, who worked closely with the director, explaining his psychology and how he would have reacted to events, as well as helping to give military training to the actors. As portrayed in the *Making of* included in the DVD *Days of Santiago*, the real life veteran is a thin, short, limping young man with Andean features. Méndez underlines that during the filmmaking, Santiago acted out many of the veteran film scenes with great realism and enthusiasm. However – and here we return to the politics of visibility – the director selected a Euro-descendent middle-class actor from Lima, Pietro Sibille, to represent the veteran in the film. Sibille trained for the leading role in a gym. He acquired the physical fortitude of a great Hollywood-style soldier, in contrast with the actual veteran's smaller, less able body. This portrayal denies the reality of the loss of physical (not only mental) well-being in veterans extracted (often by force) from poor sectors of the Peruvian population. Any reference to Santiago's hurt body is erased in the film. The contrast between Sibille's strong able body and the actual Santiago's limping body is evident in the *Making of* documentary, when the actor and the veteran walk side by side on the beach. *Days of Santiago* includes an Andean-descendent veteran in the filmmaking process, yet excludes images of anyone resembling him or his community from the film. During the film, the public is encouraged to identify with the strong 'whiter' soldier's struggles. But because Andean faces and bodies are missing from the film, the empathy generated towards the plight of the returned veteran in the film will not easily transfer into empathy towards darker-skinned, lower-class Andean veterans encountered in Lima.

Conclusion

A handful of Peruvian films aim to critically depict the traumas of violence and racism towards lower-class Andean descendants in Peru, who continue to be treated as foreign or even threatening to the nation, in spite of constituting a majority that has historically done most of the work to enrich, feed, and construct the country. Most of these films are unable to completely escape the violent patterns of representation of Peruvian cinema. By erasing the persons and bodies of the poor, and re-creating their image using richer and 'whiter' actors, the films I analyse tend to contradict their stated intent, purposefully or not. The ethical and ethnic repercussions of a 'casting fetishism' that eliminates Indigenous-looking faces from the screen in films that are supposedly about historical Indigenous trauma are serious, especially considering that for almost five centuries the official discourse has excluded this population while justifying their exploitation or annihilation. This violence has taken place in the name of progress and prosperity reserved for a non-Indigenous minority that is still dominant. The fact that the filmmakers, Chaski Group, Lombardi, and Méndez, belong to the non-Indigenous minority gives them power to portray historical Peruvian traumas, and also an artistic responsibility that is contingent on the traumatic memories of both victims and perpetrators. If discourses have contributed to the production of national traumas, films can contribute culturally to the creation of new discourses that assist in working through traumas that have been continually denied or erased. Films can help restore healing processes in society, and perhaps 'open up a space for transformation of the viewer', by promoting 'inter-cultural compassion and understanding' (Kaplan and Wang 2008, 10). In order to promote inter-cultural empathy, though, filmmakers need to surpass a limited point of view and be aware that their casting choices may be influenced by their ethnic and class prejudices. Otherwise, as in the films I examine, their filmic work will contribute to the erasure of the traumatic memories of the Indigenous groups that have been the main sufferers of trauma in Peru.

Acknowledgements

Initial research and travel to the "Interrogating Trauma: Arts & Media Responses to Collective Suffering International Conference" at Perth, Western Australia (2–4 December 2008) was funded by a Uellon Postdoctoral Fellowship, University of Pennsylvania (2007–2009).

Notes

1. Between 1940 and 1980, Peru's urban population grew from 2.4 million (35% of the population) to 11.6 million: 65% of the Peruvian population became urban (Soto et al. 1987, 7–8).
2. I use the term 'whiter' instead of 'white' to allude to the complex ethnic hierarchies in Peru, in which lighter-skinned Peruvians of Euro-descendent or mixed Euro, Andean and/or Afro-descendent heritage are considered 'white' or 'whiter' than others, and therefore 'racially' superior (even though these Peruvians might not be considered 'white' in a European context).
3. According to Francisca da Gama, 'Sendero was based on Maoist ideology and a reclaiming of Peruvian Marxist José Carlos Mariátegui. By appropriating the work of Mariátegui, Sendero could emphasize its localized application of Maoism and create its own "indigenous" Marxism. It launched its People's War in 1980 just when organized international communism was in retreat.' The exclusion of the Indigenous population in Peru 'allowed Sendero to operate amongst the rural indigenous peasantry' (Gama 2007, 1).
4. All translations from Spanish are my own, unless otherwise indicated.
5. Even though racism is not 'legal', the minimum height and 'physical presence' required to enter the air force and the navy exclude Indigenous or mixed-descent Peruvians from those forces, permitting their participation only in the lower ranks of the army (Manrique Gálvez 2002, 341). Peruvian military service was compulsory since the 1823 Constitution and until 2000. Compulsory military service and the illegal *leva* or forced recruitment was applied only to lower-class and rural communities (Abad 1999, 38).
6. The National Police Force of Peru alludes to its 'involvement in socio-economic problems heightened by the phenomenon of narco-terrorism and its chilling and bloody sequels'; it also asserts that in the 1980s and 1990s the police confronted 'serious alterations to the Internal Order' and that the police contributed to 'the defeat of terrorist organizations: MRTA, Shining Path, as well as dismantling international drug trafficking organizations' (Policía Nacional del Perú 2009).
7. *Gloria* [Glory] evaporated milk publicity has won anti-prizes in Peru for its racist advertising schemes that exhibit rich white families and urge Peruvian children to grow taller by drinking the canned milk (García 2005; Flores 2008). This expensive product is typically marketed and sold to lower-class families, which mix the concentrated drink with boiled water. For more information on the history of the *Gloria* milk industry in Peru, see the documentary *Peru: Neither Milk nor Glory* directed by Grupo Chaski (1986). Most Peruvians (70–90%) are lactose intolerant (Maurer 2007).
8. See Dori Laub (1995) on the three levels of witnessing (witness of an experience, witness of a testimony, and witness of the process of witnessing) (61).
9. In 1972, the Velasco regime enacted the Law for the Promotion of the Film Industry in order to promote an 'authentic national cinema' that would reflect the Peruvian reality and transmit a revolutionary message (Bedoya 1992, 188–9). At the end of the 1970s, films centred first on the problems of peasants in rural Peru, and then on urban problems because most professional filmmakers were in and of the capital city (Lombardi 1989, 61; Huayhuaca 1989, 82). Velasco's Film Law gave a boost to Peru's film industry by encouraging local productions, requiring compulsory screening of Peruvian cinema, and offering tax incentives for local producers. President Alberto Fujimori (1990–2000, currently in prison for human rights violations and corruption) eliminated the Film Law in 1992 together with other state cultural policies. 'Systematically adopting neo-liberal economic and social policies, Fujimori's government saw

culture in general, and film in particular, as one more commodity that needed to compete within local and global market forces without state participation' (Martínez 2008, 11).
10. See Sebastián Salazar, *Lima la horrible* [Lima the horrible] (1964), for a deconstruction of the myth of Lima as a modern city with democratic opportunities.
11. Five thousand five hundred Peruvian *campesinos* were killed between 1983 and 1984 (Manrique Gálvez 2002, 20).
12. The film's distribution under the Film Law allowed a prolonged exhibition in Peruvian theatres with artificially low ticket prices, which allowed access to a great part of the Peruvian population (Barrow 2005, 44–57).
13. Chaski director Fernando Espinoza has explained that in choosing an actor for the role of Gregorio, the film collective searched for 'a boy who had an experience of no more that one or two years in the capital, so that he was still tied to his own culture, who was bilingual, and who could incorporate his own migrant experience in the film process' (1989, 230).
14. Other human rights violations of this period include: the Accomarca massacre (August 1985), where 47 peasants were gunned to death by the Peruvian armed forces; the Cayara massacre (May 1988) in which 30 were killed and dozens disappeared; and the summary execution of more than 200 inmates and political prisoners during prison riots in Lurigancho, San Juan Bautista (El Frontón) and Santa Bárbara in 1986 ('Alan García' 2008).
15. President Alan García's first term in office (1985–1990) was marked by hyperinflation of 2,000,000% that profoundly destabilized the Peruvian economy; poverty increased by 13% (to 55%); and an estimated 1600 forced disappearances took place ('Alan García' 2008). García's current presidency has a 70% disapproval rating (Bamrud 2008).

References

Abad, Samuel. 1999. ¿Adiós a las levas? La difícil ruta hacia un servicio militar voluntario [Goodbye to forced recruitment? The difficult route towards a voluntary military service]. *Revista del Instituto Legal de Defensa* 120: 38. http://www.idl.org.pe/idlrev/revistas/120/pag38.htm (accessed 24 July 2009).

Alan García. *Wikipedia*. 27 November 2008. Wikimedia Foundation. http://en.wikipedia.org/wiki/Alan_Garc%C3%ADa (accessed 24 July 2009).

Bamrud, Joachim. 2008. Leader of the year: Alan Garcia. *Latin Business Chronicle*, 23 December 2008. http://www.latinbusinesschronicle.com/app/article.aspx?id=2975 (accessed 24 July 2009).

Barnard, Rita. 2000. Contesting beauty. In *Senses of culture: South African culture studies*, ed. Sarah Nuttall and Cheryl-Ann Michael, 344–62. Oxford: Oxford University Press.

Barrow, Sarah. 2005. Images of Peru: A national cinema in crisis. In *Latin American cinema: Essays on modernity, gender and national identity*, ed. Lisa Shaw and Stephanie Dennison, 39–58. Jefferson, NC: McFarland.

Bedoya, Ricardo. 1992. *100 años de cine en el Perú: una historia crítica* [One hundred years of film in Peru: A critical history]. Lima: Universidad de Lima-Instituto de Cooperación Iberoamericana (ICI).

Brown, Laura S. 1995. Not outside the range: One feminist perspective on psychic trauma. In *Trauma: Explorations in memory*, ed. Cathy Caruth, 100–12. Baltimore and London: Johns Hopkins University Press.

Burneo Labrín, José. 2001. La creación de la Comisión de la Verdad en el Perú [The creation of the Truth Commission in Peru]. *Reforma y gobernabilidad. Palestra de Estado: Portal de asuntos públicos de la Pontificia Universidad Católica del Perú*, 13 August 2001. http://palestra.pucp.edu.pe/pal_est/?file=verdad/burneo.htm (accessed 24 July 2009).

Caruth, Cathy. 1995a. Trauma and experience: Introduction. In *Trauma: Explorations in memory*, ed. Cathy Caruth, 3–12. Baltimore and London: Johns Hopkins University Press.

———. 1995b. Interview with Robert Jay Lifton. In *Trauma: Explorations in memory*, ed. Cathy Caruth, 128–47. Baltimore and London: Johns Hopkins University Press.

Collyns, Dan. 2009a. Peru furore over museum donation. *BBC News*, 28 February. http://news.bbc.co.uk/2/hi/americas/7916203.stm (accessed 24 July 2009).

———. 2009b. Peru U-turn on war museum funds. *BBC News*, 6 April. http://news.bbc.co.uk/2/hi/americas/7986180.stm (accessed 24 July 2009).

Comisión de la Verdad y Reconciliación (CVR). 2002. Audiencias Públicas en Ayacucho – Audiencia Pública en la ciudad de Huamanga – Primera Sesión, día 08 de abril del 2002 (de 08:00 a 13:00 horas) [Public Hearings in Ayachucho – Public Hearing in the city of Huamanga – First Session, day 8 of April of 2002 (from 8:00 to 13:00)]. *Informe Final de la Comisión de la Verdad y Reconciliación*. http://www.cverdad.org.pe/apublicas/audiencias/sumillahuamanga01.php (accessed 24 July 2009).

———. 2004. *Hatun willakuy: versión abreviada del Informe Final de la Comisión de la Verdad y Reconciliación* [The great story: Abbreviated version of the Final Report of the Truth and Reconciliation Commission]. Lima: Comisión de Entrega de la Comisión de la Verdad y Reconciliación.

Days of Santiago [Días de Santiago]. Dir. Josué Méndez. Chullachaki Producciones, Cachoeira Films and MilColores Media, 2004. DVD. Lions Gate, 2005.

Ejército del Perú [Peruvian army]. 2009. El Ejército del siglo XX [The army in the twentieth century]. *Portal Institucional: Dirección de Informaciones del Ejército (DINFE)*. http://www.ejercito.mil.pe/index.php?option=com_content&view=article&id=491&Itemid=288 (accessed 24 July 2009).

Erikson, Kai. 1995. Notes on trauma and community. In *Trauma: Explorations in memory*, ed. Cathy Caruth, 183–99. Baltimore and London: Johns Hopkins University Press.

Espinoza, Fernando. 1989. Grupo Chaski. In *El cine peruano: visto por críticos y realizadores* [Peruvian cinema: As seen by critics and filmmakers], ed. Balmes Lozano Morillo, 225–33. Lima: Cinemateca de Lima.

Franco, Jean. 1999. High-tech primitivism: The representation of tribal societies in feature films. In *Critical passions*, 181–95. Durham, NC and London: Duke University Press.

Flores, Julio. 2008. Cómprale al Perú [Buy Peruvian]. Kaotic.minD, 16 April. Blogger. http://kaotic-mind.blogspot.com/2007/04/cmprale-al-per.html (accessed 24 July 2009).

Fuerza Aérea del Perú [Peruvian air force]. 2008. Historia de la Fuerza Aérea del Perú [History of the Peruvian armed forces]. http://www.fap.mil.pe/historia.htm (accessed 24 July 2009).

Gama, Francisca da. 2007. Filming the war with Sendero. *Jump Cut: A Review of Contemporary Media* 49: 1–3. http://www.ejumpcut.org/archive/jc49.2007/daGama-Sendero/index.html (accessed 24 July 2009).

García, Alberto. 2005. Activistas de derechos humanos dan 'premio' a publicidad racista [Human rights activists give 'award' to racist publicity]. *La República Online*, 22 March. http://www.larepublica.com.pe/component/option,com_contentant/task,view/id,71645/Itemid,0/ (accessed 24 July 2009).

García, María Elena. 2004. Rethinking bilingual education in Peru: Intercultural politics, state policy and indigenous rights. *Bilingual Education and Bilingualism* 7, no. 5: 348–67.

Giroux, Henry. 2002. *Breaking into the movies: Film and the culture of politics*. Malden, MA and Oxford: Blackwell.

Gregorio. Dir. Fernando Espinoza, Stefan Kaspar, and Alejandro Legaspi. Grupo Chaski, 1984. VHS. New York Video Archives, 1984. DVD. Distribuidora Digital Chaski, 2008.

Hirsch, Joshua. 2008. Post-traumatic cinema and the Holocaust documentary. In *Trauma and cinema: Cross-cultural explorations*, ed. E. Ann Kaplan and Ban Wang, 93–121. Hong Kong: Hong Kong University Press.

Huayhuaca, José Carlos. 1989. Para hacer cine, ir al cine [To make films, go to films]. In *El cine peruano: visto por críticos y realizadores* [Peruvian cinema: As seen by critics and filmmakers], ed. Balmes Lozano Morillo, 71–85. Lima: Cinemateca de Lima.

Instituto Nacional de Estadística e Informática. 2007. *Informe técnico: la pobreza en el Perú en el año 2007* [Technical report: Poverty in Peru in the year 2007]. http://siteresources.worldbank.

org/INTPERUINSPANISH/Resources/InformeTecnico_Pobreza2007.pdf (accessed 24 July 2009).
Kaplan, E. Ann. 2008. Traumatic contact zones and embodied translators: With reference to select Australian texts. In *Trauma and cinema: Cross-cultural explorations*, ed. E. Ann Kaplan and Ban Wang, 46–63. Hong Kong: Hong Kong University Press.
Kaplan, E. Ann, and Ban Wang. 2008. Introduction: From traumatic paralysis to the force field of modernity. In *Trauma and cinema: Cross-cultural explorations*, ed. E. Ann Kaplan and Ban Wang, 1–22. Hong Kong: Hong Kong University Press.
Kukuli [Dove]. Dir. Luis Figueroa and Eulogio Nishiyama. Kero Film, 1960.
LaCapra, Dominick. 2001. *Writing history, writing trauma*. Baltimore and London: Johns Hopkins University Press.
Laub, Dori. 1995. Truth and testimony: The process and the struggle. In *Trauma: Explorations in memory*, ed. Cathy Caruth, 61–75. Baltimore and London: Johns Hopkins University Press.
Lincoln, Sarah L. 2008. This is my history: Trauma, testimony, and nation-building in the 'new' South Africa. In *Trauma and cinema: Cross-cultural explorations*, ed. E. Ann Kaplan and Ban Wang, 25–43. Hong Kong: Hong Kong University Press.
The Lion's Den [La boca del lobo]. Dir. Francisco Lombardi. Producciones Inca Films, Tornasol Films, and Televisión Española, 1988. VHS. Cinevista Video, 1999.
Lombardi, Francisco. 1989. Cine peruano, posibilidades y perspectivas [Peruvian cinema, possibilities and perspectives]. *El cine peruano: visto por críticos y realizadores* [Peruvian cinema: As seen by critics and filmmakers], ed. Balmes Lozano Morillo, 59–64. Lima: Cinemateca de Lima.
Lowenstein, Adam. 2008. Allegorizing Hiroshima: Shindo Kaneto's *Onibaba* as trauma text. In *Trauma and cinema: Cross-cultural explorations*, ed. E. Ann Kaplan and Ban Wang, 145–61. Hong Kong: Hong Kong University Press.
Making of. 2005. Chullachaki Producciones. *Días de Santiago*. DVD. Lions Gate, 2005.
Manrique Gálvez, Nelson. 2002. *El tiempo del miedo: la violencia política en el Perú, 1980–1996* [The time of fear: political violence in Peru, 1980–1996]. Lima: Fondo Editorial del Congreso del Perú.
Mariátegui, José Carlos. [1928] 1974. *Siete ensayos de interpretación de la realidad peruana* [Seven interpretive essays on Peruvian reality]. Lima: Empresa Editora Amauta.
Marina de Guerra del Perú [Peruvian navy]. 2009. Marina actual: la Marina de Guerra del Perú desde 1969 a la actualidad [The Peruvian navy from 1969 to the present]. http://www.marina.mil.pe/marina_actual.htm (accessed 24 July 2009).
Martínez, Gabriela. 2008. Cinema law in Latin America: Brazil, Peru and Colombia. *Jump Cut: A Review of Contemporary Media* 50: 1–28. http://www.ejumpcut.org/archive/jc50.2008/LAfilmLaw/index.html (accessed 24 July 2009).
Maurer, Geraldine. 2007. Del consultor: a tener cuidado con la leche [From the consultant: Be careful with milk]. *El Comercio*, 23 April. http://www.elcomercio.com.pe/EdicionImpresa/Html/2007-02-01/ImEcVidayFuturo0662359.html (accessed 24 July 2009).
Mazzotti, José Antonio. 2002. *Poéticas del flujo: migración y violencia verbales en el Perú de los 80* [Poetics of the flow: Migration and verbal violence in Peru of the 80s]. Lima: Fondo Editorial del Congreso del Perú.
McClennen, Sophia A. 2008. The theory and practice of the Peruvian Grupo Chaski. *Jump Cut: A Review of Contemporary Media* 50. http://www.ejumpcut.org/archive/jc50.2008/Chaski/index.html (accessed 24 July 2009).
Nieto Degregori, Luis. 2004. Ensayo sobre la ceguera [Essay on blindness]. In *Pachaticray (El mundo al revés): Testimonios y ensayos sobre la violencia política y la cultura peruana desde 1980* [Pachaticray (Upside down world): Testimonies and essays on political violence and Peruvian culture since 1980], ed. Mark R. Cox, 19–21. Lima: Editorial San Marcos.
Nugent, José Guillermo. 1992. *El laberinto de la choledad* [The labyrinth of 'cholitude']. Lima: Fundación Friedrich Ebert.
Pagán-Teitelbaum, Iliana. 2008. El glamour en los Andes: la representación de la mujer indígena migrante en el cine peruano [Glamour in the Andes: The representation of indigenous migrant women in Peruvian cinema]. *Revista Chilena de Antropología Visual* 12, no. 2: 1–30. http://www.antropologiavisual.cl/pagan.htm (accessed 24 July 2009).
Peru: Neither milk nor Glory [Perú: ni leche ni Gloria]. 2008. Dir. Alejandro Legaspi, Stefan Kaspar, and Homero Rivera. Grupo Chaski, 1986. DVD. Distribuidora Digital Chaski.

Policía Nacional del Perú [National Peruvian Police]. 2009. *Historia* [History]. http://www.pnp.gob.pe/historia.html (accessed 24 July 2009).

Quiroz, Carlos A. 2007. Qué bien me veo en la TV peruana [I look great on Peruvian TV]. *Peruanista*, 19 February. Blogspot. http://peruanista.blogspot.com/2007/02/que-bien-me-veo-en-la-tv-peruana.html (accessed 24 July 2009).

Salazar Bondy, Sebastián. [1964] 2002. *Lima la horrible*. Concepción, Chile: Editorial Universidad de Concepción.

Santner, Eric L. 1990. *Stranded objects: Mourning, memory, and film in postwar Germany*. Ithaca, NY and London: Cornell University Press.

Shohat, Ella, and Robert Stam. 2004. *Unthinking Eurocentrism: Multiculturalism and the media*. London and New York: Routledge.

Soto, Hernando de, et al. 1987. *El otro sendero: La revolución informal* [The other path: The informal revolution]. Bogotá: La Oveja Negra.

Stern, Steve J. 1998. *Shining and other paths: War and society in Peru, 1980–1995*. Durham, NC: Duke University Press.

Valdez Morgan, Jorge. 2005. La sociedad filmada: apuntes sobre la historia del Perú a través de tres películas (1933, 1961, 1977) [Filmed society: Notes on Peruvian history through three films]. *Histórica* 29, no. 2: 1–30. http://www.scribd.com/doc/12588855/La-sociedad-filmada-Apuntes-sobre-la-historia-del-Peru-a-traves-de-tres-peliculas-1933-1961-1977 (accessed 24 July 2009).

———. 2006. Cine peruano y violencia: realidad y representación. Análisis histórico de *La boca del lobo* [Peruvian cinema and violence: Reality and representation. A historical analysis of *The Lion's Den*]. *Contratexto: Revista de la Facultad de Comunicación de la Universidad de Lima* 14: 1–5. http://www.ulima.edu.pe/revistas/contratexto/v4/art10.htm (accessed 24 July 2009).

Vargas Llosa, Mario. 1992. El nacimiento del Perú [The birth of Peru]. *Hispania: The Quincentennial of the Columbian Era* 75, no. 4: 805–11.

Vilanova, Núria. 1999. *Social change and literature in Peru (1970–1990)*. Lewiston, NY: Edwin Mellen Press.

Walker, Janet. 2005. *Trauma cinema: Documenting incest and the Holocaust*. Berkeley, Los Angeles and London: University of California Press.

———. 2008. The vicissitudes of traumatic memory and the postmodern history film. In *Trauma and cinema: Cross-cultural explorations*. Ed. E. Ann Kaplan and Ban Wang, 123–44. Hong Kong: Hong Kong University Press.

Dictatorship memories: Working through trauma in Chilean post-dictatorship documentary

Antonio Traverso

School of Media, Culture and Creative Arts, Curtin University, Perth, Australia

This essay discusses the representation of traumatic memory in Chilean post-dictatorship documentary. It argues that Chilean political memory documentaries of the post-dictatorship period, beyond their necessary depiction of the traumas and suffering of victims and survivors, consistently reveal productive attributes of life under dictatorship, such as the people's creative capacities of agency, resilience and imagination. In order to illustrate this proposition the essay offers an encompassing critical review of post-dictatorship documentaries directed by Chileans both in Chile and abroad between 1990 and 2007, focusing in particular on the films' representation of strategies of working through that counterbalance the *acting out* of suffering and damage that is characteristic of trauma cinema.

Introduction

Film production in Chile has been sustained since the early twentieth century. Locally made cinema became part of a national project of industrialization with the foundation of the state-owned film company *Chile Films* in 1941, which provided resources for large studio productions, yet collapsed by the end of the 1940s. National cinema production was reinvigorated again from the late 1950s to the early 1970s, mainly through the activities of two university film departments that achieved notable outcomes until the advent of the military regime in 1973.[1] Since the return of parliamentary democracy in 1990, the activities of independent Chilean filmmakers, both in Chile and abroad, have been supported with the establishment of Fondart (the National Fund for the Arts) in 1992,[2] the Film and Audiovisual Development Law in 2004,[3] and the National Film Archive in 2006.[4] Government financial support combined with private investment and sponsorship have resulted in an ever-increasing number of fiction and documentary films and videos made each year, with an approximate 100 programmes made in 2008 alone.[5] Alongside this exponential increase in the number of films produced in the past 20 years, there has been a growing literature in Spanish, currently establishing the scholarly coordinates of what may become the field of Chilean national cinema studies.[6]

As demonstrated by Alicia Vega (2006) and Jacqueline Mouesca (2005), the documentary tradition in Chile has always been a strong and prolific one.[7] At the same time, documentary makers have shown a recurrent interest in the depiction of national historical traumas. The most representative social documentaries of the 1960s and early 1970s, for example, focused on the suffering and resilience of Chileans in the face of structural poverty, political violence, and environmental disasters. This interest has continued in recent documentary films that address the traumatic memory of the military coup of 11 September 1973, and the 16-year dictatorship that followed. In considering Chilean documentary's engagement with the history, experience and memory of the military dictatorship, this essay expands the negligible critical scholarship on this topic available in English.[8] The essay argues that, rather than repetitively *acting out* fixed traumatic memories – often the mark of trauma cinema[9] – post-dictatorship documentary in Chile encourages strategies of representation that *work through* the memory of the damage and suffering caused by the military regime.[10]

In order to illustrate the above claim, this essay offers a critical overview of documentaries directed by Chileans both in Chile and abroad between 1990 and 2007, some of which are both well known and well theorized – Patricio Guzmán's in particular (Ruffinelli 2001, 2008; Chanan 2007; Rodriguez 2007; Cisneros 2006) – while others have never been written about. Owing to length considerations, this encompassing survey does not involve in-depth analyses of the films. Rather, it seeks to delineate a general view of the way in which Chilean documentaries have worked through the traumatic memory of the dictatorship since 1990. Prior to the critical review of Chilean films, in the next section I briefly address some of the theoretical implications of the use of methods of acting out and working through by trauma texts.

Acting out and working through in trauma texts

The political debates unleashed every time an important political memory text has reached the public in post-dictatorship Chile are not dissimilar to the debates over representation held in most post-conflict societies. Indeed, in addition to the problem of political factions arguing over the most accurate version of the past or the most correct interpretation of the meaning of historical facts that can be denied no longer, there are ethical questions that concern the purported right or capacity of writers, artists, and filmmakers to represent, or at least attempt to represent, the inexpressible suffering of victims and survivors. As E. Ann Kaplan and Ban Wang state in this regard: 'Narratives and images designed to represent traumas are viewed with suspicion, for they seem to have the seductive power to gloss over the horrendous fact and distort the literal truth of the trauma' (2004, 8). It is therefore possible to discern a dialectic between a tendency to speak out the trauma and one that compels victims to remain silent, perhaps themselves motivated by the desire, on the one hand, to move beyond trauma and, on the other, to remain within it. This dialectic is observable both at the macro level of social processes and at the micro level of therapy conducted with, for example, torture survivors and relatives of missing political detainees, such as those in Chile (see Agger and Jensen 1996; Kornfeld 1995). In classic psychoanalytic terms the objective of therapy is to help the sufferer to come to terms with the reality of the traumatic experience, while detaching themselves from it through a process of cathartic acting out and subsequent symbolization. According to Carolina Garland, Freud believed that 'if the original events are brought into consciousness and put into words (the 'talking cure'), especially if they are accompanied by the original intense feeling they provoked, then the symptoms will disappear' (2005, 249). However, Garland stresses that what makes this process problematic is the fact that sufferers use defence mechanisms when overwhelmed by traumatic symptoms. Defence mechanisms often involve physical actions, such as risky and threatening behaviour and self-destructive or self-effacing acts, which at the same time strengthen the subject's identification with or inhabitation of their trauma and produce a temporary sensation of agency and mastery over the source of threat. In therapy, this type of action mechanism is contrasted with and complemented by thought mechanisms, such as imagining, remembering, considering, reflecting, and deciding, all of which can be achieved through verbalization (250–1). The ultimate aim of therapy is, therefore, to help the sufferer 'to get his or her experiences into a form in which they can be held in the mind, *thought about* and worked over in symbolic form' (250). In other words, psychoanalysis seeks to break the cycle of repetition of the trauma by creating symbolic representations that *stand for* the traumatic events.

In studies of trauma culture a similar kind of opposition has been discussed in relation to cultural texts that seek to represent historical trauma. According to this debate, some texts (writings, art, films, performances) would tend towards the production of re-enactments of the trauma – through depictions of violence, terror, pain, confusion, and fragmentation – while others would tend towards thought and *distantiation* mechanisms – through reflective engagement with memories, fantasies, silences, and desires. Often this is referred to as the opposition between acting out and working through.[11] Kaplan and Wang explain: 'Acting out is a melancholy possession of the subject by the repressed past, on the model of the dissociated self. Dialectically, working through is an attempt of breakout' (2004, 5–6). In a widely cited essay, Dominick LaCapra produces a lengthy and detailed critical analysis of Claude Lanzmann's Holocaust documentary *Shoah* (1985), in which he argues that the Israeli director uses a *re-traumatizing* method of treating the memory of the Holocaust by almost obsessively prompting survivors and other witnesses to act out traumatic symptoms in front of the camera.[12] Lanzmann's strategy, argues LaCapra, is evidenced by the director's careful selection, and concomitant omissions, of interview subjects, who seem to appear on screen in so far as they can act as 'objects of transferential identification' (1997, 260). In this sense, for LaCapra, *Shoah*'s ultimate aim appears to be 'the incarnation, actual reliving, or compulsive acting out of the past – particularly its traumatic suffering – in the present' (1997, 4). Alternatively, LaCapra favours texts that tend to work through the trauma of the past and, in so doing, encourage the release of witnesses and audiences from the cycles of trauma transmission. In opposition to views that reject efforts to move *beyond* trauma as an implicit betrayal of the memory of a traumatic event, LaCapra clarifies at the conclusion of his essay the meaning of the concept of working through that he proposes for trauma culture. He explains: 'Working-through, of which mourning is one prominent form, should not be conflated with utopian optimism or total liberation from the past and its melancholic burdens; instead, it should be seen as a supplement and counterforce to melancholia and acting out' (269). Similarly, Garland explains that 'recovery' in psychoanalytic terms should not be understood as 'achieving a pre-trauma condition once more, but achieving a state of mind in which the event is not felt to be the only or the most significant experience in that individual's life as a whole' (2005, 246).[13] Thus, LaCapra stresses that acting out and working through are inseparable terms of the same process and that while to a degree acting out is inevitable 'it should not be isolated, theoretically fixated on, or one-sidedly valorized' (1994, 205).

Broadly speaking, most films, and other kinds of text, which deal with historical trauma tend to perform or act out traumatic memories – whether through stylistic approach, dramatization, and/or confessional or performative interviews – while to a lesser extent do they seek to work through painful memories and histories. Elsewhere I engage in a close analysis of a recent Chilean documentary that, despite inheriting much of the approach established by Lanzmann in *Shoah*, through its articulation of a dialectics between strategies of acting out and working through, arguably contributes to the process of cultural release of the cycle of historical trauma in Chile (Traverso 2009).[14] In that essay I describe that film's use of methods of acting out and working through in the following terms:

> [W]hereas acting out seeks to bring forth the reality of the trauma, for example, by asking a witness to remember what they prefer to leave as forgotten or to speak out what cannot be conveyed in words, working through consists of on-screen strategies of memory work that elaborate the witness' traumatic memory through imaginative play that reworks not only the witness' identification with their trauma but also their position in relation to a community of others who similarly suffer and seek release. (215)

Following from that earlier piece, my proposition in this essay, as expressed in the introduction, is that most Chilean documentaries of the post-dictatorship period act out not only witnessing and acting out traumatic memories but also, often by linking subjective and social experiences as well as emphasizing productive attributes of the survivors (such as agency, resilience and creativity), encourage a cultural process of working through the traumatic past of this South American nation.[15]

Indeed, since 1990 documentary cinema in Chile has contributed to the nation's broader project of recovering historical memory.[16] In these films the history of the military regime, a period that painfully ended or injured the lives of thousands, is made to intersect with the subjective memory of direct witnesses, and often the traumatic memories of the films' subjects are worked through in front of the camera.

Moreover, in these films the figure of memory is used as the link between individual suffering, which is mostly lived intimately, and the broader political culture in which the subjects are located. The films work through traumatic memory via the use of a range of strategies: speaking to people – who either knew a missing or dead person or know essential information about them – in the presence of survivors and relatives; talking to survivors and relatives at locations where they used to spend time with the missing or dead person, and/or at sites where atrocities were experienced; and having the subjects look at photographs while discussing both what they depict in the past and what memories they elicit in the present.

Therefore, a core attribute of these documentaries, as will be shown below, is the convergence between the suffering of direct witnesses of atrocity and the wider political context. As a result, the acting out of trauma that often occurs in private testimony is in these films elaborated in the process of working through traumatic memory, which is often triggered by collective political activism. An open form of collective memorialization is thus articulated in the films' depictions of public acts, in which we see members of the community embracing the painful experiences of the victims and their families.

The features of Chilean documentary described above are illustrated below in relation: firstly, to two video documentaries made in 1990, during the transition from the military regime to the first democratically elected government since 1970; secondly, to the films of two prominent Chilean documentary directors living abroad, namely, Patricio Guzmán and Patricio Henriquez; and, thirdly, to six feature-length documentaries directed by Chileans living in the country.

Political memory in Chilean video documentary

With the emergence of public political demonstrations against the dictatorship in the early 1980s, in conjunction with the new relatively easy access to video technology, numerous independent media collectives were formed in Chile.[17] As a result, countless low-budget, anti-dictatorship video documentaries were produced, which provided evidence not only of the violence of the military and the suffering of the population but also of the people's active challenge to military rule. Two video documentaries by the Proceso group, namely Andrés Vargas's *Huellas de sal* (1990) and Pablo Tupper and Patricia del Rio's

La verdadera historia de Johnny Good (1990), illustrate the deep changes affecting Chilean society by 1990. These documentaries reflect the public climate during a year in which the armed forces left the institutions of government and the new civilian president was appointed. Stylistically simple and rudimentary in terms of production, the potency of these films is in the treatment of their content, namely, the *desaparecidos* (missing political prisoners). *Huellas de sal*, for example, contains the testimony of a small group of grieving widows and mothers, who, for over a decade, have searched the dry sands of the Calama desert in northern Chile. The women have been looking for the missing remains of their husbands and sons, secretly executed by the infamous *caravana de la muerte* (death convoy) in October 1973.[18] In addition, the film goes on to depict street demonstrations in which crowds hold iconic banners with portraits of the missing, and the question *Dónde están?* (Where are they?), concluding with a public performance by a group of mothers and widows who dance the *cueca sola* (*cueca* alone).[19] *La verdadera historia de Johnny Good* (hereafter referred to as *Johnny Good*), meanwhile, displays authentic footage of the unearthing of human remains, corresponding to 20 political prisoners of the Pisagua concentration camp, who were summarily shot and buried in unmarked graves by the *caravana de la muerte*. The film also includes the testimony of relatives of the victims and of ex-prisoners of the Pisagua camp. Through the account of two former prisoners, who speak to the camera as they stand on the stage of a derelict theatre located within the camp's ruins, we understand that the film's title derives from the name of a comedy show – *El gran amor de Johnny Good* [Johnny Good's greatest love] – which was produced by a group of prisoners by order of the camp's commander to 'lift up the spirit of the rest of the camp's dwellers'. In the documentary's final scene we see images of the belated public funeral of the victims of Pisagua, in which a mass of people slowly march on the streets of the northern port-city of Iquique in 1990, carrying the 20 coffins and holding banners with the photographs and names of the dead.

The return of parliamentary democracy to Chile in March 1990 marked the commencement of a new period in the history of Chilean cinema, which can be denominated post-dictatorship cinema. *Huellas de sal* and *Johnny Good* are located on each side of the boundary between anti-dictatorship and post-dictatorship documentary, as their production took place, respectively, only months before and after the end of the military regime. Significantly, the amalgamation of past and present is a key element in these two documentaries. In fact, even though the unlawful executions of prisoners were carried out by the military in late 1973, it was only possible for the Chilean courts to effect the exhumation of remains after the military were no longer in power in 1990. This transitional element is expressed in the films' content and structure, where a contrast is visible between the present pain of survivors and victims' relatives and the belatedness implied in this looking at events that took place almost 17 years earlier. In the films, the tragedy of survivors and relatives of the missing, whose suffering never ceased in the void of denial and untruths – for example, as represented in *Huellas de sal* by the depiction of their directionless wandering in the desert – is resolved dramatically in the finding, unearthing, and re-burial of the dead.

Political memory in exilic Chilean documentary: Patricio Guzmán and Patricio Henriquez

Patricio Guzmán's *Chile: Memoria obstinada* (1997), *El caso Pinochet* (2001), and *Salvador Allende* (2004) constitute prime examples of post-dictatorship documentary made by Chileans living abroad. *Chile: Memoria obstinada* (hereafter referred to as

Memoria obstinada.) expresses its self-conscious engagement with the theme of memory not only by including the word *memoria* in its title but also by vividly documenting the recollections of witnesses and survivors. This is indeed a deeply involved on-screen exercise in working through traumatic memory. The film's first five minutes, for example, depict the dramatic clash of sensations that occur when a traumatic memory is contrasted with direct perception as a survivor returns to the site of the traumatic event after an extended period. The opening scene, in fact, contains not one but an agglomeration of returns: of the director, of his subject, and also, so to speak, of the film itself. Indeed, it is not coincidental that the film's title has been complemented with the sub-heading *La batalla de Chile IV*. In other words, this is no new film, but the continuation of Guzmán's three-part documentary epic of the early 1970s. Thus, figuratively speaking, this is the same film that returns to the site of trauma to continue from where it left off more than two decades earlier. In doing so, the film – like director Guzmán, his subjects, and a section of his audience – appears to remember its own past. To facilitate this process of remembering, *Memoria obstinada*'s memories are depicted on the screen via the regular insertion of black and white sequences from *Batalla de Chile*, which are dissolved to similar colour images in the present. For example, in the first scene after the film's opening we see Juan, an ex-member of Allende's personal guard and a survivor of the coup, wandering about inside La Moneda, Chile's presidential palace. At one point, Juan stands on the presidential balcony (from where Allende used to salute the crowds) and looks towards Plaza de la Constitución. The camera emulates his action, revealing the street below with a few passing cars and pedestrians. In the shot's immediate foreground, we see a small ornament that tops one edge of the balcony's metallic protection. Here the film dissolves into a black and white shot from *Batalla de Chile*, which is identical in its framing: we see the same balcony ornament in the middle of the frame. However, down in the Plaza, instead of the empty pavement there is a compact mass of demonstrators standing shoulder to shoulder, jumping and chanting. The archival shot is punctuated by silence and a melancholic and somewhat eerie flute-like sound that emphasizes the scene's evocation of distance and loss. Then the film dissolves back to the previous colour shot of the balcony ornament and the empty Plaza below. The technique of dissolving between archival and contemporary shots of the same location, in which angle and framing have been replicated, is used by Guzmán throughout his films time and again. The visual transition signifies a movement in time that shows both the changes and continuities of the location or subject, and that also refers more broadly to the theme of traumatic memory.

While the main theme of Guzmán's *El caso Pinochet* (hereafter referred to as *Caso Pinochet*) is the extended house arrest of the former dictator in London during 1998 and 1999 and the attempts made by a Spanish judge to have him extradited to Spain to face charges of crimes against humanity, an equally central focus is the film's witnessing of the testimonies of some of the dictatorship's survivors. The film's beginning is, in fact, strongly reminiscent of the above-mentioned *Huellas de sal* and *Johnny Good*, with wide-angled shots showing the dry Chilean desert and people walking on the sand. Yet, in addition to the relatives of the *desaparecidos*, who painfully convey their testimonies directly to the camera, in this case the group also includes a Chilean judge, forensic police, anthropologists, and other witnesses. All of them have congregated here as part of the legal procedures directed to the identification of the human remains, believed to be buried in an unmarked grave in the vicinity. In this sense, from the onset *Caso Pinochet* works through the traumatic features of witness testimonies by framing these in the context of a legal process, that is, by reinterpreting the history and memory of an unfathomable injustice in terms of the concrete possibilities of a criminal investigation. This dialectic between acting out and working through trauma is also visible in a section of the film that contains a series of interviews with survivors of atrocity. As much as these direct witnesses act out the trauma experienced, they also give expression to the agency that can be involved in suffering, which, in their testimonies, is perceived in the insightfulness, creativity, resilience, hope and dignity with which they have been able not only to survive but also to live into the future.

Salvador Allende continues the exploration of political memory in Chile found in Guzmán's earlier documentaries. In one of the film's early scenes we see a hand that peels off and then with a rock hits the external layer of grey paint on a wall beside a highway, increasingly revealing the blue colour underneath. This image is presented as a visual metaphor for Guzmán's own subjective forgetting and remembering. Then, Guzmán's film cuts to images of political mural and graffiti art from the early 1970s, covered under layers of paint and time on Santiago's street walls. Using these images metaphorically to evoke the link between an individual's trauma and a collective political memory, the film seems to imply that the partial erasure and layering of images and materials caused by time and the elements does not destroy but, on the contrary, both constitutes and enables memory, thus thwarting the dictatorship's painful but fruitless attempts at erasing the past.

Not as well known as Guzmán but definitely as prolific, Patricio Henriquez is a Chilean director who, establishing himself in Canada, has produced a long list of political documentaries dealing with issues and events of global significance. Some of Henriquez's most important titles focus on the memory of the Chilean dictatorship and, not unlike Guzmán's documentaries, rather than dwelling in the pure remembrance of traumatic experience, they emphasize the political project of establishing the truth about the dictatorship's crimes and making those responsible accountable for their actions. Among key titles by this director are: *11 de septiembre, 1973: El último combate de Salvador Allende* (1998); *Imágenes de una dictadura* (1999); *Desobediencia* (2005); and *El lado oscuro de la dama blanca* (2006). Like the other documentaries discussed in this essay, the films of Henriquez largely articulate the historical through subjective witness testimony, and always energize their material through the tension between the depiction of oppression and suffering, and the portrayal of the people's will to continue to struggle. In this sense, they constitute important documentary contributions to the process of working through traumatic memory in Chile.

El lado oscuro de la dama blanca (hereafter referred to as *Lado oscuro*) focuses on the best known of the Chilean navy's ships: the training vessel *La Esmeralda* (The Emerald). This is a large, strikingly white sailing ship, nicknamed by the sailors as *la dama blanca* (the white lady). Henriquez's film looks at 'the dark side' of the history of this ship, establishing that: '97 men and 58 women were imprisoned and tortured [aboard] in 1973' and that '[b]y 2006 no individual has been identified or charged for these acts'. As in his other documentaries, as well as focusing on the testimonies of direct witnesses to articulate the history and experience of these events, in *Lado oscuro* Henriquez pays attention to the current attempts by a group of survivors and relatives of victims to make the Chilean navy acknowledge the whole truth about the atrocities that took place aboard *La Esmeralda*, bring those responsible to justice, and offer a formal public apology to the victims and their families. Besides exploring the macabre details of the trauma of those giving testimony – in fact, throughout the film, dark, expressionist depictions of the survivors' traumatic memories are persistently contrasted with the daylight shots of *La Esmeralda* – Henriquez's *Lado oscuro* emphasizes acts of resilience, solidarity, and creativity by individuals who have survived unspeakable suffering and continuing offence at the hands of a hermetic and powerful military institution.

Political memory documentary made in Chile

Like Guzmán and Henriquez, numerous Chilean filmmakers living in Chile have addressed the theme of the memory of the dictatorship experience, exploring, on the one hand, the violence and atrocities of the Chilean military and, on the other, the people's capacity to overcome, to struggle, and to be creative. Among the most important documentaries are Silvio Caiozzi's *Fernando ha vuelto* (1998), Carmen Luz Parot's *Estadio Nacional* (2002), Pachi Bustos and Jorge Leiva's *Actores secundarios* (2004), Sebastián Moreno's *La ciudad de los fotógrafos* (2006), Lorena Giachino's *Reinalda del Carmen, mi mamá y yo* (2006), and Niles Atallah's *Memoria desierta* (2007). With their specificities and differences all these films foreground the recollections and testimonies of witnesses in order to contribute to a project of recovering historical memory while working through Chile's traumatic past.

Silvio Caiozzi's award-winning documentary *Fernando ha vuelto* focuses on the finding and identification of the remains of one of the dictatorship's *desaparecidos*. Fernando Olivares became a missing political prisoner soon after the coup, when he was 27 years of age, after being taken from his home in front of his family. In 1991 a large number of human remains were found in an unmarked mass grave at Cementerio General, Santiago's main public graveyard. After four years of work forensic scientists were able to identify Fernando's remains. Although Caiozzi's documentary carefully explores the irreversible impact that Fernando's long-lasting disappearance has caused on his extended family – this includes painful testimonies by Fernando's widow, elderly mother, and son – the film constitutes an attempt to work through this family trauma by making a film about it, thus shifting the tragedy's register from the private to the public realm.

Meanwhile, Carmen Luz Parot's *Estadio Nacional* focuses on the experience of survivors of this infamous concentration camp. Estadio Nacional (National Stadium), Chile's principal sports centre, was used by the army to imprison and interrogate more than 12,000 men and women, of whom approximately 7000 were tortured and an undetermined number summarily executed. Parot's film retraces the history of the former concentration camp through a combination of archival footage and the testimonies of several former prisoners. Following a strategy of memory work used in other Chilean documentaries, this film marks memory passages by editing together old and new footage of the same object or scenario. For example, soon after the start of the film, current aerial colour footage of the sports centre slowly dissolves into archival black and white footage of the same venue in 1973, in which we see groups of prisoners on the benches behind a wire fence. From a shot of one of the stadium's light towers, the film dissolves from the black and white archival footage to a colour shot of exactly the same light tower in the present. Following another strategy of memory work established as an attribute of post-dictatorship documentary, in *Estadio Nacional* testimonies are prompted by paying on-screen visits with the survivors to the specific spaces of confinement, interrogation, and torture within the stadium's installations. In addition, while the witnesses narrate the immediate recollections triggered by the locations, their accounts are supported by archival stills and film footage. In one scene, for example, an ex-prisoner of the stadium takes the filmmaker to the section where he was kept captive. Archival footage is inserted that replicates the same dark corridors. He points at the walls, recalling that they used to be covered with stories, thoughts, and loose expressions carved by the prisoners with sharp objects, stones, or their own fingernails. He wonders if they would not be found underneath the layers of paint. In fact, soon he finds and reads visible inscriptions, mostly initials and dates, underneath the beige paint. Significantly, this scene makes this film resemble

Memoria obstinada, where director Guzmán, like an archaeologist of political memory, scratches a wall's paint to reveal old layers with graffiti from the 1970s. At one point *Estadio Nacional* dwells in the acting out of trauma by including the testimonies of men and women who survived torture and rape. Acting out in these sequences refers to the moment of bodily revelation of the trauma or horror by the witness in front of the camera, often manifested in the breakdown of the capacity for logical thought and linguistic expression. However, the film soon opens up to a mode of elaboration of (or working through) the traumatic recollections, consisting in playful, collective dramatizations of past traumatic events, followed by group discussion and personal reflection.

Pachi Bustos and Jorge Leiva's *Actores secundarios* is another formidable example of Chile's culture of political memory, through which political communities remember their experience of the dictatorship and, in this way, work through their common traumatic past. As an audiovisual document, Bustos and Leiva's film contributes to Chile's process of recovering its historical memory by foregrounding the crucial role of high school students as a prime, rather than *secondary*, social actor in the struggle against the dictatorship during the decade of the 1980s. The film thus bears witness to the fearless and idealistic disposition with which masses of teenagers wearing school uniform and carrying notebooks under their arms fought face to face against anti-riot police on central city streets. Since the film's writer-directors were themselves high school activists during that period, they focus on the history of this movement through the testimonies of many of their immediate peers, as well as through abundant archival video and photographs. The film's way of approaching its topic from the perspective of collective memory rather than simply as a historical report is exercised mainly through interviews with men and women who remember their times as teenage activists almost two decades earlier. In addition, most of the interviews are done not with individuals but with small groups of three or four friends who reminisce as they walk through their old school or sit at what used to be one of their usual cafés. In some cases, friends have not seen each other since leaving high school and so the film captures the current excitement of the reunion, which at the same time intensifies the memory work in front of the camera. Not unlike the re-enactment scene in *Estadio Nacional*, as referred to above, in one of the final sections of *Actores secundarios*, a large group of former high school students gather on the street outside their old school and symbolically re-stage a historic school occupation, to the extent of one of them giving instructions through a megaphone, as they did all those years ago. After this action they sit on the street outside the school and talk to the camera and to each other, while remembering the details of that day. Scenes such as these in *Estadio Nacional* and *Actores secundarios* effectively constitute ritualized memorial acts that work through the nation's traumatic past.

Likewise, Sebastián Moreno's *La ciudad de los fotógrafos*, whose central theme is political photography taken during the peak of the dictatorship in the 1980s, depicts the traumatic aspects of military repression, but consistently places the emphasis on the bellicose response of Chilean activists on street demonstrations. Meanwhile, Lorena Giachino's *Reinalda del Carmen, mi mamá y yo* is structured as a first-person documentary narration in which the director turns the camera on her own mother.[20] Giachino's film follows a personal trajectory that moves from traumatic memory through a belated mourning and towards the promise of healing and renewal. However, this is not a private document for the family's perusal alone but a powerful public document that addresses the historical and political dimensions of the relationship of the film's subjects to the dictatorship period, and encourages a process of working through this traumatic past.

Finally, Niles Atallah's *Memoria desierta* is a short, low-budget documentary that pays attention to the memory of the Chacabuco concentration camp, a site located in Chile's northern desert, where hundreds of people were kept as political prisoners in the aftermath of the coup.[21] Following strategies already established by earlier documentaries, Atallah's film explores the memory of the former camp through the testimonies of ex-prisoners, who recall both their traumatic and creative experiences. For example, in a scene reminiscent of *Memoria obstinada* and *Estadio Nacional*, one of the witnesses tries to find the marks and inscriptions that prisoners used to make on the walls. Like other documentaries, *Memoria desierta* contributes to Chile's project of recovering its historical political memory by exploring a specific and hardly known chapter of the dictatorship period. However, also following a general direction in post-dictatorship documentary rather than dwelling on the repetition of traumatic recollections, it accentuates the creativity, resilience and commitment of survivors to work through their traumatic experiences in the present.

Conclusion

This essay has considered the attention given by Chilean post-dictatorship documentaries to the history, experience and memory of the period of the military regime. It has argued that where Chilean documentaries may appear to be fixated with acting out traumatic memories of the military dictatorship, more often than not they work through the memory of the pain and suffering of that period. In order to illustrate its claim the essay has delineated a broad critical review of documentaries directed by Chileans both in Chile and abroad between 1990 and 2007.

The essay has expanded the scarce scholarship available in English about the continuing attention devoted by Chilean cinema to the traumatic memory of the military period. In doing so, it is hoped that the essay contributes to Chile's public process of working through, as the nation deepens its attempts to come to terms with its traumatic past. Although length restrictions have not made it possible to address the important issue of the reception of these films by Chilean audiences (the discussion has necessarily focused on the films as text), an analysis of the question of spectatorship in relation to these documentaries may suggest that the films invite their audiences to a public, open process of release from cycles of transmission of cultural trauma by elaborating multiple modalities for witnessing and working through the nation's traumatic past.

Notes

1. On the history of the film school of Universidad de Chile, see Salinas and Stange (2008); and on the history of the film institute of Universidad Católica, see the fourth chapter in Cavallo and Díaz (2007).
2. In 2009 the audiovisual section of Fondart allocated funds to the tune of one thousand million pesos (approximately, US$2.5 million) to eleven feature film projects, five of which are documentaries; see Fondart's website (Spanish): www.consejodelacultura.cl/fondosdecultura/
3. Ley del Fomento del Cine y el Audiovisual (No. 19.981, November 2004); see full text of the law (Spanish) at: www.leychile.cl/Navegar?idNorma=232277
4. Cineteca Nacional: www.cinetecanacional.cl; www.ccplm.cl
5. See online a recent economic and demographic report on Chile's cultural industries, *Cultural Industries Profile – Chile*, prepared for the Department of Canadian Heritage by Rafael Otano and Patricia Hidalgo at: Chile_culturl_industries_jan_2007-eng[1].pdf
6. For a succinct summary (Spanish) of the essential historiographic studies of Chilean cinema, see Vásquez (2000).

7. Besides the titles by Mouesca (2005) and Vega (2006), see the following Spanish sources on Chilean documentary: Ruffinelli (2001, 2008), Corro et al. (2007) and Donoso (2007).
8. For sources in English see Pino-Ojeda and Ortega (2009), Traverso (2009), Chanan (1976, 2007), Rodriguez (2007), Cisneros (2006), Wayne (2001), Pick (1987) and Coad (1980).
9. I am using the expression coined by Janet Walker in her influential 2005 book.
10. Unless otherwise indicated, in the remainder of the essay 'documentary' is used to denote 'Chilean post-dictatorship political memory documentary', that is, political documentary films and videos made in 1990 and after, that thematize the experience of the military period.
11. On *acting out* and *working through* see the conclusion in LaCapra (1994); the introduction in Kaplan and Wang (2004); Walker (2005); and Hirsch's essay in Kaplan and Wang (2004).
12. Several scholars have disagreed with LaCapra's critique of *Shoah* (see, for example, Hirsch's essay in Kaplan and Wang 2004). The counter-argument can be broadly summarized thus: even though the film clearly engages in prompting traumatic acting out, its broader cultural and historical function is one of encouraging a process of working through the trauma of the Holocaust, which until then had been misrepresented, silenced, or denied. LaCapra's essay, however, anticipates such criticism by acknowledging the crucial significance of the film, both historical and aesthetic, and explaining in detail the rationale of his criticism.
13. Aor. Konrad Brendler defines *working through* as 'the gradual assimilation of overwhelming conflicttype [*sic*] experiences which the psychic organism initially rejects and in the long run suppresses if there is no adequate psychic basis and support for processing the impressions' (1995, 250).
14. Also see Traverso (2008), where I propose a similar argument in relation to two Chilean narrative films.
15. The material for this and my two previously cited essays is drawn from an in-progress monograph provisionally entitled 'Dictatorship screens: Chilean cinema, politics, and traumatic memory', where I analyse both documentary and narrative films that thematize Chile's military dictatorship period.
16. While the main events are fairly well known, here is a summary for the uninitiated: socialist president Salvador Allende was ousted by a US-backed military coup lead by General Augusto Pinochet in 1973. Allende and many of his supporters died on the day of the coup and for the next 16 years of dictatorship an estimated 3000 political opponents died, while hundreds of thousands suffered state-sponsored exile, imprisonment, violence, and torture. Pinochet's regime ended in 1990, with the beginning of the current period of parliamentary democracy; see Dorfman (2003) and Constable and Valenzuela (1991).
17. Among the most prolific media collectives of the 1980s were: Ictus, Proceso, Eco, Canelo de Nos, Más Media, and Nueva Imagen. While most groups disappeared soon after the end of the military regime in 1990, among the successful survivors are: Ictus, one of Chile's principal theatre companies originally founded in 1955 (http://www.teatroictus.cl/); and Nueva Imagen, founded towards the end of the dictatorship in 1989, which has become one of Chile's most important independent film and television production houses (http://www.nuevaimagen.cl/). Also see the U-Matic Project website (http://www.umatic.cl/index.html), which contains a comprehensive list of independent video productions made in Chile from the 1970s to 1990s, including a selection of clips.
18. The phrase *caravana de la muerte* was coined in Chile to refer to a group of military officers led by General Sergio Arellano who travelled by helicopter after the coup, visiting concentration camps, summarily executing prisoners whose names appeared on a death list, and then hiding or destroying their remains.
19. This is a well-known organization of mothers and widows of the *desaparecidos*, similar to Argentina's *Madres de la Plaza de Mayo*, who as a way of drawing public attention to the issue of missing political detainees in Chile danced the *cueca*, the Chilean national dance (traditionally danced by a couple), without a partner. The British pop singer Sting famously dedicated the song 'They Dance Alone' to them.
20. See my in-depth analysis of *Reinalda del Carmen* in Traverso (2009), from which this paragraph is adapted.
21. *Memoria desierta* was produced as part of a cultural memory project called *The Chacabuco Project* (www.chacabuco.org). Another documentary, *La sombra de don Roberto* (2007), also looks at the memory of the Chacabuco camp through a slow-paced conversation amidst the camp's ruins with one of the survivors, Roberto Zaldívar.

References

Agger, Inger, and Soren Jensen. 1996. *Trauma and healing under state terrorism*. London and Atlantic Highlands, NJ: Zed Books.

Brendler, Aor. Konrad. 1995. Working through the Holocaust: Still a task for Germany's youth? In *Beyond trauma: Cultural and societal dynamics*, ed. Rolf Kleber, Charles Figley, and Berthold Gersons, 249–75. New York and London: Plenum Press.

Cavallo, Ascanio, and Carolina Díaz. 2007. *Explotados y benditos: mito y desmitificacion del cine chileno de los 60*. Santiago: Uqbar Editores.

Chanan, Michael, ed. 1976. *Chilean cinema*. London. British Film Institute.

———. 2007. *The politics of documentary*. London: British Film Institute.

Cisneros, James. 2006. The figure of memory in Chilean cinema: Patricio Guzmán and Raúl Ruiz. *Journal of Latin American Cultural Studies* 15, no. 1: 59–75.

Coad, Malcolm. 1980. Rebirth of Chilean cinema. *Index on Censorship* 9, no. 2: 3–8. Repr. in Ruth Petrie, ed. 1997. *Film and censorship: The index reader*. Washington, DC and London: Cassell.

Constable, Pamela, and Arturo Valenzuela. 1991. *A nation of enemies: Chile under Pinochet*. New York: Norton.

Corro, Pablo, Carolina Larraín, Maite Alberdi, and Camila Van Diest. 2007. *Teorías del cine documental chileno 1957–1973*. Santiago: Pontificia Universidad Católica de Chile.

Donoso, Catalina. 2007. *Películas que escuchan*. Buenos Aires: Corregidor.

Dorfman, Ariel, et al., eds. 2003. *Chile: The other September 11*. London: Global.

Garland, Carolina. 2005. Trauma and the possibility of recovery. In *Introducing psychoanalysis: Essential themes and topics*, ed. Susan Budd and Richard Rusbridger, 246–61. London and New York: Routledge.

Kaplan, E. Ann, and Ban Wang, eds. 2004. *Trauma and cinema: Cross-cultural explorations*. Hong Kong: Hong Kong University Press.

Kornfeld, Elizabeth. 1995. The development of treatment approaches for victims of human rights violations in Chile. In *Beyond trauma: Cultural and societal dynamics*, ed. Rolf Kleber, Charles Figley, and Berthold Gersons, 115–31. New York and London: Plenum Press.

LaCapra, Dominick. 1994. *Representing the Holocaust: History, theory, trauma*. Ithaca, NY: Cornell University Press.

———. 1997. Lanzmann's *Shoah*: 'Here there is no why'. *Critical Inquiry* 23, no. 2: 231–69.

Mouesca, Jacqueline. 2005. *El documental chileno*. Santiago: LOM Ediciones.

Pick, Zuzana. 1987. Chilean cinema: Ten years of exile (1973–83). *Jump Cut: A Review of Contemporary Media* 32 (April): 66–70.

Pino-Ojeda, Walescka, and Mariana Ortega. 2009. Latent image: Chilean cinema and the abject. *Latin American Perspectives* 36, no. 5: 133–46.

Rodriguez, Juan Carlos. 2007. The post-dictatorial documentaries of Patricio Guzman: *Chile, Obstinate Memory*; *The Pinochet Case* and *Island of Robinson Crusoe*. PhD diss., Duke University.

Ruffinelli, Jorge. 2001. *Patricio Guzmán*. Madrid: Cátedra/Filmoteca Española.

———. 2008. *El cine de Patricio Guzmán: en busca de las imágenes verdaderas*. Santiago: Uqbar Editores.

Salinas, Claudio, and Hans Stange. 2008. *Historia del cine experimental en la Universidad de Chile 1957–1973*. Santiago: Uqbar Editores.

Traverso, Antonio. 2008. Contemporary Chilean cinema and traumatic memory: Andrés Wood's *Machuca* and Raúl Ruiz's *Le domaine perdu*. *IM: Interactive Media* 4. http://nass.murdoch.edu.au/nass_im_ejournal.htm

———. 2009. Working through trauma in post-dictatorial Chilean documentary: Lorena Giachino's *Reinalda del Carmen*. In *People, place and power: Regional and international perspectives*, ed. Dawn Bennett, Jaya Earnest, and Miyume Tanji, 262–90. Perth, WA: Black Swan Press.

Vásquez, David. 2000. El cine chileno en sus libros: breve panorama histórico. *PCLA* 1, no. 4. http://www2.metodista.br/unesco/PCLA/revista4/artigo%204-1.htm

Vega, Alicia. 2006. *Itinerario del cine documental chileno 1900–1990*. Santiago: Universidad Alberto Hurtado.

Walker, Janet. 2005. *Trauma cinema: Documenting incest and the Holocaust*. Berkeley: University of California Press.

Wayne, Mike. 2001. *Political film: The dialectics of third cinema*. London: Pluto.

Filmography

11 de septiembre, 1973: El último combate de Salvador Allende [11 September 1973: The last battle of Salvador Allende]. Directed by Patricio Henríquez. Canada/France: produced by Macumba International and Méditerranée Film Production, 1998.

Actores secundarios [Secondary actors]. Directed by Pachi Bustos and Jorge Leiva. Chile: produced by Ensenãnza Media and Fondart, 2004.

La Batalla de Chile [The battle of Chile]. Directed and produced by Patricio Guzmán. Chile/Cuba, 1975–1977.

El Caso Pinochet [The Pinochet case]. Directed by Patricio Guzmán. France/Spain: produced by Renn Productions and Patricio Guzmán Producciones, 2001.

Chile: Memoria obstinada. La batalla de Chile IV [Chile: obstinate memory. The Battle of Chile IV]. Directed by Patricio Guzmán. France/Canada: produced by Les Films d'Ici and the National Board of Canada, 1997.

La Ciudad de los fotógrafos [City of photographers]. Directed by Sebastián Moreno. Chile: produced by Películas del Pez, 2006.

Desobediencia [Disobedience]. Directed by Patricio Henriquez. Canada: produced by Macumba International, 2005.

Estadio Nacional [National Stadium]. Directed by Carmen Luz Parot. Chile: produced by Fondart and CORFO, 2002.

Fernando ha vuelto [Fernando is back]. Directed by Silvio Caiozzi. Chile: produced by Andrea Films, 1998.

Huellas de sal [Trails of salt]. Directed by Andrés Vargas. Chile: Grupo Proceso, 1990.

Imágenes de una dictadura [Images of a dictatorship]. Directed by Patricio Henriquez. Canada: produced by Macumba International, 1999.

El Lado oscuro de la dama blanca [The dark side of the white lady]. Directed by Patricio Henriquez. Canada: produced by Macumba International, 2006.

Memoria desierta [Deserted memory]. Directed by Niles Atallah. Chile: produced by Diluvio, Ministerio de Relaciones Exteriores and Goethe Institut, 2007.

Reinalda del Carmen, mi mamá y yo [Reinalda del Carmen, my mum and I]. Directed by Lorena Giachino. Chile, 2006.

Salvador Allende. Directed by Patricio Guzmán. France/Spain: produced by JBA Production and Patricio Guzmán Producciones, 2004.

Shoah. Directed by Claude Lanzmann. France: produced by Films Aleph and Historia Film, 1985.

La Sombra de don Roberto. Directed and produced by Hakan Engstrom and Juan Diego Spoerer. Chile/Sweden, 2007.

La Verdadera historia de Johnny Good [The true story of Johnny Good]. Directed by Pablo Tupper and Patricia del Rio. Chile: produced by Grupo Proceso, 1990.

Index

Page numbers in **Bold** represent figures.

Emotions and Human Mobility

This book provides insights into the emotional dimensions of human mobility. Drawing on findings and theoretical discussions in anthropology, sociology, cultural studies, philosophy, linguistics, migration studies, human geography and political science, the authors offer interdisciplinary perspectives on a highly topical debate, asking how 'emotions' can be conceptualised as a tool to explore human mobility.

Emotions and Human Mobility investigates how emotional processes are shaped by migration, and vice versa. To what extent are people's feelings about migration influenced by structural possibilities and constraints such as immigration policies or economic inequality? How do migrants interact emotionally with the people they meet in the receiving countries, and how do they attach to new surroundings? How do they interact with 'the locals', with migrants from other countries, and with migrants from their own homeland? How do they stay in touch with absent kin? The volume focuses on specific cases of migration within Europe, intercontinental mobility, and diasporic dynamics.

Critically engaging with the affective turn in the study of migration, *Emotions and Human Mobility* will be highly relevant to scholars involved in current theoretical debates on human mobility. Providing grounded ethnographic case studies that show how theory arises from concrete historical cases, the book is also highly accessible to students of courses on globalisation, migration, transnationalism and emotion.

This book was originally published as a special issue of the *Journal of Ethnic and Migration Studies.*

Maruška Svašek is Reader at the School of History and Anthropology, Queens University, Belfast, and Co-Director of the Cultural Dynamics and Emotions Network (CDEN). Her research interests include emotions, migration, material culture and ageing. Recent publications include *Moving Subjects, Moving Objects: Transnationalism, Cultural Productions and Emotions* (2012), *Anthropology, Art and Cultural Production* (2007), and *Postsocialism: Politics and Emotions in Central and Eastern Europe* (2006).

Emotions and Human Mobility

Ethnographies of Movement

Edited by
Maruška Svašek

Routledge
Taylor & Francis Group
LONDON AND NEW YORK

First published 2012
by Routledge
2 Park Square, Milton Park, Abingdon, Oxon OX14 4RN

Simultaneously published in the USA and Canada
by Routledge
711 Third Avenue, New York, NY 10017

Routledge is an imprint of the Taylor & Francis Group, an informa business

This book is a reproduction of the *Journal of Ethnic and Migration Studies*, volume 36, issue 6. The Publisher requests to those authors who may be citing this book to state, also, the bibliographical details of the special issue on which the book was based.

British Library Cataloguing in Publication Data
A catalogue record for this book is available from the British Library

ISBN13: 978-0-415-50760-8

Typeset in Garamond
by Taylor & Francis Books

Publisher's Note
The publisher would like to make readers aware that the chapters in this book may be referred to as articles as they are identical to the articles published in the special issue. The publisher accepts responsibility for any inconsistencies that may have arisen in the course of preparing this volume for print.

MIX
Paper from responsible sources
FSC www.fsc.org FSC® C004839

Printed and bound in Great Britain by the MPG Books Group

Contents

Notes on contributors

Petra Andits recently completed her PhD in the School of Philosophy, Anthropology and Cultural Inquiry at the University of Melbourne, Australia.

Aleksandra Galasińska is Senior Research Fellow in European Studies at the University of Wolverhampton, UK.

Alexandra Hall is Lecturer in the Department of Politics at the University of York, UK.

Timm Lau recently completed his PhD in Social Anthropology at King's College, Cambridge, and has been awarded a Postdoctoral Fellowship at the University of Calgary, Canada, by the AXA Research Fund.

Naoko Maehara is PhD Candidate in the School of History and Anthropology at Queen's University, Belfast.

Katy Radford is Research Fellow in the School of Sociology, Social Policy and Social Work at Queen's University, Belfast.

Maruška Svašek is Reader in the School of History and Anthropology at Queen's University, Belfast, and Co-Director of the Cultural Dynamics and Emotions Network.

Amanda Wise is Senior Research Fellow at the Centre for Research on Social Inclusion, Macquarie University, Australia.

Emotions and Human Mobility: Key Concerns

Maruška Svašek

This introduction discusses some of the major developments in the study of emotions, and suggests ways in which various theories and perspectives might be relevant to the study of migration. It looks in particular at the study of social interaction between migrants and members of local communities, and to the study of interaction within transnational families. It addresses a number of questions, namely: What are emotions? How are emotional processes shaped by migration? To what extent are these dynamics influenced by structural possibilities or constraints such as immigration policies or economic inequality? How do migrants interact emotionally with the people they meet in reception countries, and what is the nature of the attachments they make with their new surroundings? How do they maintain contact with their absent kin? In what ways do migrant organisations and institutions frame migrant experiences, provide support, increase their sense of belonging, or influence and implement government policies? In summarising current debates, this introduction will outline the different approaches used by contributors to this volume, while also drawing on research conducted by the author on the Sudeten Germans. It concludes with some suggestions for further research.

This edited volume contributes to a growing field of interdisciplinary research that explores how emotional processes shape human mobility and vice versa. Recent research on the emotional dimensions of human mobility has covered a wide variety of topics,[1] raising a number of significant questions. Fundamentally, how can we conceptualise emotions that are in essence both physical and metaphysical, to create a better understanding of human mobility? To what extent are the emotions of migrants influenced by structural constraints, for example by immigration policies or economic inequality? How do migrants interact emotionally with the people they meet in their adopted countries? To what extent do migrants stay attached to their homeland? How do migrant organisations provide emotional support for their clients, or increase their sense of belonging in their new, unfamiliar environment? What role do religious and educational institutions play in the emotional interactions both within and between migrant groups, or between migrants and locals?

A few examples from my own fieldwork conducted in Northern Ireland help to illustrate the power of emotional dynamics at play in migrant lives. The decision to emigrate can trigger very different feelings in those who have opted to leave and those who are left behind. Conflicting emotions, including excitement, anger, fear, guilt, hope and joy, can arise prior to leaving as demonstrated by the statement of a 23-year-old female Polish migrant worker whom I interviewed in Belfast in 2007:

> [When I told my parents I wanted to move to Ireland] they were shocked and worried. Though I'm an adult they said I was too young. I just said 'I'm going'. My mother tried to talk me out of it but my father and uncle said I should go because I could have a better life.

In this Polish case, the emotional interactions occurred within the context of kin relations in which the different actors attempted to influence each other's feelings, demonstrating that emotional processes are often central to sociality. As Brian Parkinson (1995: 170) noted, '[o]ur emotional attitudes to one another are part of the continual redefinition of ongoing relationships'.

The following quote from a 37-year-old female Singaporean migrant, who recently settled with her husband in Northern Ireland, illustrates how migrants confronted with anti-foreign sentiment might respond emotionally to such experiences:

> I once walked with my husband in the city centre. We met some girls, Goths, and they called me 'Chinese prostitute'. I was furious. They are not only ignorant but are also making a public display of it. Why would they try to ruin someone else's life with that? (2007)

The experience of discrimination triggered a strong emotional reaction. This individual, a university graduate who had completed an English literature degree in Australia, and who was outspoken about issues such as emancipation and oppression, clearly felt insulted and outraged once again at the mere recollection of the event. As a member of a minority group in Northern Ireland, it was not easy for her to raise public awareness of such xenophobic attitudes, but it did in fact motivate her to produce a documentary about racism in Northern Ireland that was broadcast on national television. Translating her own emotional distress into a public statement about discrimination, she succeeded in engaging with what has been called 'the politics of emotions' (Lutz and Abu-Lughod 1990; Svašek 2006).

The need to keep good relationships with relatives in the homeland can also require conscious emotional management. A 37-year-old female Chinese migrant from Beijing, who has lived in England and Northern Ireland for over 10 years, noted in 2007:

> When we go to China I must make sure to keep all the relatives happy, so we always visit my own and my husband's family. I always buy them exactly the same gifts.

In order to avoid accusations of favouritism, she used identical forms of gift-giving as a way of demonstrating equal appreciation for relatives on both sides of the family, identifying herself as 'fair and loyal kin'. In this case, emotional practice clearly functioned as an identity claim, reinforcing a specific moral discourse of proper transnational kinwork. Migrants often invest much time and effort in the 'emotion work' (Hochschild 1983) necessary to maintain reciprocal exchange relations and sustain a 'sense of family' across distance (Baldassar 2007: 392; see also Baldassar 2008; Baldassar et al. 2006; Ramirez et al. 2007; Ryan 2008; Velayutham and Wise 2005; Wilding 2006).

The three case studies presented earlier show that emotional processes are part and parcel of human mobility. Even though we should be careful not to designate

'migrants' as an exclusive kind of mobile people, as mobility-related feelings are of course shared by migrants and non-migrants alike, it should nevertheless be acknowledged that certain emotional processes are caused by migration-specific issues (Skrbiš 2008; Svašek 2008: 215). These processes do not take place in the isolated minds/bodies of migrants, but arise in the interaction of individuals with their human and non-human surroundings.

This book will explore two major processes, namely the often multiple emotional attachments of migrants to their homelands and new places of residence, and the emotional interactions between migrants and members of local communities. As the contributions that follow will demonstrate, these two themes are strongly connected and should be analysed in tandem. There are many ways in which these two levels of analysis may be interlinked. Encounters between locals and newcomers may, for example, stimulate or discourage migrant from identifying with their new surroundings. Migrants with a strong 'ethnic' presence in their adopted country may also anger, frighten or attract particular members of the local population, resulting for instance in avoidance, attacks, intermarriage or other such emotionally charged acts.

Emotional Processes in a World of Movement

Before discussing the individual contributions to this book, I shall further outline its theoretical position in the field of ethnic and migration studies. The central assumption of all contributors is that, if we want to unravel and understand the social, economic, political and experiential complexities of human mobility and belonging, it is necessary to include a focus on emotional dynamics. As argued by David Conradson and Deirdre McKay (2007: 172; see also Aranda 2003; Gray 2008), '[f]ar from being a secondary or unimportant dimension of mobility [. . .] affect and emotion are central aspects of international migration'. Yet what are emotional dynamics? How can we define emotions and use the perspective to create better insights into migration-related issues?

In earlier work, I have argued that it is useful to regard emotions as dynamic processes through which individuals experience and interpret the changing world, position themselves vis-à-vis others, and shape their subjectivities (Svašek 2005, 2006, 2008; Svašek and Skrbiš 2007). The self, in this perspective, is regarded neither as a closed container of passions nor as an entity that simply reacts to forces from outside, but rather as a mobile, multiple, relational being-in-the-world that is captured by his or her surroundings, engaging with past, present and future situations. Taking 'the affective turn' (Clough and Halley 2007), scholars such as Giles Deleuze, Félix Guattari, Brian Massumi and Baruch Spinoza have employed the notion of 'affect' to explore how bodies, things and other phenomena, conceptualized as field of intensity and impact, work on one another. In the Spinozian understanding of affect, there is 'no longer a subject, but only individuating affective states of an anonymous force' (Spinoza, quoted by Alliez 2004: 27). Agreeing with Nigel Thrift (2008: 13), however, I would argue that while the idea of fixed selves, living in predetermined stable environments must be replaced the notion of mutually constituting forces, it would be unproductive to completely loose a focus on the human subject (see Svašek 2005).

Interested in the dynamics of human mobility and emotions, David Conradson and Deidre McKay (2007: 236) have suggested making a distinction between 'affect' and 'emotion', defining emotions as 'the self-conscious recognition, experience and

interpretation of various bodily affects'. As will become clear in the following chapters, the contributors to this book take various perspectives on emotional dynamics, with some appropriating the concept of 'affect', and others employing other theoretical frameworks. Crucially, the overall approach in this book acknowledges that emotional encounters are not only shaped by direct interaction with others, but also by memories and imagination (Casey 1987; Tonkin 2006). Certain events in the past, such as a happy childhood or the experience of bullying at school, can have a long-lasting impact on one's self-image and attitude towards others. Traumatic events, such as rape or torture, can result in mental and physical breakdown, social isolation, memory loss or compulsive memory, and may become central to a group's identity politics (Kramer et al. 1984; Krystal 1995; Leydesdorff 1992; Leys 2000; Svašek 2005). The 'others' in emotional encounters are not only other human beings, but might also include animals, landscapes, material objects, images or events that affect people emotionally. From an experiential point of view, engagements with other human beings are, of course, in many ways different to interactions with non-human phenomena. The multi-sensorial and interactive experience of spending the night with a lover, for example, cannot easily be compared with the mainly visual experience of adoring a beautiful painting. Even though material things such as cars or paintings may have secondary emotional agency and a real emotional impact on the user or viewer (Gell 1998; Walker 1999) they have no autonomous mind or will, lack the ability to communicate through speech, and are mostly unable to move independently. Yet objects, images, tastes and smells may come to 'stand for' particular human others, for example when a daughter wears the jewellery of her deceased mother. Multi-sensorial engagement with 'things from home' may be an important way for migrants to have inner dialogues with the absent homeland and create a sense of belonging (Burrell 2008; Fortier 2000; Svašek 2008: 221).

In this context, it is vital to realise that individuals do not need to share space or time to react emotionally to one another's existence. A man may meet his best friend in a restaurant, or a girl may play enthusiastically with her pet hamster. In both cases, physical co-presence is part and parcel of the event. Yet someone may get nervous about meeting an opponent the next day, anticipating problems, or may get butterflies in the stomach just thinking about a lover. In both cases, the 'target' of emotional engagement is absent and active as 'inner presence'. The experiential differences between actual, remembered and imagined emotional encounters must, of course, be acknowledged (see Svašek 2000). This is also crucial in the analysis of migration where, in transnational social networks, the tension between physical proximity and physical absence is an important part of the experience. In addition, in the case of local/newcomer dynamics, the distinction between emotional processes based on ideas about others, and experiences of actual interaction must also be made clear. As some of the contributions to this volume will demonstrate, local people's ideas of migrant others and migrants' ideas of local others may be informed by misinformation or one-sided press reports. Such misunderstandings may be reinforced or undermined through actual engagement.

Emotions as Discourses, Practices and Embodied Experiences

It can be useful to define emotional processes as discourses, practices and embodied experiences (Svašek 2005, 2008). At an empirical level, these theoretical perspectives are of course interrelated, but for analytical purposes it is helpful to separate them as they emphasise distinct processes (Svašek and Skrbiš 2007). The perspective of 'discourse' outlines how cultural categories of emotions, and the notion of emotivity itself, produce knowledge about the world and the self that is often historically and group specific. The viewpoint of 'practice' draws attention to the performative nature of emotions, in terms of both unconscious, learned behaviour and the more deliberate politics of emotions. The outlook of 'embodied experience' explores physical aspects of emotional experience, in particular the perceptual process of bodily sensation and interpretation, and the interaction of bodies in space (Csordas 1994; Lyon 1995). Various authors have stressed that emotions can be physically overwhelming, and may be hard to manage or control in certain circumstances. This implies that the experiential reality of, for example, overpowering fear, devastating grief, or irresistible attraction cannot be fully explained through discursive analysis alone, nor by an exploration of performed rules that are group specific (Bourdieu 1977; Leavitt 1996; Lock 1993).

I shall illustrate this approach with an example from my research on ethnic Germans who were expelled from Czechoslovakia after the Second World War in 1945–47, namely the Sudeten Germans.[2] As will also be further explored in Chapter 9, many Sudeten Germans, in particular those old enough to vividly remember the expulsion, have produced emotional discourses that construct the 'lost homeland' as an object of love, longing, and suffering (Fendl 2002), as demonstrated by the following poem entitled 'Far lies the land':[3]

Far lies the land that used to be my homeland,	*Fern liegt das Land, das meine Heimat war,*
The hand of war broke the holy altar	*Des Krieges Hand zerbrach den heiligen Altar,*
That my forefathers, in the course of time,	*Den meine Väter in der Zeiten Lauf*
Built for me and the future.	*Bauten für mich und alle Zukunft auf.*
Destitute lies the village, silenced is the language	*Verödet liegt das Dorf, verstummt das Wort,*
Given to me by my mother for consolation.	*Das mir die Mutter gab zu Trost und Hort,*
My father's house shot at and burnt,	*Mein Vaterhaus zerschossen und verbrannt,*
And strangers live in the homeland.	*Und Fremde hausen auf dem Heimatland.*
I love people and all creatures,	*Ich liebe Mensch und alle Kreatur,*
Nature gave us all equal rights,	*Zu gleichem Recht gebar uns die Natur,*
But my heart cries out intensely to heaven,	*Doch daß mein Herz zum Himmel brünstig schreit*
This time owes us justice and freedom!	*Um Recht und Freiheit, schuldet diese Zeit!*
I hear the song of the forests in the homeland,	*Ich hör' der Heimat Wälder Wipfellied,*
That reaches deep into my soul;	*Das bis zu mir in meine Seele zieht;*
My child, do you hear the ancient sound?	*Mein Kind, hörst du den urweltlichen Klang?*
So join in with my song of freedom!	*So stimmt mit ein in meiner Freiheitssang!*

This poem, written by the expellee Emil Magerl in 1947, was published in 1949 in the *Tachauer Pfraumberger Heimat*.[4] The monthly 'homeland letter' (*Heimatbrief*) was published in the Bavarian city of Weiden by expellees from the Egerland area.

In general, the *Heimat* (homeland) discourse in the publication makes a strong connection between love, longing and suffering, exemplified by the poem. Love for the homeland, in this case, is imagined as a natural attachment between people and territory, a legitimate and sacred connection that is fundamental to their sense of belonging. According to this logic, separation from the homeland is unnatural and immoral and causes painful longing and intense suffering. Interestingly, the homeland is also depicted as a suffering entity that similarly longs for the return of the expellees. Characteristic of blood-and-soil (*Blut und Boden*) ideology, the poem personifies the homeland, blurring subjec–object distinctions between 'the land' and 'the people'. The forests are said to be 'singing' to the expellees, urging them to come back home.

Love-for-the-homeland discourses, central in expellee poetry, have often been politicised, offering a highly selective account of the past by depicting the Sudeten Germans as a collective group of victims. They tend to leave out references to the historical reasons for the expulsion: the widespread Sudeten German support for, and active involvement with, the Nazi regime during the annexation of the Sudetenland and the events that followed during the Second World War. Tellingly, the poem refers only vaguely to 'the hand of war', avoiding a more critical perspective and historical details. The expulsion is simply depicted as a wrong which should be righted by divine intervention ('my heart screams to heaven'). As such, the poem creates a space for readers to feel 'love-longing-suffering' as a timeless and natural urge to return to a perceived halcyon age.

During the past five decades, claims for compensation and the return of Sudeten German property have been reinforced through concrete emotional practices, for example during orchestrated rituals that have celebrated Sudeten German heritage and commemorated the victims of the expulsion. Speeches by influential German politicians such as Edmund Stoiber have framed and supported the claims. These practices have included conscious, strategic emotional performances of love and anger, as well as less conscious dynamics inherent in people's emotional habitus. In the Sudeten German case, the celebrations have allowed (a declining number of) expellees and their offspring[5] to express, manage and perform a complexity of feelings. As described in more detail in earlier publications, these feelings include grief, resentment and hatred, as well as, at least in some cases, hope for reconciliation with the Czechs (Svašek 1999, 2000, 2002, 2005; see also Fendl 2002; Giegold and Otto 1994). It is important to note that, through such public practices, particular homeland discourses have been enacted, reinforced and sometimes criticised.

The third level of embodied experience is also crucial. Many expellees whom I met during my fieldwork were visibly moved by their personal attachment to their homeland. Talking with tears in their eyes about their lost place of birth, with emerging anger about their 'stolen' possessions, or with horror about the acts of violence they (as both individuals and 'Sudeten Germans') had experienced, they interpreted these

feelings as proof of homeland attachment.[6] In 1999 I conducted an interview by phone with an elderly man who had witnessed several killings. He led a comfortable life in Austria, he said, but was still strongly attached to the Sudetenland. He wanted to talk to me, he explained, even though recounting his memories was extremely painful. 'I will have nightmares again the coming week', he said, 'just because of talking to you, but I want people to know how we were treated after the war was officially over'. Like numerous other expellees who have been involved in campaigning for *Heimatsrecht*,[7] he wanted acknowledgement and compensation for his suffering, and demanded restitution of his lost property. The example shows that by reliving past events by recounting their memories to one another, grief and anger continued to shape their self-perception and their understanding of the world around them.

As noted earlier, this book will explore connections between the often multiple emotional attachments of migrants to their homelands and new places of residence, as well as the emotional interactions between migrants and members of local communities. Such connections were obvious in the Sudeten German case. My research mainly focused on expellees from Egerland who had resettled in eastern Bavaria, not far from their places of birth. Building a new life in postwar Germany was not easy, as the economic conditions were hard and many Bavarian locals saw them, at least initially, as outsiders who had 'foreign' cultural traits and spoke an incomprehensible dialect. In many cases, the experience of being outsiders increased Sudeten German feelings of distinctness, simultaneously reinforcing their attachment to the lost homeland. Identification as a collective group of expellees was also fed by their conviction that the postwar Czechoslovak government would sooner or later allow them to return to the Sudetenland. The reality of the unfolding Cold War, however, forced many Sudeten Germans to form a more permanent connection to their new place of residence. As ethnic Germans, integration through mixed marriages with Bavarian spouses was relatively easy. Building their own houses, numerous informants told me, rooted them in their new surroundings. In addition, their children who were born in Bavaria often defined themselves primarily as Bavarians. As the Cold War persisted, many members of the older generation nurtured a greater sense of belonging to their new place of residence, yet without giving up their deterritorialised Sudeten German identity. Through active expellee politics, their love for the homeland was politicised and redefined as a 'right to return'. Political support for this *Heimatrecht* was relatively strong in Bavaria. The new West German central government, however, strongly discouraged the claims, seeking instead to close the book on its Nazi history and redefine the nation's collective identity in terms of its '(West) European' alliance.

This shows the complexities of multiple identification and emotional attachment in the Sudeten German case. Contextually specific interactions among the expellees, and between the expellees and 'the locals' (including German spouses, neighbours, local politicians, religious leaders and national representatives), fed perceptions of belonging and non-belonging, and helped to construct deterritorialised and reterritorialised identities (Svašek 2002). While rising economic standards in West Germany secured a comfortable lifestyle for many expellees, which strengthened positive feelings of belonging to the country, the Sudeten German background remained for many an alternative source of active emotional attachment.

Emotional Encounters within Structured, Professionalised Settings

In the previous section, I focused on Sudeten German expellees, a group of forced migrants whose lives have been affected in different ways by historically specific dynamics. The category of 'migrants' is, however, much more diverse, including people who leave their country of origin for a wide variety of reasons, settling temporarily or more permanently in other states. 'Migrants' include, for example, migrant workers, illegal immigrants, refugees, victims of people smugglers, and retiree migrants, whose emotional ties to the homeland may have different forms and intensities.

Arriving at their new destination, all migrants are confronted with local residents, and their first encounter is often with officials at border crossings. In cases of expulsion and forced migration, first interactions are often still in the homeland with members of the occupying armed forces who organise and oversee the eviction. The behaviour of employees who work within particular spaces of departure and arrival, such as expellee camps and airports, is commonly shaped by culturally and professionally specific emotion rules. As Arlie Hochschild (1983: 11) noted, those who work in jobs that involve dealing with people need to manage their own emotions, and are required to handle the feelings of the people they encounter through their work. The chapters that follow will demonstrate that in the context of migration-related professions, job-specific requirements often construct migrants in specific ways that push particular modes of emotional interaction. Officers working at passport control for example, scrutinise incomers as 'potential cheats' who need to be exposed before they endanger their fellow citizens. The discourse of 'threat', in other words, influences the emotional interaction between migrant and official. As objects of inquisitive gazes, body scans, and possibly invasive searches, migrants may experience fear, anger or simply feelings of annoyance.

In Britain, unwanted foreigners who cannot be deported immediately are temporarily placed in immigration removal centres. In the next chapter, Alex Hall explores everyday practices in one of these centres, focusing in particular on officers who are responsible for the care and control of detainees awaiting court rulings on their asylum applications. What she analyses are, in essence, rationalised processes of control interlaced with complex emotional dynamics. Hall argues that through emotions we are connected to the world around us, and as objects of emotion the detainees are invested with value. These types of emotional process often entail moral judgement. Hall's analysis emphasises, however, besides the more metaphysical aspects of the informant's psychological experiences, the sensory immediacy of emotional processes. She argues that emotions themselves should not be regarded simply as mental evaluations or judgements, but also as the very physically embodied experiences they also evoke, which are, in turn, partly shaped by processes of appraisal. The officers' perception and treatment of the detainees is strongly informed by mistrust and fear, 'construals' that are strengthened by government discourses of migration policy as the management of risk. Through strict observation and control, they attempt to transform inconvenient, potentially dangerous migrant bodies into manageable subjects. The transformation of people into objects of control is facilitated by contempt, an emotion that helps construct the detainees as morally inferior beings. Balancing her pessimistic view on the treatment of detainees in the immigration removal centre, Hall ends on a more positive note, arguing that, during her fieldwork, there were several occasions when officers empathised with individual detainees, acknowledging their status as fellow human beings.

As with Hall, the contribution by Kathy Radford explores the emotional interaction between newcomers and locals in highly structured settings, namely immigration reception centres and related healthcare services in the Republic of Ireland. In Chapter 3, she shows how local professionals who work in the healthcare system (medics and death attendants) often fail to deal with the culturally specific emotional needs of migrants and asylum-seekers, partly because the system does not stimulate cross-cultural understanding and empathy. Ethnocentric and misinformed reports in the media about 'alien' practices such as circumcision only add to their misconceptions. This is not surprising, as ideas about the treatment of the body are culturally specific, and there may be conflicts about the correct execution of, for example, male circumcision within particular migrant groups. Radford calls for a policy that provides healthcare personnel with knowledge and skills that will give them insights into such issues, and enable them to better address immigrants' emotional needs.

These following two chapters clearly demonstrate that government policies and structural possibilities and constraints that are intrinsic to institutional settings in the migrant-receiving countries impact on migration-related emotional dynamics, shaping interactions between locals and newcomers. The emotional needs of incoming asylum-seekers are frequently denied or misunderstood, partly as a result of professional codes that favour emotional detachment and fail to provide appropriate training programmes. Not surprisingly, the lack of empathy increases the incomers' experience of non-belonging.

Anti-Immigration Sentiments, the Media and Everyday Experience

Referring to the Irish context, Claire Healy (2007a, 2007b) has argued that anti-immigration feelings among residents in their adopted countries have been under-researched due to misplaced political correctness. Scholars have avoided touching the subject out of fear of being accused of racism. In addition, Irish researchers have felt a moral obligation to protect migrants because of Ireland's own history of emigration. In Healy's view, the sources of anti-immigration sentiments should be critically explored, and a distinction drawn between evidence-based fears/resentment and speculative fears/resentment.

To get a better picture of how emotional tensions may arise between long and short term residents of particular localities, the sensorial reality as well as the mental experience of living-together-in-space must be explored. In Chapter 4, Amanda Wise analyses 'sensory multiculturalism': the experiential and multi-sensorial dimensions of ethnic coexistence in a suburb of Sydney. Apart from the older Anglo-Celtic population, the area has been inhabited by Greek, Italian, Polish, Lebanese and Turkish migrants, and more recently by Indian and Chinese migrants. Wise concentrates in particular on the experience of long-term elderly residents of European descent who have settled in the suburb in large numbers over the past decade. She argues that her informants feel uncomfortable with the Chinese, as the latter have transformed the environment in terms of smell, taste, sight, touch and sound, turning it into an alien place. The Chinese were also perceived to be unkind and impolite, as they failed to show affective responses deemed 'appropriate' by the longer term residents. This shows that discourses of emotion are reproduced through practice and embodied experience, and that living together or close to people who have internalised different rules

influencing their emotions can generate feelings of alienation, non-belonging and resentment.

Wise's chapter makes clear that negative perceptions about migrants can be fed by emotional discourses, practices and embodied experiences. Discourses of risk and fear present an image of the local self as highly vulnerable, potentially harmed by dangerous outsiders. Such discourses were also apparent in the analyses by Hall and Radford. Images of others as harmful and polluting forces may be reinforced through practices of fear, expressed through strategies of physical avoidance. In an ethnically diverse society, however, complete avoidance is often not possible, as demonstrated by Wise's article. The multi-sensorial dimensions of interaction in shared public spaces may add force to a sense of mutual otherness. As Wise shows, this process of affective distancing is not necessarily based on racist ideology. In her case study, it is rather rooted in embodied emotional dispositions.

Historical Processes and Enfolding Life Trajectories

Longer term residents are not only confronted with newcomers of different national backgrounds, but also with compatriots. As Aleksandra Galasínska demonstrates in Chapter 5, since the Second World War, Poles have settled in Britain in different time periods and, even though the individual groups acknowledge one another as Poles, differences are emphasised and played out through communicative and affective practice. Galasínska distinguishes between Poles who immigrated after the Second World War, those who left Poland between 1989 (the end of state socialism) and 2004 (Polish entry into the European Union), and those who arrived in Britain after 2004. The different historical conditions that have framed their experiences as migrants have influenced their sense of self. The analysis explores gossip as an important emotional performance through which individual Polish immigrants have distanced themselves from each other, drawing boundaries between specific groups. It shows that their stories about each other function as moral evaluations of sociality, creating distinct notions of 'superior Polish self' within specific social contexts. In these stories, expressions of anger and resentment encode and perform subjectivity, a process that is influenced by similarities and differences in individual life trajectories.

The course of individual life histories is also central in the contribution by Naoko Maehara, who explores the multiple emotional attachments of Japanese wives of Irish husbands in Chapter 6. The analysis follows three women in their changing roles as wives, mothers, daughters and daughters-in-law. The women often feel ambivalent, trying to juggle their various loyalties and emotional needs within their transnational family networks. In an attempt to manage their own ambivalence, they create certain narratives about themselves and others to justify difficult choices. The notion of Japanese husbands as men who are solely devoted to their work, a mirror image of their own Irish husbands, for example, features in their stories as an emotional justification for their choice to live abroad. Such images are reinforced through communication within virtual and actual communities of Japanese women in Ireland.

Narrative performance is clearly an area in which emotions are managed and enacted, as shown by both these contributions. In the case of migrant narratives of self, issues about the ambivalence of transnational belonging clearly come to the fore. Such

ambivalences may strengthen or weaken the emotional bonds within migrant communities, and may complicate continuing identification with the homeland.

Multiple Attachments, Belonging and Space

In the next two contributions, the issue of multiple belonging is also a central concern. In Chapter 7, Timm Lau discusses the multiple emotional attachments of Tibetan refugees who are based in India. Defining attachment as 'a sense of possessing that affects subjectivity', he looks at how Tibetan discourses of harmony encode norms concerning family life that reflect and produce strong links to the homeland. Attachments to the homeland are enacted through the idealisation of dominant marriage practices in Tibet, a belief in strong fraternal ties, and expressions of family loyalty. Yet the refugees live in Indian society, and are almost unavoidably influenced by Indian cultural practices. A discourse of love that attracts young Tibetans in particular is the one propagated by popular Bollywood films. The desires enacted in, and triggered by these films, strongly impact on their imagination, serve to inspire a greater sense of attachment to their place of settlement. The popularity of the films causes tensions between younger and older generations of Tibetans, as the notion of romantic ties between two lovers is radically different from the traditional Tibetan ideal of fraternal polygamy, where two or more brothers marry the same woman. Torn between two attachments, the Tibetan youngsters are confronted with feelings of double-belonging, which demonstrates how Tibetan migrant subjectivity is both ambiguous and inconsistent.

Petra Andits' focus in Chapter 8 is on changing attitudes within the Australian–Hungarian community towards the Hungarian state after the fall of communism in 1990. Initially, many Australian–Hungarians, who for various reasons had felt alienated from communist Hungary, hoped that democratisation would restore their sense of belonging to Hungary. Hope, in other words, became the expression of a desire to be reintegrated into an imaginary Hungary that would transcend the geological distance and national borders that separated them from their roots. Underlying the politics of hope was a moral claim to having saved or protected authentic Hungarian culture in the Australian diaspora, while those in Hungary had undermined Hungarian identity through Communist ideology. Not surprisingly, these Antipodean claims to a 'purer' Hungarian identity were criticised and ridiculed in Hungary, and many attempts by the émigrés to gain influence in their homeland were undermined or simply ignored. As the desire for new subjectivity was not realised, the émigrés were disappointed and disillusioned. Their resulting resentment and anger had clear moral dimensions.

Both chapters demonstrate the importance of memory and imagination to emotional dynamics. While in the case of the Hungarian émigrés, high expectations of reintegration lead to a sense of disillusionment when compatriots in Hungary fail to welcome them with open arms, in the Tibetan case, idealised memories of family life in the homeland compete with images of love expressed in Indian Bollywood movies.

In the last contribution by Maruška Svašek, the focus on mnemonic processes is connected to an exploration of politics and experiences of space. As with Andit's contribution, this final chapter explores negotiations of identity in the post-Cold War period in a new political era, especially in the light of past mobility. It seeks to explain how, during and after the disappearance of the Iron Curtain, Czech and German

citizens, politicians, priests and Sudeten German postwar expellees made claims to past and present emotions within specific socio-spatial contexts, not only to reflect on specific histories of migration and forced migration, but also to actively pursue political aims. The analysis demonstrates that distinct geopolitical situations in border areas may have a specific influence on border people's social and emotional life. As border inhabitants live relatively close to inhabitants of potentially hostile neighbouring states, they often feel more vulnerable than those who live in state centres. The proximity of the border may however also be an incentive for the establishment of close cross-border contacts, a policy stimulated with the European Union. This creates a complex situation on which emotions are easily politicised.

Conclusion: Emotional Attachments in a World of Movement

Emotions connect individuals to society as well the physical environment they live in, thereby shaping their engagement with the world. To understand this process it is useful to take a multi-layered approach, examining not only how people define and talk about particular emotions and attachments, but also exploring how sociality is shaped by emotional interaction, or how attitudes and interactions are informed by people's emotional judgements and habitus through time and space. It is also crucial to examine the ways in which individuals and groups manage emotions when following, or refusing to follow, group-specific emotion rules, and to explore their involvement in the politics of emotions. In addition, the bodily dimensions of emotional experience must be analysed, and attention must be paid to the ways in which memories and expectations influence emotional encounters in concrete settings.

As in any social context in which settled groups and newcomers confront each other, feelings are often consciously managed by individuals in an attempt to control or change the situation. Relations of dominance and subordination may be played out through emotional practice, justifying or challenging social, economic and political disparity. Professional codes may inform this process, as is often the case in institutionalised settings. As some of the chapters suggest, further research on emotions and human mobility should therefore include a focus on power, and explore how emotional processes may stimulate or undermine specific forms of inequality.

Some emotional processes, such as love, desire and admiration, draw individuals towards the object of their focus. The eight contributions to this book demonstrate that in a mobile world these objects might consist of many different phenomena, including 'a well-paid job', 'an ideal romantic relationship' or 'an idealised homeland'. Discourses construct these phenomena as sources of longing and aspiration, creating knowledge that is often reinforced through engaged social and bodily interaction. The perspective of 'concern-based construals' defines this practice as a form of perception and engagement that is partly shaped by normative discourse. While this process is generally strongly grounded in people's emotional habitus, reinforcing learned and internalised attitudes and preferences, there is also space for change. As self-conscious individuals, moving through different life stages and faced with new experiences, people may change their perception of particular others, and come to feel differently about them.

This complex process of being in, moving through, and relating to the world, explains why individuals from long-settled communities as opposed to recent migrants, might like or dislike one another. Evidently, socioeconomic factors play an important

role, as competition for scarce resources such as jobs, housing and funding opportunities can create or exaggerate feelings of jealousy and hatred. Unsurprisingly, negative emotions often stimulate patterns of avoidance. Paradoxically, however, feelings of irritation, anger or anxiety also project others in the self, as objects of intense emotional engagement. The resulting negative feelings may be strengthened and lead to actual violence when managed through a conscious politics of emotions, instigated by provocative media reports, political speeches and policies that seek to justify such behaviour.

The chapters that follow show that, in a world of mobility, personal attachments to people and places are multiple and changing. In the case of migrants, the type and strength of emotional connectivity at any particular moment in time clearly depends on a wide variety of factors. While an unfriendly welcome in the adopted country might serve to increase feelings of belonging to the homeland, positive experiences with members of local communities can result in positive emotional investment in new relationships. Emotional processes, however, are complex and often contradictory. As Bhatia and Ram (2004: 229) have pointed out, the contradictions, complexities and shifts of immigrant identification must be examined carefully, because 'the voices involved in communication with oneself or others are [not] always in harmonious accord with each other'. In many ways, this is equally valid for locals who are exposed to different levels of immigration in their communities. So as to avoid uninformative generalisation it is therefore necessary to conduct in-depth ethnographic research and to explore not only the social, economic and political dimensions of human mobility, but also its psychological complexity.

Acknowledgments

Earlier versions of the chapters by Alex Hall, Katy Radford and Aleksandra Galasínska were presented at the conference Emotional Interaction: Migrants and Local Communities (17 November 2006 at Queen's University Belfast). I would like to thank the AHRC for their financial support (Diasporas, Migration and Identities Research Networks and Workshops scheme) which enabled me to organize this conference (as well as two related conferences) and develop my approach to emotions and human mobility. I am also grateful to Dimitrina Spencer with whom I co-organised the session Emotional Attachments in a World of Movement at the 2006 EASA conference. Our ongoing discussions about politics and emotions have stimulated me to formulate some of my ideas. A final thanks to Justin I'Anson-Sparks for very helpful suggestions and his invaluable editorial input.

Notes

1 Recent publications include discussions of emotional interaction within transnational families (Baldassar 2007; Baldassar et al. 2006; McKay 2007; Yeoh et al. 2005), the effects of communication technologies on long-distance interaction (Panagakos and Horst 2006; Wilding 2006) and emotional return journeys to the homeland (Baldassar 2001; Lambkin 2008; Ramirez et al. 2007). Other scholars have analysed the emotional costs of labour migration in terms of gender, ethnicity and power (Ehrenreich and Hochschild 2005), or practices of homemaking and diasporic belonging in migrant communities (Ahmed et al. 2003; Burrell 2008; Fortier 2000). Individual chapters and articles have appeared in numerous books and journals. Furthermore, journals such as *Mobilities* (Conradson and

McKay 2007), *Identities: Global Studies in Culture and Power* (Svašek and Skrbiš 2007) and the *Journal of Intercultural Studies* (Svašek 2008) have produced special issues on emotions and human mobility.

2 As also discussed in Chapter 9, the Sudeten Germans formed the second-largest ethnic group in Czechoslovakia when it was established after the First World War, which brought an end to the German-dominated Habsburg Empire. When Hitler gained power in Germany, many Sudeten Germans supported him and welcomed the incorporation of 'the Sudetenland' (border areas belonging to Czechoslovakia) into the Third Reich in 1938, as well as the Nazi occupation of the remaining parts of Moravia and Bohemia in 1939. After the end of the Second World War, President Beneš signed a number of decrees and sided with the Potsdam Agreement. As a result, the majority of the over 3 million Sudeten Germans were expelled to Germany and Austria.

3 Thanks to Dirk Schubotz for helping me to translate the poem from German into English.

4 Magerl was expelled from Wusleben and resettled in the Bavarian village of Hohlweiler. Before the expulsion, around 300 Sudeten Germans lived in Wusleben, situated close to the Czech–German border. In 1949, it became part of a restricted military zone on the Czech side of the Iron Curtain. (http://www.zanikleobce.cz/index.php?lang-d&zdroj-427, last accessed 07 March 2008); see also Hamperl (1997) for more detailed information.

5 For obvious reasons, the number of Sudeten Germans with first-hand experience of the expulsion is decreasing. To most of their children, grandchildren and great-grandchildren, their ancestral Sudeten German background has little or no relevance.

6 Evidently, the physical dimensions of emotions can also be consciously managed, for example, through the body politic and the careful orchestration of rituals, when people are gathered in a space as one collective, when sad music is played after moments of quiet reflection, or when acts of celebration are accompanied by colourful processions, as happened during some of the expellee events. The fear of loss and separation is so ingrained in human nature that I myself, while critical of Sudeten German expellee politics, felt strongly moved by the rituals.

7 Sudeten German organisations have been calling for *Heimatsrecht* since the expulsion, demanding support from the West German government (the issue was taboo in East Germany) and, since 1990, from the German government. They have also raised the issue at the European Parliament and the American Senate (Svašek 2002).

References

Ahmed, S., Castañeda, C., Fortier, A. and Sheller, M. (eds) (2003) *Uprootings/Regroundings: Questions of Home and Migration*. Oxford: Berg.

Alliez, E. (2004) *The Signature of the World: What is Deleuze and Guattari's Philosophy?* London: Continuum.

Aranda, E. (2003) 'Emotional adaptation: bringing emotions into the study of transnational migration'. Atlanta, GA: Atlanta Hilton Hotel, paper presented at the annual meeting of the American Sociological Association, 16 August 2003.

Baldassar, L.R. (2001) *Visits Home. Migration Experiences Between Italy and Australia*. Melbourne: Melbourne University Press.

Baldassar, L.R. (2007) 'Transnational families and the provision of moral and emotional support: the relationship between truth and distance', *Identities, Global Studies in Culture and Power*, *14*(4): 385–410.

Baldassar, L.R. (2008) 'Missing kin and longing to be together. emotions and the construction of co-presence in transnational relationships', *Journal of Intercultural Studies*, *29*(3): 247–66.

Baldassar, L., Wilding, R. and Baldock, C. (2006) 'Long-distance caregiving: transnational families and the provision of aged care', in Paoletti, I. (ed.) *Caregiving of Older Disabled*. New York: Nova Science, 201–27.

Bhatia, S. and Ram, A. (2004) 'Culture, hybridity and the dialogical self: cases from the South Asian diaspora', *Mind, Culture and Activity*, *11*(3): 224–40.

Bourdieu, P. (1977) *Outline of a Theory of Practice*. Cambridge: Cambridge University Press.

Burrell, K. (2008) 'Managing, learning and sending: the material lives and journeys of Polish women in Britain', *Journal of Material Culture*, *13*(1): 63–83.

Casey, E.S. (1987) *Remembering: A Phenomenological Study*. Bloomington, IN: Indiana University Press.

Clough, P.T. and Halley, J. (2007) *The Affective Turn. Theorizing the Social*. Durham and London: Duke University Press.

Conradson, D. and McKay, D. (2007) 'Translocal subjectivities: mobility, connection, emotion', *Mobilities*, *2*(2): 167–74.

Csordas, T.J. (ed.) (1994) *Embodiment and Experience. The Existential Ground of Culture and Self*. Cambridge: Cambridge University Press.

Ehrenreich, B. and Hochschild, A.R. (eds) (2005) *Global Woman: Nannies, Maids, and Sex Workers in the New Economy*. New York: A Metropolitan and Own Book.

Fendl, E. (ed.) (2002) *Zur Ikonographie des Heimwehs. Erinnoringskultur von Heimatvertriebenen*. Freiburg: Johannes-Künzig-Instituts für ostdeutsche Volkskunde.

Fortier, A. (2000) *Migrant Belongings: Memory, Space, Identity*. Oxford: Berg.

Gell, A. (1998) *Art and Agency. An Anthropological Theory*. Oxford: Clarendon Press.

Giegold, H. and Otto, G. (1994) *Nachbarn im Gespräch. Tschechen und Bayern*. Regensburg: Buchverlag der Mittelbayerischen Zeitung.

Gray, B. (2008) 'Putting emotion and reflexivity to work in researching migration', *Sociology*, *42*(5): 935–52.

Hamperl, W. (1997) *Vertreibung und Flucht aus dem Kreis Tachau im Egerland: Schicksale in Berichten, Dokumenten und Bildern*. Altenmarkt: published by the author.

Healy, C. (2007a) 'Turning point: reception and perceptions of newcomers in Ireland since 1996'. Belfast, paper presented at the conference Emotional Interaction. Migrants and Local Communities, 17 November.

Healy, C. (2007b) 'A nation of emigrants or immigrants? The challenge of integration in Ireland and Portugal', *Irish Migration Studies in Latin America*, *5*(2): 117–20.

Hochschild, A.R. (1983) *The Managed Heart. Commercialization of Human Feeling*. Berkeley: University of California Press.

Kramer, M., Schoen, L.S. and Kinney, L. (1984) 'The dream experience in dream-disturbed Vietnam veterans', in van der Kolk, B. (ed.) *Post-Traumatic Stress Disorder: Psychological and Biological Sequelae*. Washington: American Psychiatric Press, 81–95.

Krystal, H. (1995) 'Trauma and aging: a thirty-year follow up', in Caruth, C. (ed.) *Trauma: Explorations in Memory*. London: Johns Hopkins University Press, 76–99.

Lambkin, B. (2008) 'The emotional function of the migrant's "birthplace" in transnational belonging: Thomas Mellon (1813–1908) and Andrew Carnegie (1835–1919)', *Journal of Intercultural Studies*, *29*(3): 315–30.

Leavitt, J. (1996) 'Meaning and feeling in the anthropology of emotions', *American Ethnologist*, 23(3): 514–39.

Leydesdorff, S. (1992) 'A shattered silence: the life stories of survivors of the Jewish proletariat of Amsterdam', in Passerini, L. (ed.) *International Yearbook of Oral History and Life Stories, Volume I. Memory and Totalitarianism*. Oxford: Oxford University Press, 145–64.

Leys, R. (2000) *Trauma: A Genealogy*. Chicago: University of Chicago Press.

Lock, M. (1993) 'Cultivating the body: anthropology and epistemologies of bodily practice and knowledge', *Annual Review of Anthropology*, 22: 133–55.

Lutz, C.A. and Abu-Lughod, L. (eds) (1990) *Language and the Politics of Emotion*. Cambridge: Cambridge University Press and Paris: Editions de la Maison des Sciences de l'Homme.

Lyon, M.L. (1995) 'Missing emotion: the limitations of cultural constructionism in the study of emotion', *Cultural Anthropology*, *10*(2): 244–63.

Magerl, E. (1949) 'Fern liegt das Land . . .!', *Tachauer Pfraumberger Heimat. Heimatbrief*, 5: 114.

McKay, D. (2007) 'Sending dollars shows feeling: emotions and economies in Filipino migration', *Mobilities*, *2*(2): 175–94.

Panagakos, A.N. and Horst, H.A. (2006) 'Return to Cyberia: technology and the social worlds of transnational migrants', *Global Networks*, *6*(2): 109–24.

Parkinson, B. (1995) *Ideas and Realities of Emotion*. Routledge: London and New York.

Ramirez, M., Skrbiš, Z. and Emmison, M. (2007) 'Transnational family reunions as lived experience: narrating a Salvadoran auto-ethnography', *Identities, Global Studies in Culture and Power*, *14*(4): 411–32.

Ryan, L. (2008) 'Navigating the emotional terrain of families "here" and "there": women, migration and the management of emotions', *Journal of Intercultural Studies*, *29*(3): 299–314.

Skrbiš, Z. (2008) 'Transnational families: theorising migration, emotions and belonging', *Journal of Intercultural Studies*, *29*(3): 231–46.

Svašek, M. (1999) 'History, identity and territoriality. redefining Czech–German relations in the post-Cold War era', *Focaal: Journal of Anthropology*, 32: 37–58.

Svašek, M. (2000) 'Borders and emotions. Hope and fear in the Bohemian-Bavarian frontier zone', *Ethnologia Europaea: Journal of European Ethnology*, *30*(2): 111–26.

Svašek, M. (2002) 'Narratives of "home" and "homeland". The symbolic construction and appropriation of the Sudeten German *Heimat*', *Identities: Global Studies in Culture and Power*, *9*(4): 495–518.

Svašek, M. (2005) 'The politics of chosen trauma. Expellee memories, emotions and identities', in Milton, K. and Svašek, M. (eds) *Mixed Emotions: Anthropological Studies of Feeling*. Oxford: Berg, 195–214.

Svašek, M. (2006) 'Postsocialist ownership: emotions, power and morality in a Czech village', in Svašek, M. (ed.) *Postsocialism: Politics and Emotions in Central and Eastern Europe*. Oxford: Berghahn, 95–114.

Svašek, M. (2008) 'Who cares? Families and feelings in movement', *Journal of Intercultural Studies*, *29*(3): 213–30.

Svašek, M. and Skrbiš, Z. (2007) 'Passions and power: emotions and globalisation', *Identities: Global Studies in Culture and Power*, *14*(4): 367–84.

Thrift, N. (2008) *Non-Representational Theory. Space/Politics/Affect*. New York: Routledge.

Tonkin, E. (2006) 'Being there: emotion and imagination in anthropologists' encounters', in Milton, K. and Svašek, M. (eds) *Mixed Emotions. Anthropological Studies of Feeling*. Oxford: Berg, 55–70.

Velayutham, S. and Wise, A. (2005) 'Moral economies of a translocal village: obligation and shame among South Indian transnational migrants', *Global Networks*, *5*(1): 27–47.

Walker, J.A. (1999) *Art & Outrage. Provocation, Controversy and the Visual Arts*. London: Pluto.

Wilding, R. (2006) 'Virtual intimacies? Families communicating across transnational contexts', *Global Networks*, *6*(2): 125–42.

Yeoh, B.S.A., Huang, S. and Lam, T. (2005) 'Transnationalizing the "Asian" family: imaginaries, intimacies and strategic intents', *Global Networks*, *5*(4): 307–15.

'These People Could Be Anyone': Fear, Contempt (and Empathy) in a British Immigration Removal Centre

Alexandra Hall

Detention is proliferating as a governmental response to human mobility in the 'war on terror'. Theoretical engagements with spaces of detention and enclosure have been influenced by Agamben's work on the camp and the sovereign exception. Such a view focuses on the abject 'bare life' that is produced by the sovereign decision. Drawing on ethnographic fieldwork among staff at a UK immigration removal centre, the paper makes the case for 'going inside' the detention centre. It examines the everyday life of detention through the lens of emotion, with a focus on fear and contempt. Exploring these emotions as forms of judgement or construal can unravel staff dispositions towards the detainees, and can demonstrate the ways in which emotion shapes the treatment the detainees receive. The paper argues for emotion as an analytical tool; in the case of detention, it can supplement abstract accounts of 'the camp'.

Introduction

In May 2008, the UK Border Agency announced plans to expand the UK's immigration removal centre estate by 60 per cent. This expansion was required, argued Liam Byrne (the then Border and Immigration Minister), because 'we now remove an immigration offender every eight minutes—but my target is to remove more, and remove them faster' (Home Office 2008a). The increased investment in immigration detention is part of New Labour's decade-long 'shake up' of the immigration system. The agenda for this reorganisation was formulated clearly in the 2002 White Paper, *Secure Borders, Safe Haven: Integration with Diversity in Modern Britain:*[1] the movement of people into Britain is at once a positive force for economic

good and a worrying threat that needs to be contained. This double conceptualisation has ushered in interventions to strategically administer different types of mobility: economically 'beneficial' migration has been enabled, but there has been a 'clamp down' on asylum, a politically contentious and moralised form of human mobility.

Detention—what the White Paper described as 'an unfortunate but essential element in the effective enforcement of immigration control'—has emerged as a crucial element of the search for a 'robust and credible' system. Practices of detention are linked in official rhetoric to deportation and what Walters (2002) calls the 'international policing of aliens': the (forcible) reallocation of people to sovereign territories. The logic of deportation is underpinned by the 'national order of things' (Malkki 1995), which creates an overarching framework through which moral and political horizons are shaped. Within this moral and political order, the person without the protection of a state (the asylum-seeker) and those with no legal immigration status ('illegal immigrants') emerge as limit concepts; the 'others' against whom the sovereign state reasserts itself (Dillon 1999).

Contemporary practices of detention are not novel, but belong to a set of historical techniques that have (spatially and socially) isolated populations deemed problematic, deviant, dangerous or polluting (see Bashford and Strange 2003; Foucault 1977; Sibley 1995). Indeed, the relegation of anomalous people and those charged with their care to designated places and enclosures, with associated barriers, prohibitions and regimes of expertise, has been a ubiquitous feature of modernity. Current detention procedures, then, have parallels in previous historical moments. The twentieth-century wartime internment of aliens in the West, for example, managed the vague threat and unknown risk of 'enemy aliens' through coerced isolation in ways similar to today's reliance on detention (Bashford and Strange 2002; Cesarini and Kushner 1993). In Britain, the detention of persons generally subject to immigration control was first codified in the 1920 Aliens Act, while the 1971 Immigration Act gave immigration authorities the power to detain asylum-seekers. The routine administrative detention of non-citizens under immigration law became widespread and normalised in the UK through the 1990s, a trend that is mirrored internationally (see Bloch and Schuster 2005; Malloch and Stanley 2005; Pratt 2005; Schuster 2005; Welch and Schuster 2005). On 29 March 2008 there were 2,310 people in detention in the UK, 1,640 of whom had at some stage claimed asylum (Home Office 2008b). In the first quarter of 2008, 3,740 people were removed after having been detained under Immigration Act powers, 46 per cent of whom had been asylum-seekers and 68 per cent of whom had been detained in immigration service removal centres (Home Office 2008c: 12–13).

Officially, a person may be detained if his or her identity and basis of immigration or asylum claim are in question, or if a person is seen as being likely to abscond. People are also detained as part of 'fast-track asylum procedures' (for 'straightforward' asylum claims) and in support of the removal of 'failed asylum-seekers' and others who have no legal immigration status. In practice, people are detained for a variety of (subjective) reasons, including deterrence and punishment (Weber and

Gelsthorpe 2000), and at all stages of an immigration or asylum claim. The detention of people who are claiming asylum is particularly contentious; it appears to constitute a 'penalty' and punishment, and thus goes against the terms of the 1951 United Nations Geneva Convention Relating to the Status of Refugees, the agreement on which international standards of protection for people feeling persecution are based. Asylum, then, is one of the casualties of the drive to tighten up the UK border, an example of what Genova (2002: 437) calls the 'spectacle' of enforcement, a tangible and showy display of force in response to ever-spiralling accusations of 'soft touch' Britain.

The war on terror has seen national domestic immigration politics increasingly blur with the governance of security and the management of risk (Bigo 2001). The governance of space, symbolic representation and conduct, through which the national community is imagined, increasingly draws on the 'terrorist', 'illegal immigrant' and 'bogus asylum-seeker' as foci for citizenship practices: indeed, all good citizens are called upon to become vigilant for the threatening anomaly in everyday life (Amoore 2007). Moreover, it is frequently claimed that contemporary securitisation has produced a particular kind of affective politics, one that is hinged on fear and anxiety (see, for example, Isin 2004; Massumi 2005). However, this claim is accompanied by a dearth of detailed accounts of the spatio-temporal situated emergence of nameable emotions at particular sites. The detention centre is the space where the anxieties surrounding mobility become crystallised and where the distinctions between citizen and other must be sustained in the minutiae of everyday life.

This paper explores the everyday social life of the UK immigration removal centre (IRC), using emotion as a lens of analysis. Drawing from ethnographic fieldwork among staff at a secure centre in the UK, which I will call Locksdon,[2] the paper discusses fear and contempt as a way of understanding the operation of the centre, and the treatment that is given to men accommodated there.

Locating 'The Camp'

Giorgio Agamben has been hugely influential in critical work focusing on high-profile detention facilities in the war on terror such as Guántanamo Bay (Butler 2005; Diken 2004; Minca 2005) and the various interventions of confinement and enclosure made around migration (Isin and Rygiel 2007; Nyers 2006). Agamben draws on Carl Schmitt's notion of sovereignty—'Sovereign is he who decides on the state of exception' (cited in Agamben 1998: 11)—to argue that the camp (he uses the wartime death camp as his example) is a materialisation of the state of exception. This exception is the suspension of normal rules and laws in the name of protecting (and producing) sovereign rule. The decision on the exception *constitutes* sovereign power, which is revealed to be inside and outside the rule of law. The camp is the concretisation of the exception, where rule and exception, norm and emergency, violence and law merge. Agamben makes clear that the exception is not a space

simply *excluded* from the juridical order. Rather, the exception is included in the juridical order through its very exclusion.

The camp is also where the biopolitical nature of modern politics is most clearly revealed. Foucault (1977) used 'biopower' to refer to the distinct form of power that emerged in the European eighteenth century and which sought to address the problems that emerged from conceptualising human life as a population. Biopower is constituted by an array of supervisory and regulatory mechanisms that seek to manage and order life itself: it is the investment of natural, biological life with politics. Agamben sees biopolitics to have a far longer history than Foucault suggests. Political community since ancient times *appears* to have been based on the exclusion of humankind's natural, 'bare', biological life, but, for Agamben (1998: 7), this is not a straightforward exclusion, but rather an 'inclusive exclusion (an exceptio)'. Modern politics is not novel in its interventions upon biological life and its processes. Sovereign power operates precisely in the decision on which lives count as political, and which are to be 'excepted'. Behind sovereign power's concern with health and longevity is the potential to let some people die, as the camp demonstrated. People in the camps became reduced to bare life (depoliticised, 'unencumbered' life) through the removal of their rights, political status and nationality, in such a way that 'no act committed against them could appear any longer as a crime' (1998: 174). The camp inhabitant epitomises Agamben's *homo sacer*, over whom sovereign power has ultimate power.

Agamben's camp has provided a way of thinking more broadly about spaces of internment, detention and enclosure. The contemporary sovereign decision emerges in bureaucratic pronouncements on detention (Butler 2005), for example, and humanitarian efforts to contain refugee flows. The refugee—who 'radically calls into question the fundamental categories of the nation-state' by demonstrating the precarious relationship between rights, birth and nation Agamben 1998: 134)—calls forth various strategies of containment. In the constant state of emergency that is called into being by the war on terror, these 'surplus' populations are held in a 'zone of indistinction [. . .] on the edge of the juridical order' (Walters 2002: 286). This, then, is the administration of bare life, made abject.

Nevertheless, as Isin and Rygiel (2007) argue, Agamben's ahistorical, essentialised camp paradigm cannot adequately account for the *novel* nature of contemporary 'frontiers, zones and camps'. Whereas Agamben saw the camp as a 'space of abjection' where people were denationalised and then eliminated, contemporary enclosures are better viewed as 'abject spaces' where people are treated 'neither as subjects (of discipline) nor objects (of elimination) but as those without presence' (1998: 184). Importantly, these places seek to foreclose the possibility of political action by making people invisible and inaudible, by preventing them from entering sovereign territories where they may exercise international rights, for example. Sketching a strategy for reinstating the camp as a *political* space, Isin and Rygiel argue for a closer consideration of the particularities of contemporary places of enclosure and confinement, as abject

spaces but also as 'spaces of resistance', paying attention to the 'thoughts and practices that sustain them' (2007: 185).

It is with this in mind that I make a case for going *inside* places of detention, to explore the lives that are lived within. Focusing on staff attitudes to their charges is part of an endeavour to understand how an abject status might be inscribed, and how it fails. More specifically, I ask what can be learnt by using emotion as a analytical lens. As Svašek and Skrbiš (2007: 368) argue, emotional processes and the mobility of globalisation are wholly entangled. While the secure detention centre brings to mind the rationalised, ordered regimes of the disciplinary spaces described by Foucault (1977), the mechanisms of secure detention are always shot through with affective, emotional and symbolic concerns (see Aretxaga 1997; Feldman 1991). As a distinct and fraught arena of encounter between inside and outside, citizens and others, the IRC is an environment where machinic, rule-bound working practices intertwine with disdain, fantasy, anger and empathy.

Emotion

There is, argues Roberts (2003: 7), 'a rampant disorder internal to the concept of emotion'. This disorder emerges from the varying ways that emotions have been conceptualised in philosophy, the social sciences, humanities, sciences and in demotic discourse. In the West, at least, emotions have often been contrasted with 'rationality', thought and mind; regarded as unintelligent, uncontrollable 'passions'; associated with animal-like physicality and contrasted with reasonable thought (see Parkinson 1995: 116). The ongoing 'emotional turn' of the social sciences, however, has reinstated emotion's critical potential (Ahmed 2004a; Davidson *et al.* 2005; Milton and Svašek 2005). In geography, for example, the study of emotion has been invigorated by recent debates surrounding the theorisation of affect, which has problematised the embedding of emotion in the human subject. Affect seeks an understanding of 'the emotional' as moods, intensities and excitations that circulate and are transmitted between human bodies, objects, non-human living beings, and technologies (Anderson 2006; Brennan 2004). Such an approach expands theoretical and empirical work in the area, but has been criticised for discouraging 'an engagement with everyday emotional subjectivities' (Thien 2005; see Anderson and Harrison 2006 for a reply) and for its potential to sideline inequality (Tolia-Kelly 2006).

Anthropology has been concerned with the 'living out' of emotion and with tracing the ways in which power, discourse, bodies, culture and 'the social' intertwine in the experience, expression and conceptualisation of emotion. While this project generally retains at its core an interest in the emotional (affectively capable) human subject, the concern with the cultural diversity of 'the emotional' has constantly problematised the boundaries of Western conceptualisations of the field, and has investigated affective engagements that transcend the human (see Lutz 1988; Milton 2002). Emotions emerge as 'embodied experiences and discursive practices which, on an analytical level, blur the boundary between body and mind' (Svašek 2005b: 196). Emotions are simultaneously

functional realms of action, socially constructed categories, evaluative judgements and ideological discourses reinforcing power relationships (Svašek 2005a). They are also, for some, intrinsically cultural, that is, 'structured by particular cultural systems' (Lutz 1988: 5), and inflecting that system in turn.

In anthropology, there is broad division between those who view emotions as 'physical feelings susceptible to explanation' and those who see them as social and cultural, 'ideas in the mind, a form of cognition whose social and cultural meaning is to be interpreted' (Josephides 2005: 79 in a discussion of Leavitt 1996). The learned and contextual nature of emotions, and their inter-subjective experience and expression, involves interpersonal interaction and negotiation, as well as the mobilisation of cultural representational complexes and norms. Both a concept and social practice, emotion is a way of being-in-the-world, of making claims about an identity or a situation. In this sense, emotions can be forms of 'communicative performance' (Lutz and Abu-Lughod 1990: 11) that are related to the 'elicitation' of responses from others in social life (Josephides 2005: 79). While this constructionist view draws attention to the diversity and particularity of emotions, it also threatens to ignore or downplay emotion's physical manifestation and universal possibilities. Milton (2005: 26), for example, notes that conceptualisations of emotions draw on frameworks of thought that cannot help but perpetuate the separation of mind and body, even while seeking to overcome these distinctions.

Josephides (2003: 60–1, citing Solomon 1983: 251) sees emotions as interpretations and forms of judgement that 'constitute the world of our experience', crucial to our engagement with others. Such an approach, admittedly, recasts the emotional in terms of mind and cognition. It (deliberately) focuses attention on the human subject within a political and cultural milieu and places centrally his or her understanding, perception of, and interaction with that milieu. For the study of places like Locksdon, where emotions are bound up with the working of the centre, such an approach has value for taking seriously the ways in which emotion merges with, sustains, and creates, a sense of difference. Ahmed (2004b: 121) sees emotions as working within a flow of signs about bodies, persons and things: 'the accumulation of affective value shapes the surfaces of bodies and worlds'. Emotions circulate within affective economies, she argues, 'sticking' to certain bodies, attributing meaning to them, and working to 'align subjects with some others and against other others' (2004b: 117). It becomes important to understand how emotions generate the effects they do.

In seeing emotions in this way, I follow Martha Nussbaum, who argues that emotions are responses to the perception of value, and must be recognised as an intrinsic part of our reasoning and ethical life. Nussbaum sees emotions as cognitive appraisals which 'ascribe to things and persons outside that person's control, great importance for that person's own flourishing' (Nussbaum 2001: 2, 4), a view that she qualifies by acknowledging the importance of norms, context and individual human histories. Emotions take an object of some kind and invest it with value; they are eudaimonistic, linked to a person's viewpoint. This is not to say that emotions are self-interested, but we tend to feel emotion by construing things through the

experiences, beliefs and values we already have; we are connected to the people, environments and situations around us, and our emotional experience is the crystallisation of this connection. Nussbaum (2004: 27, 29) argues that beliefs and perceptions are not equivalent to emotions, but are an important part of what the emotion itself *is*.

This is partly similar to Roberts' paradigm for considering emotions as 'concern-based construals' (2003: 64). This is not a matter of suggesting that people 'see' things in a certain way and then feel something, nor of suggesting that the construal is illusory, or subject to change on reflection (though it might be). Rather, a person's emotions are construals in that they have an immediacy reminiscent of sense perception. A construal, then, is an organisation of the senses, a kind of perceptual experience of something in certain terms. Subjective, contradictory and not necessarily conscious (he argues it is possible to feel anger without knowing it), emotions are construals 'imbued, flavoured, coloured, drenched, suffused, laden, informed or permeated with concern' (Roberts 2003: 70–3, 76–9). Concern forms part of the perception in such a way as to 'characterise the appearance of the object' and to become a term of the construal (2003: 80, 145). Emotions are not judgements in the sense of embracing a certain belief or appearance of a person, object or situation; emotions are *part* of the appearance, which may be supported by corresponding judgements.

Both Roberts and Nussbaum support an idea that emotions are essentially cognitive in nature, linked to the way in which an acting subject makes sense of the world, and shapes that sense-making process in turn. There may be limitations to such an approach—for example, neither places *centrally* the bodily aspects of emotional experience and both gloss over the social, political and cultural as things that can be folded into emotion as essentially individual experience. Nevertheless, an approach that links emotion to an evaluation of an object (socially, culturally and contextually negotiated in relationships with others) is ideally placed to tease apart the multilayered interpretations that coalesce in emotional experience and expression. More than this, it offers a way of understanding the intertwining of emotion and politics: how emotion attaches to various bodies and becoming implicated in contextual understandings of difference. In the case of Locksdon IRC, such an approach provokes a reading of the secure environment that makes it possible to relate broader concerns of the war on terror, for example, with particular affective dispositions within the centre. Understanding the immigration removal centre as a place of politics, resistance, *and emotion* supplements notions of 'the camp' as an empty, anomic space.

Locksdon Immigration Removal Centre

Immigration detention is distinguishable from imprisonment in that most detainees have not been convicted of any criminal offence. There is no limit to the period of custodial detention under the Immigration Acts (as opposed to people accused of

crimes), though a detained person can apply for bail. The analytical distinction between detention and imprisonment blurs with the use of prison service establishments to accommodate immigration detainees. Locksdon IRC is run by the prison service for the immigration authorities and staff are trained prison officers.

Locksdon is a functional, well-maintained building, but was never designed to accommodate immigration detainees. It is surrounded by a high perimeter fence and barbed wire, with a single gate entrance for people and vehicles. Inside the secure enclosure there is an administrative building, a Visits Centre, a Multifaith Centre, a sports field and the main Centre building, which comprises the reception area, dormitories, gymnasium, dining hall and kitchen, education department, health department and offices for on-site Immigration Officers and Locksdon staff. Moving around the establishment entails unlocking and re-locking a series of gates, some on a time delay lock.

As well as the officers, there are administrative workers, estates staff, nurses, immigration officers, a Chaplain and education staff from a nearby Adult Education College. Locksdon is visited regularly by its designated volunteer Visiting Committee, an independent body which monitors conditions at Locksdon for staff and detainees. There is also a volunteer visiting group that befriends detainees and a Detainee Consultative Committee where problems with the regime can be addressed. Detainees can also put their grievances personally to the Manager, on application. Locksdon officers tend to come from 'working-class' or 'lower-middle-class' backgrounds; most do not have tertiary education and, aside from their prison work, many have skilled manual trades. The majority of officers have served in the Armed Forces. A career in the Prison Service is a well-trodden route for men and women leaving the Forces, although Prison Service recruitment initiatives in recent years have favoured a more inclusive mix of backgrounds (see Liebling and Price 2001). The area surrounding Locksdon is not ethnically mixed and the officers are overwhelmingly 'white'.

Fear

> These people [detainees] could be anyone. We have no idea who they are and what they are doing here. I'm not saying that some of them aren't genuine, but do we know who they are? They could be ex-soldiers. We've had a few of them. One guy was interviewed by the Special Branch and got taken away—he was wanted for some war crime in Serbia or something. These guys—they may be wanted by the local mafia, they may be on the run from somewhere. They may have killed their granny, pissed off the family, the local gangs. They may have been involved in all kinds of stuff. All they have to do is get on a plane, get rid of their passport and arrive in Britain. Once they're here they just give a name and we have no way of knowing who they are. Immigration don't know. They haven't got a clue. And they wind up in here' (male officer).

The war on terror has opened a political space where asylum and immigration have increasingly become matters of security (Bigo 2001). Governance becomes a series of

interventions in issues of safety and unsafety, and political interventions to manage risk and protect the 'homeland' have become more refined, ubiquitous, far-reaching and technologised.

Ahmed (2004b: 124) argues that the discourses of fear surrounding migrants work to provoke sensations of being overwhelmed, feelings exacerbated by the impossibility of containment. Fear, she argues, has a *futurity*, emerging from the dread that the object of fear might 'pass by', and not be contained. In this way, circulating fear 'slides across' signified bodies, and sticks to some, making them fearsome. This pervasive fear mobilises a 'representation of a world that would be safer if only ambiguity, ambivalence and uncertainty could be controlled' (Amoore 2006: 337). Key to securing this safe world is the inexorable drive to *identify*. Detention, of course, is officially justified precisely when identity is in question, and the technologies of confinement are based around the idea of locating, filtering and immobilising that which is threatening or undesirable.

If the detention centre works to restrict the movement of those to whom fear 'sticks', the anxiety does not disappear within the centre, but instead becomes distilled. If trust is inversely related to fear, a provisional response to the life's contingency and unknowability (Dasgupta 1988; Misztal 1996), then trust falters and fails in Locksdon. As the officer quoted above made clear, the detainees' unknownness is intensely problematic for the officers. The physical body that officers confront at Reception (where a detainee undergoes a formalised set of inductions) does not automatically correspond to the person described in the detention warrant faxed through from the immigration authorities. Mistakes are made, warrants get muddled, names get confused, the wrong detainee is moved. Staff must be vigilant for identity mix-ups. The officers feel that the only thing they know about the detainee, for sure, is the body in front of them. A man's origins, biography and history are unknown. This deferral of trust is linked partly to the officers' experience of identity fraud in immigration contexts, and in their previous mainstream prison work with convicted criminals. Officers are acutely aware that people may not be as they seem; documents can be false, people are capable of terrible things, and they sometimes lie. The possible incongruence between stated identity and 'real' identity is always at issue.

In a 'proper' prison (as the officers recount), a newly convicted inmate or remand prisoner arrives with a full record, having been subjected to an examination in Foucault's (1977) terms and classified according to taxonomies of deviancies, pathologies and tendencies. Procedures roll out from this knowledge. The immigration detainee is just as likely to arrive with no passport, no detention history, no criminal record, and information held by immigration authorities is often not passed on efficiently. It is the case, of course, that the vast majority of detainees are wholly innocent of any criminal activity, despite falling foul of civil immigration law. It is also the case that, periodically, an individual will pass through Locksdon who has criminal convictions (some detainees arrive at Locksdon having served a prison sentence), or who is violent, carries weapons, and threatens staff or fellow detainees.

There is a constant potential for violence among frustrated, sometimes desperate, men in close confinement. The sporadic reality of violence gives tangible shape to the nebulous anxiety that pervades detention. The ill-defined fear of the other within a general mood of precariousness becomes an insistent construal of the detainee (with unknown intentions, proclivities, associations and histories) as capable of threat.

Amoore has argued that the war on terror is increasingly characterised by a pervasive 'vigilant mode of visuality', which deploys 'a precautionary principle that governs through the suspicion of a possible future threat' (2007: 216, 226). She argues that the contemporary preoccupation with screening and profiling at borders, and in the mundane routines of daily life, is connected to the desire to pre-empt a danger that is not yet fully shaped. Pre-emptive governance operates on a threat that is 'indeterminately in potential' (Massumi 2007: para. 13) and we are all, increasingly, being called upon to visualise what this threat might be. For the officers at Locksdon, the idea that risk might best be contained by anticipating an ever-emerging threat is a matter of common sense. In the IRC, the suspicion of the war on terror becomes attentiveness to individual bodies.

The anticipatory logic manifests itself as a general hypervigilance, an enhanced awareness of bodies in time and space, and the persistent interpretation of behaviour within a particular 'scopic regime' of signification that privileges suspicion. It is through this hypervigilance—generated by a concern not to lose 'the initiative'—that detainees may be transformed from unknown, unruly and risky bodies into known, manageable ones. One officer told me, 'You have to notice things about people'. Part of the officers' job, then, is the levelling of a scrutinising gaze over the detainees (and each other) for signs of 'indiscipline', such as security breaches, or more intangible signals of dangers yet to unfold, such as insolence or abuse. Staff note suspicious incidents in the 'Obs (Observations) Book', an ongoing inscription of suspicion (that shapes that suspicion in turn) which simultaneously forms the initial containment of risk, and from which active security reports are generated. Threat and disorder can be managed with the correct procedural vigilance:

> We are trying to build intelligence, knowledge. We're trying to build a picture of what is happening in the establishment at any time (male Senior Officer, Locksdon).

In Roberts' terms, concern (to prevent harm, to maintain control) forms part of the perception of the detainees' actions in such a way as to characterise the appearance of the object and to become a term of the construal. The officers' heightened awareness of the detainees is an embodied disposition, a somatic alertness. Milton's discussion about the ecological nature of emotion is useful here. Learning and emotion are intimately interconnected, she argues, and emotions of 'interest' or 'anticipation' are states of body and mind in which we explore our environment and learn from it. Emotions are intrinsically linked to what we remember, focus on, perceive and attend to in our environment (including social environment) which in turn cyclically shapes 'how we approach our environment, which influences what we learn from it' (2005:

34). In the context of the IRC, alert watchfulness is produced from, and in turn feeds into, emotional engagement with detainee action. As a learned response and embodied attitude, apprehension (manifested as vigilance) is not just a conscious interpretation or evaluation, but a way of engaging, seeing and paying attention that has the location of danger as its goal.

Importantly for the argument of this paper, the barely-articulated suspicion which often characterises the officers' engagement with the detainees contributes to the 'making abject' of the men. As Ahmed (2004b: 128) argues, 'Fear does not involve the defence of borders that already exist; rather fear makes those borders'. In Locksdon, the officers' hypervigilance *creates* distance from the men in their care and control, and etches (and re-etches) the difference between citizens and others. The detainees become bodies in time and space, objects to be tracked and scrutinised, surfaces which emotions inscribe, and to which are attached certain traits (trouble, compliant, disruptive). The detainee as *person* falls away.

Contempt

> One Wednesday afternoon, the officers organised a five-a-side football tournament for detainees. As I walked with Sally down to the sports field, we passed a detainee from Nigeria. Sally scoffed to me that he was 'a real pain in the arse'. The man had been 'making a name for himself' since his arrival a week before and he was already unpopular with the officers. He had demanded to be sent to another IRC and had 'staged' a suicide attempt the previous night. 'It was pathetic', Sally proclaimed. 'He got his roommate to go and call us and when we got there he was lying on the bed with a sheet round his neck. When we got there, he rolled off the bed with the sheet tied to the bed post.' The man had been placed in a separate unit to be monitored for self-harm.
>
> When we reached the sports field, detainees had gathered into teams based on dorm affiliations and nationalities. There was a team of 'Eastern Europeans', another of 'Africans' and an Algerian team. Sally and I settled to watch the short games in the winter sunshine. Before too long, it was the African team's turn to play. Sally nudged me when the Nigerian man appeared. 'He looks really suicidal now, doesn't he?' she remarked as the man ran up the pitch. Before long, there was trouble amongst 'the Africans'. They began shouting at one another, and the Nigerian man seemed to be accusing his team mates of some wrong against him. He claimed the ball for himself and began an elaborate display of ballmanship, bouncing it off his chest and dribbling it excessively, ignoring the cries of his team mates. He was eventually tackled and fell over. Amidst gestures of despair and ridicule from the other players, the game continued, and the Nigerian man cursed his team mates. Sally turned to me and said: 'They just can't play in a team, they always end up screaming at each other. They're like bloody children. He couldn't wait to get the ball to himself and show off. Look at them—they're all over the place. Hopeless.'

Here, then, is a racialised stereotype, through which bodies signified as African became subsumed within a discourse that construed them as 'whingers', 'like

children'. Shorthand classificatory mechanisms circulate freely in Locksdon, sifting the men and framing officers' understandings; Jamaicans are 'trouble' and insolent, but detainees from other Caribbean islands are generally 'OK'; the Turks 'look after their own'; the Algerians organise into gangs; the Chinese keep to themselves and work hard, and so on.

The officers' general professional impassiveness is disrupted by periodic outbursts of contempt, like the one described above, directed at detainees of various nationalities. At the heart of this contempt is a hierarchically arranged understanding of citizen–other relations. In Roberts' (2003: 255–6) formulation, contempt is a matter of valuing some worth or status. Contempt arises when a person is construed as lacking this worth, yet insists on *obtruding*, and claiming an equal status. Contempt encompasses a concern for some value or status, and a concern about the object's *pretending* to equality. In Locksdon, the officers hold developed ideas about moral worth to which many detainees are compared unfavourably. The officers, observing the detainees at close hand for extended periods, are able to scrutinise their actions in everyday contexts and draw out critiques from their observations. Mundane situations become windows onto personal failings, like the football match.

In brief, the qualities admired by (though, of course, not always displayed by) the officers in their colleagues and friends include self-control or discipline, stoicism, personal responsibility, loyalty (to peers, friends, colleagues) and egalitarianism. These are generalised qualities to which men and women should aspire, and they take on heightened significance among work colleagues. Officers have to rely on one another in sometimes dangerous circumstances when personal safety is at stake. The traits of loyalty, dependability and responsibility within a team are crucial.

It is the detainees' perceived manipulation of the system that provokes contempt from the officers. A secure environment is a place where the body becomes the fraught focus of political inscription (of discipline, humiliation, violence) but also a key site of resistance. Bodily self-harm or suicide are attempts by the detainees to assert *control*. In Locksdon, acts such as these draw forth a set of official procedures and can, importantly, include a transferral to another IRC, which might have better facilities. An attempt at self-harm, then, has a double 'reading': a desperate gesture, but also, potentially, a cynical and self-interested ploy. The Nigerian man here was suspected of faking his depression (depressed men do not play football, Sally implied) and stood accused of a manipulative attempt to improve his lot and get out of Locksdon. The officers strive to maintain identical treatment for all detainees. This is treatment that in no way acknowledges (in fact actively ignores) detainees' individual, unique positions: it is a stringent egalitarianism. Attempting to ask for special, *non-identical* treatment is reprehensible, a sign of not being able to tolerate the treatment that properly belongs to the condition of being a detainee; men who are unable 'to get on with it' are worthy of scorn.

The officers' contempt emerges not from an inherent callousness or brutality, but from the state of affairs they see unfolding at Locksdon. At the heart of this state of affairs is the detainees' apparent *illegality* (in violating immigration rules or having a 'bogus'

claim). The officers have little appreciation of the productive, creative and tactical nature of the implementation of law in the immigration context, and the fluid distinctions it creates between lawful and unlawful mobility (see Heyman and Smart 1999). Rather, illegality is a fixed and moralised condition. The detainees' illegal behaviour is seen to entirely justify their confinement and Locksdon, then, becomes a 'trial' for those who want to 'be let in'. Many officers argued that the detainees' behaviour in Locksdon should be reflected in immigration decisions. Locksdon was secure, after all, they said, and the detainees should be grateful for safety and basic provision. Why should some detainees be able to manipulate the system? The detainees, on the other hand, are resentful and traumatised at their ongoing denial of liberty and the precarious state of uncertainty in which they are forcibly suspended, and mobilise all tactics of evasion and resistance available to them.

It is the detainees' refusal to comply with the officers' evaluation of their position that draws contempt from the officers; they still *obtrude.* More than this, a detainee who successfully secures a move out of Locksdon has scored a victory over the officers, disrupting the hierarchical order on which a secure regime rests. Heyman (2000: 643), in a discussion of US immigration officers' encounters with Mexican migrants, argues that they found exposure to the migrants' human complexity problematic. He argues that evidence of 'complex volition' (which I understand as autonomy and self-determination) indicated shared status in a conceptually bounded group. The expression of this 'complex volition' from Mexican immigrants was inappropriate: only fellow US citizens were truly equal (Heyman 2000: 644). Similarly, it is precisely the Locksdon detainees' displays of 'complex volition' that infuriates the officers. Claims to be recognised as unique individuals, the assertion of agency, demands to be acknowledged as having rights, efforts to resist or manipulate the system: all these contravened the 'correct' behaviour of the detainees. The officers expected passivity, subservience and gratitude: the detainees are illegal, after all, and *guests.*

Like 'the gift', the concept of hospitality is full of internal contradictions. A stance taken towards strangers we do not yet know, hospitality's meaning dissolves as we approach it (Derrida 2000). The welcome of hospitality is imbued with risk: the host has the power to exclude and the guest has the power to invade. Hospitality creates asymmetrical relationships, reinforcing the host as sovereign master of 'home', with the power to impose conditions on the guest (Dikeç 2002: 229–31). Guests are placed in debt until they can repay hospitality. In short, hospitality retains the stranger as stranger. The hospitality extended to the men who find themselves as detainees at Locksdon is one that must be repaid at every turn, and in every encounter. Those who fail to conform, or who fail to understand or accept the expectation to conform, are those who provoke contempt, and to whom the rules will be ever more stringently applied.

Conclusion: Emerging Empathy?

I have argued here that paying attention to the emotional dynamics of the IRC, and understanding emotion as a construal, or evaluative judgement, can disentangle

multilayered, often contradictory assumptions, among staff. I have also begun to make the case that the staff at the grassroots *matter* because the task falls to them to make meaningful (in mundane daily routines) the cultural, social and political distinctions between citizen and other that the UK immigration and detention system seeks to draw. This process is saturated with emotion; scornful fear and vigilant contempt emerge as pivots on which emotional engagement turns (though not the only pivots).

It is clear that detention is a *productive* strategy, which brings forth categories of illegality and undesirability as it seeks to contain them. The securitised governance of mobility has become a matter of justifying political interventions by inculcating, and responding to, fear and contempt around those who seek protection, and a new life in Britain. The logic of detention rests precisely on the confinement and removal of those who are 'illegal', or have 'abused' the system, or have 'failed' in their claim for recognition. The IRC has become a potent symbol of brutality for those who contest bordering processes. For those who work at the IRC, to whom falls the task of providing for the secure but humane accommodation of detained persons, daily life is fraught and contradictory. In the centre, the sovereign distinctions between 'abject life' and 'political citizen' are upheld and produced through emotional responses. I have shown that 'the secure' and 'the humane' are in tension.

The humane, however, periodically resurfaces and troubles the sovereign distinction. Within the seething environment of Locksdon, space is sometimes opened for something more than contempt and unease, suspicion and vigilance. Periodically, the officers have cause to recognise that the detainees—far from being wholly other, dangerous, threatening—are *just like them* (and vice versa). Glimpses of mutuality may be found in a conversation about cricket, excitement at a football match, a shared joke. More than this, the imagination of similarity can 'creep upon' detainees and staff in an emergent fragile empathy. A man who had been at Locksdon for nearly a year suddenly heard he was to be deported and officers bid farewell with compassion, telling one another it was not fair. An officer comforted a tearful detainee who was worried about his girlfriend and their baby, left alone after he had been picked on by the authorities in an early morning raid, and gave him a phone call, against policy. A man who had lived in Britain for years, but whose papers were incorrect, found himself at Locksdon and earned the sympathy of the officers. These were occasions when empathy flourished. In Nussbaum's terms, empathy is the imaginative reconstruction of another person's experience. The experience of empathy, and the accompanying possibility of compassion, have at their core the recognition of one's related vulnerability (Nussbaum 2001: 319). At heart, then, compassion involves a notion of common humanity, and thus has a radical potential to disrupt. All kinds of social barrier can erode the imaginative link to other people, of course; those who wish to foster cruelty remove the conditions for the imagination of similarity. Yet even in a social milieu like Locksdon, imbued with mistrust and ambivalence, the political hierarchies that are produced and reinforced by emotion cannot wholly preclude the periodic emergence of empathy and compassion.

Empathy has the potential to profoundly disturb the logic of the IRC and challenge the clear differentiations between 'citizen' and 'other' that the sovereign decision on exclusion seeks to draw. The distinction between citizen and other, in which so much is invested, is exposed, ultimately, as arbitrary. The emergence of empathy is an incongruous and disruptive emotional project.

The project to explore the daily life of the IRC is one that can demonstrate the importance of emotion and its entanglement with politics. That emotion is caught up with the particular politics of migration, and mobility is never more clearly shown than in Locksdon. Here, the drive for a rationalised and comprehensive system of mobility governance is revealed to be intertwined with affect, and emotional dispositions within the centre crystallise the broader concerns of the war on terror, with material effects on the way in which the detainees are treated. More than this, the camp as described by Agamben is revealed to be a more complex milieu than analyses that 'stop at the gate' might suggest. The language of the exception that pervades critical legal and political engagements with detention suggests that the bare life residing within the camp-like spaces of our political moment is abject, and cannot help but conjure a view of the camp as outside and empty. In fact, the processes through which the legal and political exception is brought into being in immigration detention permeate and shape the continuing social life therein. A focus on the processual 'making abject' reveals the incomplete nature of this state. If Isin and Rygiel (2007: 185) are right, and the way to grasp the possibilities for different logics and resistance is to understand in depth the thoughts and practices that sustain camp-like spaces, then a focus on emotion offers a way of going beyond the abject space. The camp is exposed as a place of emotion, politics and resistance, where fear and contempt are rife, but where empathy is never wholly effaced.

Acknowledgements

I would like to thank Maruška Svašek for organising the *Emotion and Migration* workshop at Queen's University, Belfast in November 2007 and for her helpful comments on a draft of this paper; thanks also to the anonymous *JEMS* reviewer.

Notes

[1] http://www.archive2.officialdocuments.co.uk/document/cm53/5387/cm5387.pdf. Accessed April 2005.

[2] All names are pseudonyms.

References

Agamben, G. (1998) *Homo Sacer: Sovereign Power and Bare Life.* Stanford: Stanford University Press.

Ahmed, S. (2004a) *The Cultural Politics of Emotion.* Edinburgh: Edinburgh University Press.

Ahmed, S. (2004b) 'Affective economies', *Social Text 79*, *22*(2): 117–39.

Amoore, L. (2006) 'Biometric borders: governing mobilities in the war on terror', *Political Geography, 25*(3): 336–51.

Amoore, L. (2007) 'Vigilant visualities: the watchful politics of the war on terror', *Security Dialogue, 38*(2): 215–32.

Anderson, B. (2006) 'Becoming and being hopeful: towards a theory of affect', *Environment and Planning D: Society and Space, 24*(5): 733–52.

Anderson, B. and Harrison, P. (2006) 'Questioning affect and emotion', *Area, 38*(3): 333–5.

Aretxaga, B. (1997) *Shattering Silence: Women, Nationalism and Political Subjectivity in Northern Ireland.* Princeton: Princeton University Press.

Bashford, A. and Strange, C. (2002) 'Asylum-seekers and national histories of detention', *Australian Journal of Politics and History, 48*(4): 509–27.

Bashford, B. and Strange, C. (2003) 'Isolation and exclusion in the modern world: an introductory essay', in Bashford, A. and Strange, C. (eds) *Isolation: Places and Practices of Exclusion.* London: Routledge, 1–19.

Bigo, D. (2001) 'The Möbius ribbon of internal and external security', in Albert, M., Jacobson, D. and Lapid, Y. (eds) *Identities, Borders, Orders.* Minneapolis: University of Minnesota Press, 91–117.

Bloch, A. and Schuster, L. (2005) 'At the extremes of exclusion: deportation, detention and dispersal', *Ethnic and Racial Studies, 28*(3): 491–512.

Brennan, T. (2004) *The Transmission of Affect.* New York: Cornell University Press.

Butler, J. (2005) *Precarious Life: Powers of Mourning and Violence.* London: Verso Books.

Cesarini, D. and Kushner, T. (eds) (1993) *The Internment of Aliens in Twentieth Century Britain.* London: Frank Cass.

Dasgupta, P. (1988) 'Trust as a commodity', in Gambetta, D. (ed.) *Trust: Making and Breaking Cooperative Relations.* Oxford: Basil Blackwell, 49–73.

Davidson, J., Bondi, L. and Smith, M. (eds) (2005) *Emotional Geographies.* London: Ashgate.

Derrida, J. (2000) *Of Hospitality: Anne Dufourmantelle Invites Jacques Derrida to Respond.* Stanford: Stanford University Press.

Dikeç, M. (2002) 'Pera Pera Poros: longing for spaces of hospitality', *Theory, Culture and Society, 19*(1–2): 227–47.

Diken, B. (2004) 'From refugee camps to gated communities: biopolitics and the end of the city', *Citizenship Studies, 8*(1): 83–106.

Dillon, M. (1999) 'The scandal of the refugee: some reflections on the "inter" of international relations', in Campbell, D. and Shapiro, M. (eds) *Moral Spaces: Rethinking Ethics and World Politics.* Minneapolis: University of Minnesota Press, 92–124.

Feldman, A. (1991) *Formations of Violence: The Narrative of the Body and Political Terror in Northern Ireland.* Chicago: University of Chicago Press.

Foucault, M. (1977) *Discipline and Punish: The Birth of the Prison.* London: Penguin.

Genova, N. (2002) 'Migrant "illegality" and deportability in everyday life', *Annual Review of Anthropology, 31*: 419–47.

Heyman, J. (2000) 'Respect for outsiders? Respect for the law? The moral evaluation of high-scale issues by US immigration officers', *Journal of the Royal Anthropological Institute, 6*(4): 635–52.

Heyman, J. and Smart, A. (1999) 'States and illegal practices: an overview', in Heyman, J. and Smart, A. (eds) *States and Illegal Practices.* Oxford: Berg, 1–24.

Home Office (2008a) *Large-Scale Expansion of Britain's Detention Estate.* Press Release: http://press.homeoffice.gov.uk/press-releases/Immigration-Detention. Accessed 15 June 2008.

Home Office (2008b) *Asylum Statistics, 1st Quarter, 2008.* Research Development and Statistics Directorate, http://www.homeoffice.gov.uk/rds/pdfs08/asylumq108.pdf. Accessed 2 August 2008.

Home Office (2008c) *Control of Immigration Quarterly Statistical Summary, United Kingdom, April 2008–June 2008*. Research Development and Statistics Directorate, http://www.homeoffice.gov.uk/rds/pdfs08/coiq208.pdf. Accessed 2 August 2008.

Isin, E. (2004) 'The neurotic citizen', *Citizenship Studies*, *8*(3): 217–35.

Isin, E. and Rygiel, K. (2007) 'Abject spaces: frontiers, zones, camps', in Dauphinee, E. and Masters, C. (eds) *The Logics of Biopower and the War on Terror*. New York: Palgrave Macmillan, 181–205.

Josephides, J. (2003) '"Being there": the magic of presence or the metaphysics of morality?', in Caplan, P. (ed.) *The Ethics of Anthropology*. London: Routledge, 55–76.

Josephides, L. (2005) 'Resentment as a sense of self', in Milton, K. and Svašek, M. (eds) *Mixed Emotions: Anthropological Studies of Feeling*. Oxford: Berg, 71–91.

Leavitt, J. (1996) 'Meaning and feeling in the anthropology of emotions', *American Ethnologist*, *23*(3): 514–39.

Liebling, A. and Price, D. (2001) *The Prison Officer*. HMP Leyhill: The Prison Service Journal.

Lutz, C. (1988) *Unnatural Emotions*. Chicago: University of Chicago Press.

Lutz, C. and Abu-Lughod, L. (eds) (1990) *Language and the Politics of Emotion*. Cambridge: Cambridge University Press.

Malloch, M. and Stanley, E. (2005) 'The detention of asylum-seekers in the UK: representing risk, managing the dangerous', *Punishment and Society*, *7*(1): 53–71.

Malkki, L. (1995) 'Refugees and exile: from "refugee studies" to the national order of things', *Annual Review of Anthropology*, *24*: 495–523.

Massumi, B. (2005) 'The future birth of the affective act'. Conference Proceedings: Genealogies of Biopolitics. Available at http://browse.reticular.info/text/collected/massumi.pdf.

Massumi, B. (2007) 'Potential politics and the primacy of pre-emption', *Theory and Event*, *10*(2): http://muse.jhu.edu/journals/theory_and_event/v010/10.2massumi.html.

Milton, K. (2002) *Loving Nature: Towards an Ecology of Emotion*. London: Routledge.

Milton, K. (2005) 'Meanings, feelings and human ecology', in Milton, K. and Svašek, M. (eds) *Mixed Emotions: Anthropological Studies of Feeling*. Oxford: Berg, 25–43.

Milton, K. and Svašek, M. (eds) (2005) *Mixed Emotions: Anthropological Studies of Feeling*. Oxford: Berg.

Minca, C. (2005) 'The return of the camp', *Progress in Human Geography*, *29*(4): 405–12.

Misztal, B. (1996) *Trust in Modern Societies: In Search of the Bases of Social Order*. Cambridge: Polity Press.

Nussbaum, M. (2001) *Upheavals of Thought: The Intelligence of Emotions*. Cambridge: Cambridge University Press.

Nussbaum, M. (2004) *Hiding from Humanity: Disgust, Shame, and the Law*. Princeton: Princeton University Press.

Nyers, P. (2006) *Rethinking Refugees: Beyond States of Emergency*. London: Routledge.

Parkinson, B. (1995) *Ideas and Realities of Emotions*. London: Routledge.

Pratt, A. (2005) *Securing Borders; Detention and Deportation in Canada*. Vancouver: University of British Columbia Press.

Roberts, R. (2003) *Emotions: An Essay in Aid of Moral Psychology*. Cambridge: Cambridge University Press.

Schuster, L. (2005) 'A sledgehammer to crack a nut: deportation, detention and dispersal in Europe', *Social Policy and Administration*, *39*(6): 606–21.

Sibley, D. (1995) *Geographies of Exclusion*. London: Routledge.

Solomon, R. (1983) *The Passions*. Notre Dame: University of Notre Dame Press.

Svašek, M. (2005a) 'Emotions in anthropology', in Milton, K. and Svašek, M. (eds) *Mixed Emotions: Anthropological Studies of Feeling*. Oxford: Berg, 1–25.

Svašek, M. (2005b) 'The politics of chosen trauma', in Milton, K. and Svašek, M. (eds) *Mixed Emotions: Anthropological Studies of Feeling*. Oxford: Berg, 195–215.

Svašek, M. and Skrbiš, Z. (2007) 'Passions and powers: emotions and globalisation', *Identities: Global Studies in Culture and Power, 14*(4): 367–83.

Thien, D. (2005) 'After or beyond feeling? A consideration of affect and emotion in geography', *Area, 37*(4): 450–54.

Tolia-Kelly, D. (2006) 'Affect: an ethnocentric encounter? Exploring the "universalist" imperative of emotional/affective geographies', *Area, 38*(2): 213–17.

Walters, W. (2002) 'Deportation, expulsion and the international police of aliens', *Citizenship Studies, 6*(3): 265–92.

Weber, L. and Gelsthorpe, L. (2000) *Deciding to Detain: How Discretion to Detain Asylum-Seekers is Exercised at Ports of Entry.* Cambridge: Institute of Criminology.

Welch, M. (2003) *Detained: Immigration Laws and the Expanding I.N.S. Jail Complex.* Philadelphia: Temple University Press.

Welch, M. and Schuster, L. (2005) 'Detention of asylum-seekers in the US, UK, France, Germany, and Italy', *Criminal Justice, 5*(4): 331–55.

'Unkind Cuts': Health Policy and Practice versus the Health and Emotional Well-Being of Asylum-Seekers and Refugees in Ireland

Katy Radford

Healthcare is the keystone of a number of complex progressive social justice issues that evoke complex emotions. As the demography of Ireland rapidly changes, the practices and expectations of some asylum-seekers and others seeking refugee status present new opportunities and challenges for health-service providers. This paper looks at some of the emotions evoked in healthcare issues. It draws on observations and interviews from empirical fieldwork carried out for the Health Research Board. The research was conducted both in the Adelaide and Meath Hospital, incorporating the National Children's Hospital, Tallaght and in a number of refugee reception centres in Ireland. At one level, honouring faith choices within a healthcare setting is a societal acknowledgement—often made to people at their most vulnerable—that the potent and cathartic transformative rituals they value are significant in mediating and managing their emotions. This paper argues that, at another level, it is a practical and symbolic communication of a statutory commitment to interculturalism and community cohesion.

Introduction

At 5 pm on Sunday 17 August 2003, Callis Osaghae, a four-week-old boy, was admitted to Waterford General Hospital after a home circumcision. He died there at 4.30 a.m. the next morning. The events surrounding Callis' death quickly became a

talking point at water-coolers and in the backs of taxis throughout Ireland. For many people, their understanding of the issues and knowledge of the events relied on the dissemination of media conjecture and editorial proclamations. The flurry of journalists' superlatives and the relish with which they were consumed by the readership demonstrated the symbiotic co-dependency of both reporters and their audience for emotive and sensational narratives. The Irish papers, both red-top and broadsheets, did not temper the subject matter with any contextualisation of the wider issues concerning recent immigration or migrant health issues. Instead, the articles were rich with controversial and poignant misinformation when describing the events and the unnamed circumcisor. This resulted in a diverse set of emotionally charged public responses to the tragedy and its unfolding details. Yet the emotions of the principal actors went unreported.

The facts of the case were simple. The third child and only son of Nigerian refugees Idehen (31) and Mabel (23), Callis suffered severe blood loss and was found by the state pathologist to have died as a result of both haemorrhaging and shock due to bleeding. One year later, Judge Kevin Haugh felt compelled to ask jurors not to bring their 'white Western values to bear' prior to the trial of Osaghie Igbinidion, a Nigerian, who, with his Irish-born wife, voluntarily presented himself to a Garda Síochána (the Irish police service) after he became aware of the child's death. Igbinedion was subsequently cleared of the charge of 'recklessly engaging in conduct in and about the circumcision in a manner which created a risk of serious harm or death'. Yet, despite being acquitted, the press continued to portray the practice of male circumcision in a disparaging light, drawing on social and economic arguments against asylum-seekers and refugees to fuel the fire of the narrative. Journalists offered pencil sketches of Igbinidion that relied on loaded imagery, based on descriptions of him as 'accompanied by a blonde girlfriend', 'being dependant on legal aid' and 'being arrested in a hostel for the homeless'. Their accounts fuelled anti-immigrant sentiments.

Migrancy and immigration issues which, for some time, had been bubbling under the public radar, rapidly surfaced to become prominent conversation pieces. The discussions focused in particular on asylum-seekers and refugees, portraying them as people engaged in strange, illegal, and potentially risky ritual practices. While the reaction and sentiments that are individually and collectively expressed around the death of any child are complex, in this instance they were further complicated for the majority white, Irish Catholics because of the relationship to the rituals and practices of the 'other', that they had not previously had to consider. Their 'customs' were imagined as completely alien to Irish medical practices. Discourses that emphasised the 'otherness' of migrant bodies were also reproduced by Irish employees who interacted with migrants in particular institutional settings, such as refugee reception centres, hospitals and health centres. Medical personnel had to screen incomers for contagious diseases, and were confronted with 'uncommon' desires in connection with the handling of sick and dying bodies. This, in combination with frequent linguistic communication problems, set migrant patients

apart from the more 'usual' hospital visitors. The news about the fatal case of circumcision, regarded by the majority of the Christian Irish population as an unneccesary or even brutal operation, strengthened the image of the newcomers as 'strangers'. The negative perception of migrant practices such as circumision was, of course, partly caused by a lack of knowledge, as the locals were not familiar with culturally specific expectations, taboos and needs. Their attitude towards the treatment of human bodies and corpses was based on Irish medical training and cultural traditions.

This article will examine some of the experiences of migrants in service provider/ user settings in the Republic of Ireland. While the first part of the analysis will examine issues related to healthcare, the second part will focus on the interaction between migrants and local employees in relation to death and mourning. The article is mainly based on my fieldwork and field notes. In 2005 and 2006, I conducted research for a project funded by the Health Research Board, examining the needs of those from minority ethnic and faith-based communities in healthcare provision. By initiating the project, the funders acknowledged that the commitments of the Department of Health and Children to advancing an equality and rights-based agenda across the health sector was not quite as advanced as they would wish it to be (see also Jentsch *et al.* 2007).

The intention was to consider whether or not there were satisfactory procedures in place, and cultural competencies being developed, within the statutory sector to provide adequate and appropriate support to those from non-Christian communities. To undertake the research, two specific constituencies were contacted: service providers and service users. In addition to conducting focus groups, interviews and seminar debates, and to shadowing medics, health practitioners, administrators and ancillary staff, the author undertook a series of clinical observations to gain information about the interaction between service providers and service users. Over the period of one year, considerable time was also spent in refugee reception centres and alongside those working in the chaplaincy service within an acute hospital setting. This provided an opportunity to engage informally with both groups of people, often within highly charged emotional environments.

Needs and Emotions in a Global Era

From an analytical perspective, it is useful to theorise the concept of 'needs' to get a better view of how, in multicultural settings, service providers and users may (fail to) come to a mutual understanding about appropriate medical and post-mortal practices. Dictionary definitions of the verb 'to need' stress the incompleteness or imperfection of a situation or process; something *must be done* to avoid deterioration or change the situation for the better.

In anthropology, the concept of 'needs' has been theorised by various authors. Malinowski (1944), for example, distinguished between 'individual needs' and 'basic needs'. He defined individual needs as biologically determined forces that secure

survival of the individual and demand universal responses. Basic needs, by contrast, lay stress on 'the total conditions necessary to individual and group survival, and not merely on individual impulses'. The latter regulated group behaviour and required cultural responses (Malinowski 1944: 77). Leaving aside the difficult question as to what extent needs are defined by biological or cultural forces, it is clear that both have an important impact on individual peoples' ability to experience feelings of well-being.[1]

In medical settings, it may seem useful to make a distinction between practical and emotional needs. While the former centre on issues such as staying clean, being fed and getting the right medicine, the latter refer to psychosocial dynamics and personal satisfaction with medical treatment and interpersonal engagement with service providers. Yet practical and emotional needs are often interrelated. A hospital patient must be washed for reasons of hygiene; at a first glance, this may seem a purely practical matter. Yet *how* a nurse will wash a patient, and *which* nurse is allowed to do so, depend on specific training that stipulates guidelines about social and emotional interaction on the work floor. The codes that define patients' needs are partly influenced by culture, as demonstrated by a recent analysis of the experiences and expectations of Chinese cancer patients in two oncology hospitals in Beijing. The study found that '[f]or Chinese patients, coping with illness and misfortune is largely a private and family affair, and most of them did not expect nurses to meet their emotional needs' (Liu *et al.* 2005: 262). As such, their preferences for support were somewhat different to those detailed in non-Chinese, Western settings (Harris 1998; Jung *et al.* 2003; Leydon 2000).

Professional codes of behaviour may not resonate with patients' emotional needs, especially when service providers and service users have different cultural backgrounds and personal experience. In view of such different perceptions, it is not surprising that a whole array of concerns may colour migrant experiences of offical healthcare institutions in their new surroundings, generating complaints about unrecognised or ignored emotional needs. To stay with the example of washing, various issues related to gender or kinship may be crucial. Can a male nurse wash a female patient? Which family member is allowed to be present while mother is undressed? These can be important questions. Taboos surrounding particular substances may also affect expectations. What kind of soap can be used? Should water be lukewarm or warm? In addition, the way in which medical workers are perceived by patients may also depend on cultural specificities. Sheba Mariam George (2005) has argued that, in Kerala, discourses of caste and gender define nurses as dirty and sexually loose, a stigma that was transnationally reinforced amongst Indians from Kerala who migrated to the United States.

The use in this paper of the term 'emotional needs' is partly inspired by a broader interest in emotional processes in a dynamic world, in which people cross national borders as tourists, expellees, migrants or refugees. As Svašek and Skrbiš (2007: 373) noted,

> [w]illingly or not, transnationally mobile people, perhaps best (although not exclusively) epitomised in migrants, 'carry along' particular memories and feelings and are to some extent conditioned by emotional discourses and practices learned in their place of origin.

The above emphasises that migrant emotional needs are informed by cultural background and personal history. In addition, new needs generally arise as a result of displacement, as the process of movement is often accompanied by loss of status and feelings of alienation and marginalisation. In a study of suffering amongst East African migrants and refugees in Western Australia, Farida Tilbury (2007: 451) found a wide variety of negative emotions that were partly caused by the experience of displacement, including 'frustration, uncertainty, hopelessness, shame and embarrassment, loneliness, disempowerment, shock, anger, loss of control, betrayal'. To improve their well-being, some turned to healthcare workers for help, and were usually diagnosed as 'suffering from depression' and given medication. Tilbury argues that the diagnosis was generally based on a universalistic understanding of emotions that failed to acknowledge cultural specificity. The discourse of depression, regarded as a mental illness, also denied the social and political embeddedness of the Africans' emotional problems. They were treated as independent bodies to be healed, unrelated to the forces of political oppression, poverty or racism.

Migrant emotional needs have to be understood in the context of wider forces that impact on individual life histories, and affect opportunities to create and maintain affectionate social relationships. The loss of direct, everyday support from networks of kin and friends in the homeland is often experienced as destabilising. Even though modern communication technology allows for emotional and moral support from a distance (Baldassar 2007), the lack of co-presence is experienced by many migrants as a real loss that cannot easily be replaced by alternatives. Newly arrived migrants who are placed in immigration removal centres, waiting for decisions to be made about their immigrant status, are unable to form new well-functioning supportive ties. This makes a more sympathetic understanding of their emotional needs amongst local service providers all the more important.

As will become clear in this article, in Ireland it is common practice for service providers to refuse empathetic emotional engagement with migrants by employing an impersonal communicational style that is marked as 'professional'. The research suggests, however, that a more meaningful practice-based model of communication should be developed in the health sector than currently exists. By encouraging health service practitioners (and other service providers) to demonstrate appropriate emotional responses to migrant emotional needs, the potential arises to bring a new dimension to professionalism. Recognising that the display of empathy has a key role to play in brokering relationships between individuals and groups turns the rhetoric of 'holistic care' into reality. It is by enabling emotions to be both expressed and shared, that productive human interaction is realised. The inclusion of sessions on cross-cultural empathy and migrant emotional needs in medical training programmes will

undermine the current practice of fixing and reifying cultures, and will acknowledge the fact that Ireland is a place of human mobility and cultural complexity.

The Republic of Ireland: Economic Change and Migration Movements

Everyday life in the Republic of Ireland is, of course, influenced by wider political and economic processes that stimulate the push and pull of human mobility. The Irish economy has moved from receiving 'final demand' notices from the International Monetary Fund in the late 1980s to becoming one of the fastest growing economies in Europe. For the past year or two, however, the country has suffered the effects of the global financial crisis. Per ratio of the population, the country for a time attracted more migrant workers since the EU enlargement of 2004 than any other country. (Frawley 2006: 44).

Ireland was one of the only three 'old' EU member-states which imposed no transition arrangements concerning admission to the labour market in 2004, although it did introduce restrictions to welfare benefits by imposing a two-year habitual residence rule. It also made a change to the categories of work for which it was possible to apply for work permits. These developments have had a phenomenal impact on the social and economic development of the country (Fanning 2007).

Furthermore, by the end of 2005, while 48,632 applications had been processed on behalf of asylum-seekers living in hostels, a total of 6,814—mainly Nigerians and Romanians—were granted full refugee status; 16,727 were granted leave to remain under a special application process for the parents of Irish-born children after the Supreme Court ruling in 2003 overturned the *status quo ante* where the parents of Irish-born children acquired indefinite residency rights. There are now at least 27,000 people legally resident in Ireland who originally arrived as asylum-seekers. Among members of these communities there are currently 167 languages in use, and figures from 2006 indicate that, at that time, there were 31,779 Muslims eligible to complete the census.

Alongside the shift in population, the Irish health system has undergone a period of organisational change and reform. Concepts of communication, participation and consultation are increasingly written into macro-social strategies and policy documents as an ideological 'goal' language (Apthorpe 1997). Hansen (1997), however, suggested that hospital policy documents and mission statements may use rudimentary language, defined by him as 'form without content', as they belie the complexities of communication processes essential to implementing effective communication.

In the past few years, increasing concerns have been raised in the Republic of Ireland about the treatment of migrants and refugees. A social inclusion care unit in the Health Service Executive, the body responsible for the provision of health and social services in Ireland, has been established to develop a national intercultural strategy recognising that staff currently have inadequate understanding of and responses to medical conditions rarely encountered in Ireland (Watt and McGaughey

2006: 117). In addition to the growing pressure of numbers, a key challenge they have identified in their service provision is one of language diversity, attitudinal barriers (on both sides of the couch), and a lack of cultural understanding. Summing up all of these issues, one consultant explained the challenge for him:

> Your diagnosis is in the history 90 per cent of times, and if you can't take a good history, then it's like trying to do a jigsaw with a third of the pieces.

Perhaps unsurprisingly, the overriding state of mind expressed by the health service providers in relation to healthcare within the context of both documented and undocumented migrants was one of professional uncertainty. Service providers suggested that it was primarily fear of being accused of systemic and individual racism, and not a felt need for increased empathy, that brokered their motivation to develop and adhere to communication policies and protocols.[2]

Emotional Experiences and Needs in a Refugee Reception Centre

The remainer of the article will focus on the emotional experiences of migrants and refugees in Irish institutional settings, exploring some of their needs and concerns. The following passage will explore these dynamics in Balseskin Refugee Reception Centre. The Centre was established in 2001 and consists of temporary buildings on a four-acre compound in Finglas, half an hour North of Dublin. It is able to accommodate 380 residents and also comprises a canteen and external play facilities for children, as well as the only medical centre in Ireland for asylum-seekers staffed by specialists from the Health Service Executive. Like the other asylum-seeker accommodation, it is managed by the Reception and Integration Agency of the Department of Justice but, unlike other centres, this one has been purpose-built.[3]

Outside the Coombe maternity hospital and sandwiched between two green double-decker Dublin buses is a white 24-seater van. Destination: Balseskin Refugee Reception Centre. Many of the women passengers, whose buggies are loaded up with plastic bags with shopping, have been attending the 'specialist clinic' at the hospital. They are all Sub-Saharan African. The reception centre is mostly home to Nigerians, Somalians and Romanians, principally single males aged 20–40, but there are a substantial number of young mothers and their children. As the men pass other's people's children over the heads of already seated passengers towards the back of the bus, English is very much the second or third language spoken, and then only for the benefit of the driver.

The reception centre is several kilometres away from regular public transport. From the outside it appears either like an open prison (but for the absence of security), or a colony for migrant workers (but for the absence of on-site recreational facilities). Here the government agency responsible has created a system of institutional dependency where the accommodation remains uncustomised by the residents and food is prepared and provided for them within set times. This is used to justify their need for only a small weekly stipend of €19.10 per adult with additional

€9.50 per child. The key agency's nomenclature, Reception and Integration, suggests that the service rests on these twin pillars—in practice these exist in name only and those seeking asylum are segregated in whatever way possible from their neighbours and actively discouraged from seeking out ways in which to engage with wider civil society.[4]

The residents' emotional need to create new networks of friendship and support is clearly frustrated, which makes them feel marginalised, as pointed out by one of the residents:

> I have not yet had a warm reception to this country. I am not integrated. I have been dumped out here.

Feelings of alienation and their undetermined status strongly affected their sense of self.[5] Attempting to define self-identity, home or community in this instance is paradoxical, as migration, transience, displacement, spiritual and physical estrangement directly affect any sense of belonging (Radford 2006: 146; Rapport and Dawson 1998).

The emotional responses of the undocumented migrants were both exacerbated and anaesthetised by their predicament, and strongly determined by the practicalities of survival. That is not to undermine the enormity of the emotional turmoil in such centres, but rather points to the urgency of questions and practicalities they report facing: 'Am I going to be here for much longer? Will I be able to get the retro-viral drugs that brought me here in the first instance? Who will she turn to for child-care support when she has to go to hospital for the new baby to be born? How will I get a message home to let them know that she has been born?'. For medical problems and check-ups the residents visit the medical centre, which is, however, ill-equipped to deal with the psycho-social needs of those in trauma. Furthermore, full clinical examinations of asylum-seekers are not undertaken and, consequently, complications during pregnancy are sometimes not addressed until women present in labour at the Maternity Hospital. Yet in the medical centre residents are screened for HIV, TB, Hepatitis B and C, Chicken Pox etc., because the reduction of public health risks is very much the focus of service delivery, much to the regret of those providing that service.

Patrick, now an on-site clinical nurse with a particular interest in traditional medicines and scarification processes, was formerly a development worker connected to a Catholic mission in Sub-Saharan Africa. He is frustrated:

> I don't have the opportunity to examine as thoroughly as I'd like to here and so issues relating to people's emotional state and their mental well-being are not always detected. There's some kind of mentoring programme that needs to be urgently put into place for young men and boys at risk of suicide, particularly when they're lost or have been separated from their families. I have about twenty at the moment who I've referred on to CCST [the Centre for the Care of Survivors of Torture, a specialist service operated under the auspices of Spirasi, the Spiritan Asylum Services Initiative].

Patrick's words show that some Irish service providers are willing to pay more attention to, and learn about, the specific medical and emotional needs of migrants, but often fail in their intention to do so because of structural limitations as much as time pressure. The Centre for the Care of Survivors of Torture was established within Spirasi in the 1990s by the Congregation of the Holy Spirit (Spiritans) Order. It was one of the first and remains the most active non-governmental organisation working for the rehabilitation, care and support of asylum-seekers and refugees in Ireland.

Discussing Male and Female Circumcision

The following field-diary excerpts make clear that the Balseskin Reception Centre is not only a place of alienation, but also a place of connection and discussion, as female residents exchange ideas about personal experiences and medical practices back home and in Ireland.

> I'm sitting on Simi's floor. Crammed into her tiny room at Balseskin which she shares with her baby are three other Nigerian women, one Cameroonian, one Kenyan and a Somali, all aged between twenty and forty. Makwena, a Kikuyu, has been here for the shortest time, three months, and Amina, who speaks virtually no English, has been in Ireland for three years. The women all have diverse professional backgrounds, one was a photo-journalist, another a social worker, a third a farmer and all have been educated at least until the age of eighteen. They come together with the support of a Dublin-based, Ireland-wide pan-African women's group to develop strategies to raise awareness about female circumcision, also known as female genital mutilation. All of them have either experienced it directly, or indirectly through family members.
>
> Though keen to point to the differences between female genital mutilation and male cultural circumcision, it is the week after Igbinidion's trial and as all of those women who have sons have had them circumcised, it is perhaps unsurprising that the conversation moves between the two modes of body scarification and mutilation, with death never far from the conversation. Yennis, 32, a Nigerian from the Delta State raised in an urban environment with her four sisters by their father, noted that, even though she knew about the baby Callis, 'it did not stop me to circumcise my [male] baby'. The women did, however, criticise the way male circumcision is practiced in Irish hospitals. They discussed the merits of having a home circumcision over a hospital-provided one. 'Back home they use rings—here they stitch them, they are very rough, you should see the way they cut it (. . .) The stitching is no good, I can show you my son, they should try and use ring. We want a professional, hygienic job—everyone wants this for their child. I am happy to pay €200 because when he wanted to wee it was very hard'.
>
> Yennis also talks of the suicidal thoughts she had during the first year after her child was born, and considers that this was rooted in her being on her own in the reception centre with a small baby. Disowned by her father, she has no contact with her sisters and no prospect of any family reunification. Despite being surrounded constantly by others, she became increasingly solitary and it was only when she was diagnosed with post-natal depression that she felt she was able to access the

> appropriate statutory support her underlying condition warranted. She resented the lack of an appropriate early response from her GP to her situation. 'My doctor just would come down and listen to what I had to say, and then she just says "OK, OK, OK" and writes out prescriptions'.

One would expect that health visitors, who take out time to visit migrant women with small babies 'at home', would have more opportunities than GPs to detect the emotional needs and mental health problems of migrant women. In a study conducted in Inner London, however, Drennan and Joseph (2005) found that health visitors who visited refugee families prioritised the need of children before those of their mothers. Pointing at a lack in their training, they complained that they were not properly educated to deal with the complexity of problems faced by refugee mothers.

The above makes clear that the women felt they had no opportunity to express their needs concerning circumcision in the Irish medical setting. It must, of course, be noted that in hospital settings, all patients, irrespective of their ethnicity, faith or immigration status, are generally expected to disengage their emotional responses and comply with the medical authorities so as to temporarily relinquish the social expectations of personal responsibility for their body.[6] Having been assigned and assumed an objectified position, patients are less able to play an active part in their own healing process. This may, however, be an essential component within non-Irish traditions.

Despite the women's criticism, it is not uncommon for migrant parents to seek circumcisions in Dublin hospitals. But while the operation is theoretically available, in practice it is often difficult for parents to access the service, and virtually impossible to do so in a time frame that enables them to adhere to culturally accepted prescriptions and norms. In part this is due to the limited number of consultants and medics available, but also as a result of many nurses being unwilling to take part in this service as they do not recognise its cultural significance. In the words of one nurse from rural Ireland,

> Jays [Jesus], there's not a chance that I'd be able for carrying out that one, so. I don't know anyone of us who would do it. There must be something that could be done about it under the law. What about the Offences Against the Persons Act or something?

Adapting to Cultural Diversity? The Gill Report

As a result of Callis' death, the Department of Health and Children was prompted to commission the Gill Report (2006). It recommends that cultural male circumcision be provided regionally on demand in the Irish Health Service by appropriately trained professionals. It suggested that 'if doctors are unwilling or unable to carry out the procedure in a timely fashion, parents would turn in greater numbers to community practitioners'. However, the report also suggested that medical staff who have an ethical objection to the procedure should be given the right not to be

asked to be involved. During her fieldwork, Radford frequently heard from both hospital staff and parents of an increasing number of presentations in A&E departments relating to excessive bleeding and infection. This was particularly evident in examples given by Sub-Saharan Africans, who are more inclined to work with community-based circumcision practitioners rather than the health service providers. This, they suggest, is because of the 'understanding' that the community practitioners bring. It is regrettable that there are no figures available through the hospital system to provide an evidence base for this trend, yet there is qualitative material that can be drawn on to illustrate this preference.

Mustafa Mahmood has been a paediatric consultant for ten years, working out of three Dublin-based hospitals. He rarely performs what he described as 'social' circumcisions through the Health Service, but does at least one a month in a private capacity, mostly for Muslim families with links to Middle-Eastern and Arabic-speaking countries. He said he was rarely called on by Nigerians, who 'have a well-established network of community practitioners that they prefer to use'. Nigerian practitioners receive much support from those who are frightened by the procedure being carried out under general anaesthetic. Yennis remembered how afraid she had been when her son was circumcised:

> I was not happy with this thing happening in the hospital. When they take him to theatre, my tears were just coming, I was so fearful. I couldn't hold them because I could see how my baby was struggling before he went to sleep. And then after the operation and before he came to life I could see that he was struggling to come to life. I would rather it was not done in a hospital.

Defending the Nigerian practitioner who was responsible for the death of baby Callis, she said:

> What happened in Waterford was just an accident because that man had done many circumcisions before; he had never had any problem. This guy, he calls himself the best circumciser in the world and if he was supported to do it, he would do it well. There are others in Dublin, in Ballinasloe and we have a woman in Athlone who has done it with never any problem—we know her now, she understands what it means to us and to have it done. But there is a danger that if the government does not recognise that people will go and have it done, there will be further problems.

The Gill report also recommended that the operation should be carried out in the first year of a child's life, preferably in the second six months. This, according to the National Consultative Council on Racism and Inter-Culturalism, is an example of the state targeting and mainstreaming diversity issues, exemplifying 'a service [that] has been initiated and provided not on the grounds of formal equality, but to reflect the specific needs of particular communities of interest' *de facto*; one that is responsive to the communities' emotional as well as practical needs. However, the response of asylum-seekers and their support organisations challenges this view. They point to the fact that the Gill team consulted with only Muslim and Jewish leaders,

and did not seek out the views of community representatives and activists from other communities that practice male circumcision before making its recommendations.

At the time of writing, the view of the Irish Refugee Council is that there is a need to advocate for the regulation of specialists from within the community to deliver a more appropriate service. Yennis concurs with this view:

> If you are pregnant you should be given a form to fill out [that] you want your child to be circumcised within seven days, and if the health service do not have resources to do so, then train up practitioners from the community. They don't understand that they should be supporting what the community wants, giving them more training, you know, and to help them to buy proper equipment. These people know how to respond to us. In the hospital they are cold, cold, cold.

The response illustrates a number of tensions between those 'assisters of integration' (Gilligan 2006: 44) whose attempts and motivation to work towards integration find that they are in conflict with those they are intending or mandated to represent. The questions posed by Malik (2005) remain in relation to how central the state is to the process of integration, and to what extent it should be developing partnerships with migrant community-led organisations to develop policy around this area.

Communication, Bodies and Death

Many of the challenges faced by service providers who work with migrants and refugees are dictated not just by existing policies and protocols but also by organisational culture and practice. This last section will focus on challenges related to the treatment of corpses.

The demands and practicalities of dealing with dying patients and mourning relatives may outweigh service providers' opportunities to provide an appropriate level of emotional support, and this is particularly noticeable in the case of new migrants. Field research showed that hospital staff responded to migrants' emotional needs and practical requests on an *ad hoc* basis, depending on the capacities and inclinations of individual service providers.

One of the social workers interviewed reacted to the death of a Vietnamese woman through professional distancing, a response that was not atypical amongst his colleagues. Remembering the emotionally charged incident, he used depersonalised language, describing it as 'a conflict between infection control procedures and death rituals'. He said:

> A Vietnamese woman from a Buddhist family died of an Aids-related illness in the intensive treatment unit (ITU). Her distraught family had flown over and brought oils and wraps, expecting to spend some time *in situ* washing and preparing the body. Meanwhile staff expected to place the body in a sealed bag for immediate transport to the mortuary as there was an Infection Control matter to be considered as she had been treated with high doses of steroids in the last weeks and this indicated to them that the body would quickly begin to release quantities of fluid. The family became most agitated, unclear about what was being proposed,

> and insisted on ministering to the body where it lay, and as we didn't want to appear to discriminate against them, they were gowned. But the process took longer than I thought it would and the ITU staff were surprised by the level of emotions and noise the family's activities created. This prompted me to call a halt and we literally had to bundle the body away to what we considered a more appropriate location. The body was quickly placed in a body bag and removed to the mortuary and the family were escorted there to continue preparing for a same-day cremation. One should not assume these accommodations would be made again if tested.

The above account demonstrates a tension between medical protocols and the emotional needs of grieving relatives. While this is common in all instances of hospital deaths, it is often exacerbated in the case of migrant deaths, as relatives are destabilised by possible language difficulties and the unfamilar practices and surroundings. In addition, the death of a person outside the homeland can be perceived as particularly tragic.

As noted earlier, ethnocentric presumptions arise when considering how a patient's body might best be respected in life. Yet considerations as to how that body is handled may take on an even greater significance at the time of death. Service users expressed anxiety about their lack of power to perform the proper rituals, and complained about the emotionally detached approach of medical staff at times of death. They were also overwelmend by practicalities. Questions such as 'How much will it cost me to bury my child here?', 'Who should I tell that she has died?' and 'How could I arrange to send the body back home?' were of major importance. Inhabiting a world populated by no affines and kin, many of the participants in the research perceived the service providers as potential enemies in the guise of doctors, social workers and teachers with control of access to much-needed material resources. The lack of emotional responses on the part of some service providers appeared to further underline the distance between 'us' and 'them'.

Service users tended to interpret emotional responses and empathy on the side of service providers as privileging humanity over bureaucracy. Many, however, did not think that the Irish could ever understand their predicament of displacement. As one person said, this was in some ways unavoidable

> because they do not feel like I do—and they cannot let themselves imagine how to feel like I do—so they do not know how to respond to me. There is no point for me to try and explain to them what it means to me.

The following field-diary excerpt makes clear that, despite the challenges to understand and empathise with people in radically different positions, some service providers try their best to address the emotional needs of mourning relatives. They work within the limits of the system, bombarded by a variety of expectations and practical problems without the proper training and sufficient time to deal with them.

> Gerry Ireland, the mortuary technician, is on the phone on behalf of a patient who has died, asking the Nigerian embassy to contact his next of kin with a view to

repatriating the body of a Nigerian refugee. The embassy is reluctant—this is the fourth call they have received from Gerry in as many weeks in relation to the same patient. Outside his office is a man from the Chevre Kadishe, the Jewish burial society, waiting to take a body from the fridge to the synagogue for preparation for burial within the 24-hour period designated by *halacha* (Jewish law). There is no formal arrangement with the Jewish community, the coroner's office or the hospital, but a tacit understanding and working relationship facilitated by the two men. Gerry hangs up the phone. From a drawer in a filing cabinet which contains different religious icons and interchangeable Protestant and Catholic crosses for use in the viewing room, he picks up a *challis* in which he will robe the body of a Bosnian construction worker whose chest and skull had been crushed by a concrete block the week before. He pulls the Velcro'd image of Jesus off the front of the fabric. The family are due in an hour to view the body in the mortuary chapel and Father Michael, one of the chaplaincy team who administered to the family when they arrived in the country, waits to talk with him. He tells of the communication difficulties that Gerry will have as none of them speaks English and there is no interpretation service available today—'I'm never sure how appropriate it is for me to work with people when I have no experience of their Church and when we can't speak together', says Michael, 'but I figure it is better that I stay with them in their sadness rather than they are alone and frightened. It's frustrating though—I could run around all day long, not listening and just flipping from one bed to another and doling out the Eucharist, but I think that my role is to develop a meaningful pastoral relationship with people, staff, patients and families—I want to be able to encourage people to touch their family member, to pray, all the things that come naturally to me at a time like that, and then, after the person has gone, I want to stay with them so that they know I am trying to support them in whatever limited way I can'. The mortuary technician agrees. Michael continues: 'I'm no counsellor, and no counsellor could be expected to take on 12 hours of solid counselling, but sometimes that's what you have to do in this job—and that's really hard when you're working with people who are scared because they haven't got a notion of what the system expects of them. I've had people in here with no families to support them, burying their only relatives in an alien country away from their own faith, and then it'll turn out that they have over 20 different agencies to deal with in a different language– and there's nothing really I can do to help that other than to share feelings and emotions with them. Particularly after my own father died, I began to think about how it must be just a very, very hard place to be'.

Conclusion

In the Irish health system, existing and developing organisational protocols concerning the treatment of migrants focus on cultural checklists in relation to diet, dress, modes of behaviour, rites and rituals. Yet there is evidence of a significant gap between the expectations of service users and service providers in relation to how emotional needs should be supported and managed, in particular at key points in the life cycle. Despite the rhetoric of 'whole-person care' that prevails throughout the health service, service providers have not been taught how to better understand and deal with their patients' emotional needs. While service providers attempt to

demonstrate their aspirational professionalism through clinical distancing, their lack of empathy was seen as a barrier to communication by service users.

The research found there to be minimal evidence of practitioners attempting to develop forms of communication that bridge the emotional gap presenting between themselves and those from differing cultural backgrounds. Consequently, the markers of professionalism in relation to patient satisfaction have been reduced to Likert-scale recordings of service delivery outputs such as waiting times, cleanliness and catering variety. It appeared that no significant attempts were being made to measure or value how engagement and concomitant relationships between staff and patients might impact on service users' emotional well-being or recovery. This was of concern given that many of the asylum-seekers felt they had entered a world populated by potential enemies, in the guise of social workers, doctors, legislators and government officials. In their opinion, these professionals had the potential to harness their perceived collective power to harm rather than to heal.

There are, however, service providers wishing to respond to the holistic needs of service users, particularly at the time of death, who can find their best intentions less than well received. It was in the emotional responses at the point of death that the service providers and their institutions were able to demonstrate a practical and symbolic commitment to interculturalism and in doing so create a sense of hospital–community cohesion. Yet the current statutory approach, which has resulted in grandiose rhetoric, has been followed by a systemic failure to deliver culturally appropriate services which are mainstreamed or bench-marked into agency work-plans. It has been suggested by seasoned migration commentators such as Mac Éinrí (2007) that poor communication and co-operation between the statutory and community sector is not necessarily due to ill-will or a difference of views but a failure on the official side to validate and fund the voluntary sector.

Acknowledgement

The author wishes to acknowledge the significant and particularly generous encouragement, advice and expertise received from Maruška Svašek in the development of this paper. She would also like to pay respect to the men and women who, contrary to their wishes, were unable to find a home in Ireland, and whose fears, aspirations and dreams contributed to the content of this article.

Notes

[1] In the field of education studies, Louis Raths (1947) has argued that children's emotional needs strongly influence their ability to learn. He identified eight important, interrelated needs, including the need 'to belong, to achieve, to have a feeling of economic security, to be free from fear, to love and to be loved, to be free from intense feeling of guilt, to share in decision making, and to understand the world' (Raths 1947: 14). Only if these needs were met, he argued, would a child achieve its full learning potential. On wider debates about cultural vs biological aspects of emotions, see Leavitt (1996); Milton and Svašek (2005).

[2] Tensions surrounding these 'problem' areas manifested themselves throughout the system in practical terms through the scheduling of appointments, hospital diet plans, catering, compliance with medical regimes, communication between individuals that crossed cultural and gendered norms, and with the material culture associated with the Catholic Church which remains a strong influence on state services.

[3] Conversely, the Mosney Centre is a conversion of an old Butlin's Holiday Camp and the material culture of that camp still exists, so that those awaiting court decisions about their immigration status eat their food in the Kosy Korner Kafe with a large, smiling clown in wood relief looking down over the entrance.

[4] See also Alexandra Hall's paper in this Special Issue.

[5] Filtered through the lens of an undetermined status, all seems subject to reinterpretation and distortion. Gone are the social expectations and ritualised behaviour that regulate 'normal' interaction. Instead new intercultural norms are developed with rules of reciprocity and emotional engagement tentatively negotiated and formulated within the confines of the temporary status. Writing about the experiences of asylum-seekers and undocumented migrants in the British detention system, Athwal and Bourne (2007: 106) suggest that the high levels of sudden death of so many 'is an unrecognised endictment of our society'.

[6] As both a cultural construct and the site of competing medical knowledge and hypothesis, the body has long been the subject of anthropological investigations (Littlewood 1997; Lock 1993; Turner 1984).

References

Apthorpe, R. (1997) 'Writing development policy and policy analysis plain and clear: on language, genre and power', in Shore, C. and Wright, S. (eds) *Anthropology of Policy: Critical Perspectives on Governance and Power.* London: Routledge, 43–58.

Athwal, H. and Bourne, J. (2007) 'Driven to despair: asylum deaths in the UK', *Race and Class, 48*(4): 106–14.

Baldassar, L. (2007) 'Transnational families and the provision of moral and emotional support: the relationship between truth and distance', *Identities. Global Studies in Culture and Power, 14*(4): 385–410.

Drennan, V.M. and Joseph, J. (2005) *Journal of Advanced Nursing, 49*(2): 155–63.

Fanning, B. (ed.) 2007 *Immigration and Social Change in the Republic of Ireland.* Manchester: University of Manchester Press.

Frawley, M. (2006) 'Irish resistance', *People Management,* 18 May: 44.

George, S.M. (2005) *When Women Come First: Gender and Class in Transnational Migration.* Berkeley: University of California Press.

Gill, D. (2006) *Cultural Male Circumcision: Report of Committee 2004–2005.* Dublin: Department of Health and Children, www.dohc.ie/publications/pdf/circumcision.pdf?direct=1

Gillligan, C. (2006) 'An unsatisfactory discussion of the process of ethnic minority integration in Ireland', *Translocations, 1*(1): 41–55.

Hansen, H.P. (1997) 'Patients' bodies and discourses of power', in Shore, C. and Wright, S. (eds) *Anthropology of Policy: Critical Perspectives on Governance and Power.* London: Routledge, 88–106.

Harris, K.A. (1998) 'The informational needs of patients with cancer and their families', *Cancer Practice, 6*(1): 39–46.

Jentsch, B., Durham, R., Hundley, V. and Hussein, J. (2007) 'Creating consumer satisfaction in maternity care: the neglected needs of migrants, asylum-seekers and refugees', *International Journal of Consumer Studies, 31*(2): 128–34.

Jung, H.P., Baerveldt, C., Olesen, F., Grol, R. and Wensing, M. (2003) 'Patient characteristics as predictors of primary health care preferences: a systematic literature analysis', *Health Expectations*, *6*(22): 160–81.

Leavitt, C. (1996) 'Meaning and feelings in the anthropology of emotions', *American Ethnologist*, *23*(3): 514–39.

Leydon, G.M. (2000) 'Patients with cancer-information needs and information-seeking behaviour: in-depth interview study', *British Medical Journal*, *320*: 909–13.

Littlewood, J. (1997) 'Care and ambiguity: towards a concept of nursing', in Holden, P. and Littlewood, J. (eds) *Anthropology and Nursing*. London: Routledge, 170–89.

Liu, J.E., Mok, E. and Wong, T. (2005) 'Perceptions of supportive communication in Chinese patients with cancer: experiences and expectations', *Journal of Advanced Nursing*, *52*(3): 262–70.

Lock, M. (1993) 'Cultivating the body. anthropology and epistemologies of bodily practice and knowledge', *Annual Review of Anthropology*, *22*: 133–55.

Mac Éinrí, P. (2007) 'Integration models and choices', in Fanning, B. (ed.) *Immigration and Social Change in the Republic of Ireland*. Manchester: Manchester University Press, 214–36.

Malinowski, B. (1944) *A Scientific Theory of Culture and Other Essays by Bronislaw Malinowski*. Chapel Hill, NC: University of North Carolina Press.

Mallik, K. (2005) 'Making a difference: culture, race and social policy', *Patterns of Prejudice*, *39*(4): 361–78. Manchester: Manchester University Press.

Milton, K. and Svašek, M. (eds) (2005) *Mixed Emotions. Anthropological Studies of Feeling*. Oxford: Berg.

Radford, K. (2006) 'It's not just bagels and bhajis: reflections on a research revolt', in Magnuson, D. and Baizerman, M. (eds) *Work with Youth in Divided and Contested Societies*. Rotterdam: Sense, 141–51.

Rapport, N. and Dawson, A. (1998) *Migrants of Identity*. London: Berg.

Raths, L.E (1947) 'A test of emotional needs', *Educational Research Bulletin*, *26*(1): 14–16.

Svašek, M. and Skrbiš, Z. (2007) 'Passions and powers: emotions and globalisation', *Identities. Global Studies in Culture and Power*, *14*(4): 367–84.

Tilbury, F. (2007) '"I feel I am a bird without wings": discourses of sadness and loss among East Africans in Western Australia', *Identities. Global Studies in Culture and Power*, *14*(4): 433–58.

Turner, B. (1984) *The Body and Society*. Oxford: Basil Blackwell.

Watt, P. and McGaughey, F. (2006) *Improving Government Service Delivery to Minority Ethnic Groups*. Dublin: National Consultative Committee on Racism and Interculturalism.

Sensuous Multiculturalism: Emotional Landscapes of Inter-Ethnic Living in Australian Suburbia

Amanda Wise

Every day, people from different backgrounds mix together, whether by design or necessity, in our multicultural neighbourhoods and cities. This article explores how senses, sensibilities, habitus and affects influence quotidian intercultural encounters in culturally diverse cities. The article is based upon ethnographic research in an Australian suburb which has seen large-scale Chinese migration to the area in recent years and experienced the associated rapid changes to the shops along the local high street. Focusing on a range of sites or 'contact zones' along the suburban high street, the paper explores the notion of cross-cultural habitus, in particular the sensuous and affective dimensions of what I term the 'haptic habitus'. It then examines the sensuous and embodied modes of being that mediate intercultural interactions between long-term Anglo-Celtic elderly residents in the area and newly arrived Chinese immigrants and their associated urban spaces. Ranging through the senses, from sight, smell, sound and the haptic system, the article reflects upon how the senses, affect, habitus, nostalgia and memory articulate with localised experiences of diversity. I develop the notion of 'sensuous multiculturism'—which foregrounds embodied experience in this scenario of cultural difference—and go on to argue that the dis-synchronisation of senses, embodied place-memory and habitus contribute to some forms of intercultural anxiety and everyday racism.

'Embracing diversity' has become a slogan for proponents of multiculturalism. Axiomatic though it seems, what does it really mean to live with difference at the deepest, everyday level? This has been the enduring theme of my ongoing

ethnographic research in the culturally diverse Sydney suburb of Ashfield, exploring forms of locality, belonging, affinity and disjuncture among local residents, in relation to what I call 'multicultural place-sharing'. I wanted to understand the rhythms and rhymes of urban diversity through forms and sites of interaction across difference, the production of everyday forms of belonging and of material, social and symbolic networks.

This article[1] is about the role of emotions, affect and habitus in the experience of cultural diversity among mainly White Anglo-Celtic[2] senior citizens of the 'host' community. It seeks to fill a key gap in the literature regarding this sub-group, who figure prominently as holding more racist views and tend, stereotypically, to be less comfortable with cultural difference (Forrest and Dunn 2007). The paper explores how Anglo-Celtic and other long-term elderly migrant residents of Ashfield are experiencing urban cultural change brought about by the recent arrival in the neighbourhood of large numbers of migrants from China. It does not attempt to explore the everyday lived realities of multiculturalism from the perspective of Chinese living in the local area.

Since the postwar migration boom, Ashfield, in Sydney's inner west, has become an extremely diverse area. Originally a fairly working- and lower-middle-class Anglo-Celtic population, Ashfield is now home to a myriad of ethnic groups, with the Chinese, Indian and Italian representing the largest communities. What most characterises Ashfield today is the Chinese commercial presence along its main shopping strip on Liverpool Road. Once dominated by Anglo, Italian and Greek shops, the change to the visual landscape of Ashfield's high street has been quite rapid, and has largely occurred since the mid-1990s. Today, Ashfield is home to a variety of Chinese small businesses, predominantly restaurants and small supermarkets selling Asian groceries, which constitute around four-fifths of the shops in the area (see Figure 1).

The paper is based on more than two years of ethnographic research in the area between 2002 and 2004, particularly spending time in the local shopping mall and on the high street, participating in various clubs, including local lawn bowls clubs, the church, and seniors' groups. Ethnographic participant observation also involved shopping with elderly Ashfield ladies, and spending time with them in their homes and at local fairs and fêtes. The study also involved some 40 in-depth open-ended interviews with Anglo-Celtic senior citizens, as well as a smaller number with local Chinese, Greek, Italian, Indian and Lebanese residents to explore their relationships to the suburb and to other residents.

A key finding in the study was the extent to which the Anglo-Celtic elderly were local in their orientation. The majority of elderly Anglo-Celtic participants have lived in the Ashfield area for more than fifty years. A large number have lived in the suburb, and even the same street, their entire lives. Most importantly, and unsurprisingly, the older they get, the less mobile they become; they no longer drive or have the energy to go far. The less able they are to travel, the more their daily lives become confined to Ashfield. Local shopping is often the main social activity for women of that generation, and so Ashfield shops have been an important part of their social lives.

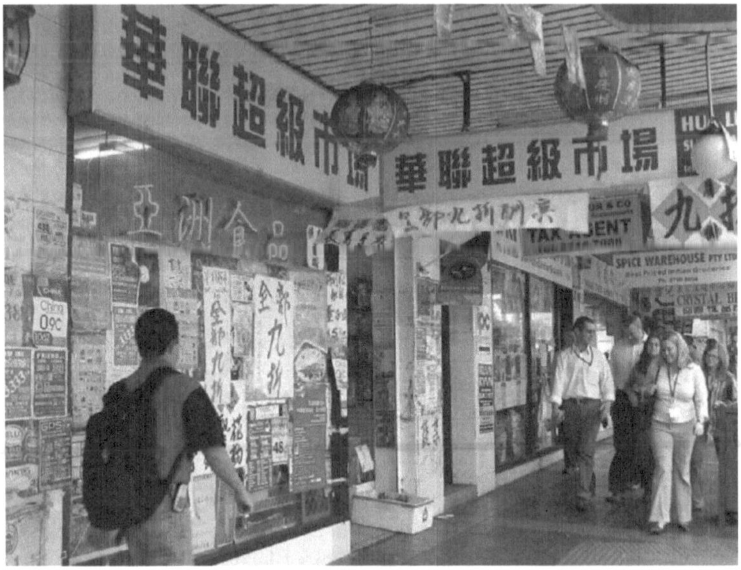

Figure 1. Hua Lin chinese grocery store on Liverpool Road. Photo by A. Wise (2005).

Non-Chinese participants in the study were overwhelmingly uncomfortable with the changes that have taken place along the Ashfield shopping strip in the last few years. Negative sentiments were particularly apparent among the long-term elderly Anglo-Celtic residents who expressed a deep-seated sense of displacement and disorientation. Similar sentiments were common among several other ethnic groups, where length of residence seems to be the determining factor. What was most interesting was how embodied and deeply emotional this sense of disequilibrium seemed to be. In this article, I argue that 'encultured' senses, habitus and bodily hexis contribute in important ways to people's orientation and/or disorientation (Rodaway 1994) in diverse urban spaces, and that these frame the appreciation of the qualities of such environments (Urry 2000: 79).

Displacing/Replacing/Displacing

The following vignette encapsulates some of the complex emotional layers of place-sharing in multicultural suburbia. Part of the study involved a group of elderly European postwar migrant women, exploring how their patterns of interaction and belonging relate to and differ from the elderly Anglo-Celtic residents. During one of our focus-group discussions which took place during their weekly social gathering, some extraordinary emotions emerged. So powerful and complicated were their feelings about Ashfield's changes, they asked me to keep their specific ethnicity a secret. For this reason I refer to them in the following pages simply as 'European'.

It was International Women's Day 2004 and, to celebrate, the council had sponsored a multiethnic event for senior women in Ashfield involving lunch and entertainment,

which was proposed and organised by the local Chinese women's community group. Being International Women's Day the Chinese women felt it important to invite, in solidarity, women from other local ethnic communities, including the European and Anglo-Celtic senior women. Held in the local Town Hall, the audience was primarily Chinese, as was the entertainment and food. There were a few tables set aside for the non-Chinese women along one side of the hall.

The European and Anglo-Celtic women arrived close together. The European women entered first, looked around the room and saw that it was all Chinese women. There was Chinese music playing and the room was decorated in Chinese colours of red and gold. They stood at the entrance to the room, not sure what to do. The Chinese women were seated already and no-one was there to greet the new arrivals. A Chinese woman came by, but with little English just nodded her head and said 'Hello' before walking on. The European and Anglo women waited about for a few minutes but no-one came over to welcome them or direct them to a table. One of the European ladies asked a passing woman where they should sit, to which the response was 'No, no, no' and a shake of the hand to indicate no English, before hurrying away. By this time the European and Anglo women were feeling lost and annoyed; eventually, the European women decided that enough was enough and they turned and left, followed closely by the Anglo women.

Speaking of this failed attempt at intercultural womanly solidarity a few days later, one of the European women in the group of fifteen or so I was with became terribly upset and animated. She said to me and the group,

> Oh my God, this was the worst day of my life. This was the worst day of my life. They say the day was International Women's Day but it was all Chinese, only for Chinese, the food, the music. You could tell they weren't interested in us. This Ashfield is so hard to live here now.

The speaker began to cry and ran off a whole gamut of daily difficulties she felt she faced in the new Ashfield. The rest of the group became equally emotional, some crying, some clearly angry and frustrated. They poured out feelings about 'rude' Chinese in the shops, being pushed in queues, rushed in front of for the bus, overlooked by perceived unfriendly Chinese shopkeepers serving Chinese first, distress at being unable to read all the signs and no longer being able to shop along the high street. They spoke emotionally of *unsmiling* Chinese faces, unfriendly neighbours, pushy bodies, dirty and dark shops. Their dystopic description of the new environment contrasted sharply with the Ashfield they said they knew before. They compared the Chinese shops unfavourably to the earlier Southern European and Anglo shops that were in Ashfield until recent years, and spoke with pride that European shop signs were always in English. One lady said that in her family-owned fruit shop she had a policy never to speak their own language in front of customers from other backgrounds because they didn't want to make others uncomfortable.[3] They were distressed that all their familiar shops had gone and in their place were new ones they felt to be so unwelcoming they

would no longer go there. All this came out in a big emotional rush, as if they'd been bottling it up for years and had never voiced it to anyone, particularly not to outsiders.[4]

And then something extraordinary happened. One of the much older ladies—a widow dressed in black who, until now, had been quiet—began to yell back at the group. First she was recounting in tears, with all her body engaged in the telling, her misery at how her Chinese neighbours let their children wee in her front garden. She described having fishy water hosed on her feet at the bus stop in front of the fish shop. The room was charged with emotion. But then she turned, almost on herself, and began to berate herself and the group . . .

> My God, what are we saying? We can't say about the new people what the Australians used to say about us. How can we do this to them, how can we make the same pain for them? This is not right to say such things. These Chinese just want to feel a little bit at home, make this place a little bit more home. We don't like them but how can we take their home away from them?

And there was much animated and emotional group discussion, many repeating their distress at the changes, others realising they'd been slipping into the same kind of racism that had been directed at them. They seemed to be arguing as much within their own selves as with one another, and there was literally crying, shouting at one another, flailing hands. Two women walked out in anger at the widow who'd stood up. The group seemed torn that there was no language but seemingly racist language to express the discomforts they were clearly feeling—though because of the pain they carried from their own experiences of racism they were deeply affected at having such negative feelings toward the new group. And then the old widow said to me:

> You cannot use this. You cannot say to the government, to the people, that this is what our community thinks. What would happen to us, people would think it is right what happened to us when we came. *We have a lot of pain* . . .

And so, after some more discussion, I handed them my tape and promised I would keep their ethnicity a secret. We talked for a while about why I thought they shouldn't feel ashamed at having such feelings, explored a bit more how their own painful experiences of racism in the early days might be similar to that experienced by the Chinese community, and how sometimes everyday cultural difference is not easy to negotiate. The description of the discussion above is a true (perhaps even understated) reflection of the intensity of what took place that day, so much so that I left feeling shaken and emotional and had to sit in my car in the underground car park for some time to take in what had just happened. I felt I could almost physically touch their pain, so strong were the emotions circulating in that room. So present were their painful memories of displacement and racism when they arrived as immigrants, their pain, after finally feeling at home 'here', at having to re-negotiate anew an entirely foreign urban cultural landscape, and the palpable emotion of shame permeating the room when they found they had no acceptable language to express what they were feeling.

My account of this event and the women's emotions surrounding the changes in the local area need to be placed in some context. The community to which this group of women belong was subject to a great deal of racism in the postwar years until the 1980s (and occasionally still today). Until the 1970s Australia was a completely Ango-Celtic-dominated place; 'Europeans' were seen as 'wogs' who ate 'smelly' food and spoke with funny accents. Children were regularly teased and bullied at school. Much of the teasing was around issues of bodily hexis which, to Anglo-Australians of the time, was rather too 'expressive' for their liking, and differing food cultures—which ironically have been embraced as 'mainstream' in today's Australia.

I want to briefly flag three issues this story raises for me. The first is that the story shows how important it is to really localise and get into the ethnographic depths of racism before we can begin to grasp its complexity. The second point is that this story reminds us that multiculturalism is something that occurs in-place. In certain circumstances it is about a politics of very localised place-sharing, yet little recognition is given to the fact that living with otherness is not something that is always entirely easy. Rather, it inevitably involves varying levels of discomfort. Yet there seem to be few possibilities in the use of everyday language to explore this discomfort that do not involve racist evaluations. And my third point is that although there was a lot of anger in the European women's story, it is also a story of hope, because it shows how habituation and belonging to place is a process that evolves and changes over time.

Habitus and Difference

Habitus, as Bourdieu describes it, is 'embodied history, internalized as second nature and so forgotten as history'. It is 'the active presence of the whole past of which it is the product' (Bourdieu 1990: 56). It refers, in essence, to the embodied dispositions that 'internalise our social location and which orient our actions', a kind of mastery of the implicit principals of the social world (Noble and Watkins 2003: 522). Embodiment of our social location manifests 'in our actions, our modes of appearance and through a bodily *hexis* or bodily bearing—posture, manners, ways of speaking—for example' (Noble and Watkins 2003: 522). This mastery of the social world can be called a 'feel for the game' which Bourdieu describes as the almost 'miraculous encounter between the *habitus* and the field, between incorporated history and objectified history, which makes possible the near-perfect anticipation of the future inscribed in all the concrete configurations on the pitch or board' (Bourdieu 1990: 66). Borrowing from Proust, Bourdieu evocatively suggests that 'one might say that arms and legs are full of numb imperatives' (1990: 69). It is precisely because of their embodied nature that habitus and hexis have the capacity to induce in us affective responses to inter-subjective encounters with those around us and to interactions with our environment.

Longer-term elderly residents of Ashfield (those for whom habitus is most deeply sedimented) were struggling to feel comfortable with the changes occurring there. Their discomfort was clearly embodied and experienced through the senses, which are in themselves a product of habitus, and the resulting disequilibrium manifested

emotionally and affectively. In this view, it can be argued that a sense of homeliness in part derives from what Hage (1997) has described as a 'well-fitted habitus'. In the following pages, I show, through a series of sensuous lenses, how Ashfield's new environment has produced a rupture, or disjuncture in the previously 'well-fitted habitus' of its long-term elderly residents.

Bodies and Other Bodies

The European women's experience at International Women's Day had very much to do with habituated expectations of other bodies in certain social fields. Drawing on Bourdieu's grammar of 'miraculous encounter' (1990: 66), when one encounters a similarly habituated body or bodies they more often than not respond in certain magical or miraculous ways to interactions with our own bodies in given situations. For example, in the right circumstances if I move my head or facial muscles in a certain way, the face of the body in front of me is likely to move, contra-mine, in fairly predictable ways.[5] If I enter a certain kind of space I can expect other bodies to arrange themselves around me in particular ways; to stand at a certain distance, to make certain expressions, to respond to moments of uncertainty within a fairly set repertoire of possibilities, to make hand movements that are responsive to mine.

The European women's experience in the foyer on International Women's Day disrupted this magic, a magic that under ideal circumstances connects bodies to the world in a kind of continuum of self–other inter-subjective commensality. Under similarly habituated circumstances the European and Anglo women would have arrived, and magically another body would appear. Its facial muscles would crease into a smile, its eyes would perhaps open in a certain way, its hands might gesture toward a table, guide the visiting bodies to it, and perhaps explain some of the things that might happen in the ensuing hour or two. Other bodies at the table might look at the new arrivals with certain facial expressions which communicate that it is OK to sit down; there might be some shuffling or re-arranging of chairs as a sign of making space for the newcomers. All of these bodily gestures (remember they are culturally habituated) are on the one hand anticipatable yet almost invisible; they function to guide bodies onto the next moment, to hint at what might be to come, to open up the space for the next moment.

Archer (2000) argues that memory is 'the bodily sedimentation of accomplished acts, which gives us a past and a future' (quoted in Noble and Watkins 2003: 533). What then of acts not successfully accomplished? Of those moments when our particular cultural magic fails to work? When other bodies don't respond as anticipated, a distinct feeling of temporal and bodily disjuncture occurs.

The Chinese women who organised this event were not interviewed to explore 'their side' of this story. But it is possible to speculate numerous reasons as to why the expected 'welcome' ritual did not occur. It may have been about cultural differences, or about shyness due to language barriers, nervousness due to previous racist encounters with European or Anglo women, or some other misunderstanding involving the role of

the host. What is important is that it was experienced as a disruption of familiar bodily ritual by the European and Anglo women and the discomfort caused (and recounted) needs to be seen in the context of their wider experience in the local area where 'failed encounters' such as these were common. The following disjunctional moment is fairly typical of interactions I have witnessed over the years conducting fieldwork in the area.

> This happens ... with Chinese or Asians behind the counter .... One of the things that they do is the change, when they give you the change, they put it on the counter. When they take your credit card when they've finished on the receipt they put it on the counter. Now that for me is absolutely rude. They're supposed to hand it to you, in your hand or put the change in your hand. There are times that I tell them, 'This is the way you do it'. That is the way, the culture of the Chinese (Sunil, South African Indian man, resident since 1975).

This brief narrative example refers to the confusion, and sometimes insult, felt when there are mismatched expectations around everyday social rituals. As Goffman points out, rituals are a fundamental part of all social interaction, and failed rituals produce embarrassment. 'In forming a picture of the embarrassed individual, one relies on imagery from mechanics: equilibrium or self control can be lost, balance be overthrown. No doubt the physical character of flustering in part evokes this imagery' (Goffman 2005: 100). This grammar of embarrassment signals the embodied affect of shame, which Sylvan Tomkins (in Sedgwick and Frank 1995) describes as intimately associated with interest. One only feels shame before one's object (person) of interest. Shame and embarrassment manifest physically: eyes lowered or averted, perhaps a blush, or momentary flustering. Shame produces a 'breaking off'. I suggest that these failed social rituals are experienced as moments of embarrassed 'flustering', which seem to produce emotions such as indignation and irritation.

These kinds of disjunctural interaction in shops were a frequently recurring motif. Sometimes they have to do with other bodies in a queue, with how a shopkeeper physically responds at the counter, or with the sorts of words used. Here are two more examples that have to do with cultural differences around bodily expectations in customer–shopkeeper interactions as they relate to a more generalised sense of 'welcome':

> The Chinese I find very, very arrogant in the shops. They'll push you out of the way, there's no 'Please' or 'Excuse me' (Bill, English migrant, resident 38 years).

> I regarded Ashfield as my suburb, my shopping centre. These are my shops, you had a friendly face. Today my shops have been replaced by other shops where I'm not welcome. Mostly you go into the shops as a non-Chinese, and the attention is curt, off-hand, unhelpful. ... Rather than cause any unpleasantness, all you can do is just walk out, and go further afield to do your shopping (Rajan, Anglicised Indian, former Ghurka, resident 30 years).

These narratives show the kinds of disjuncture that emerge when ideas about what a 'welcoming body' should do differ, and indeed ideas about where welcoming bodies

should be found and how they should respond at particular moments. These expectations are of course bounded by socially and culturally inscribed repertoires of emotional display (Abu-Lughod and Lutz 1990; Csordas 1994) and grammars of etiquette. We 'learn to interpret certain bodily manifestations *as* emotions' (Svašek and Skrbiš 2007: 371). In this case, a welcoming body is expected to display emotions such as pleasure and interest; to signal a 'pleased to see you'. For these participants, the ritual breakdown is experienced as a lack of welcome. As 80-year-old Margaret says, 'It's not as though you know in advance that you're going to be welcome there'. There are also simply bodily mis-readings, a hand gesture missed, an expectation of a shared look or smile on one side but not the other.

However, interviews with Chinese shopkeepers suggest that they consider the most polite way to deal with customers is with a brisk and efficient manner, and that it would be the height of rudeness to hold up others in the queue for a 'chat' with a customer. There is also often shyness about engaging in conversation because of language difficulties so to avoid embarrassment they tend to avoid eye contact.

From a Eurocentric perspective, Simmel (1997) describes the 'look' (eye contact) as the most direct and 'purest' interaction between two people, producing a momentary intimacy because, he says, 'one cannot take through the eye without at the same time giving', thereby producing the 'most complete reciprocity of person to person, face to face' (quoted in Urry 2000: 81). The message in the look is returned through the expressive meaning of the face. The style and nature of the reciprocal look and facial response have the capacity to generate different kinds of self–other relationship. However, in cross-cultural encounters the scope for misreading is enormous. The look is not only ethnicised, it is classed, gendered and contextual as well. Because of its intimacy, the potentials and dangers are many; making eye contact when you shouldn't, not making it when it is perceived you should, moving or not moving the facial muscles in certain ways. Many of those generic feelings of 'unwelcome' reported above to some extent relate to differing expectations around the 'look', around shopkeepers' bodies and their gestures, and in turn the failure of generative bodily magic to produce certain outcomes.

These interviewees expressed a sense of palpable moral indignation, which I suggest comes from the breakdown of everyday rituals of recognition. As Goffman points out, 'rules of conduct impinge upon the individual in two general ways: directly, as *obligations*, establishing how he [*sic*] is morally constrained to conduct himself; [and] indirectly, as *expectations*, establishing how others are morally bound to act in regard to him' (Goffman 2005: 49; see also Urry 2000: 81). As Bourdieu has shown, such codes are imprinted in one's habitus. A well-fitted habitus (Hage 1997) produces a sense of ontological comfort (Noble 2005) because 'native membership in a field implies a feel for the game in the sense of a capacity for practical anticipation of the "upcoming" future contained in the present, everything that takes place in it seems *sensible*: full of sense and objectively directed in a judicious direction' (Bourdieu 1990: 66). A temporal disequilibrium is produced when one has lost the feel for the game. This sense of 'not feeling welcome' results, I suggest, from a false sense of the future produced by

mis-matched habitus. As Bourdieu suggests, 'the presence of the past in this kind of false anticipation of the future performed by the *habitus* is, paradoxically, most clearly seen when the sense of the probable future is belied' and when ill-adjusted dispositions 'are negatively sanctioned because the environment they actually encounter is too different from the one to which they are objectively adjusted' (1990: 62).

However, context is also important and recognised as such by most Ashfield locals. While most of the non-Chinese customers in my study would not expect interaction of any kind in a supermarket, the social field of small shops is different, as these are traditionally places where interaction and a little exchange are commonplace. For many of the elderly in Ashfield it is not so much difference *per se*, but the very presence of difference in a formerly comfortable and familiar environment to which they were habituated:

> It's not so much the food. I can go to Chinatown, for *yum cha*, but I'm talking about this is where we live. This is how it's *affecting* us (Margaret, Irish migrant, resident 40 years).

For Margaret, the mismatched look, the failed miracle of encounter between the similarly habituated, are much more of an issue in her home suburb than if she were to make a journey to the place she perceives to belong properly to the Chinese: Chinatown. When she says so emphatically, 'I'm talking about this is where we live, this is how its *affecting* us', she is communicating the importance to her of a comfortable habitus in the creation of homeliness. For her, it is comfortable to accept difference when travelling, but at home there is a sense that homeliness requires an anticipatable outcome. Travelling to Chinatown (for it is a touristic undertaking as a general rule) is an act of deliberate stepping out of one's habitus (or comfort zone, in common parlance). In other words, Margaret *anticipates* discomfort in Chinatown.

Bodies in space—how they move, and their distance from one another in certain contexts—are as important as facial expressions and bodily gestures. Cultural differences around the use of bodily space and perceived crowding are one of the most common discomfort points in cross-cultural encounters. Cultural geographer Paul Rodaway (1994) describes such bodily encounters as experienced through our haptic sense system. Our haptic senses involve our tactile, kinaesthetic and proprioceptive (body in space) senses. The haptic sense system makes the surface of our bodies porous and permeable. It allows us to perceive things such as weight, pressure, balance, temperature, vibrations, presence of people and things (Fisher 1997), and orients us in space. It also involves 'interoception' where we perceive the 'visceral workings and felt intensities of our interior bodies' (Fisher 1997: 5). For these reasons, touch is one of the most intimate and reciprocal of senses, for 'to touch is always to be touched' and, importantly, it can evoke a whole gamut of emotions and associations from desire, caring and love, to disgust, revulsion and hate (Rodaway 1994: 41). Western bodies often feel deeply uncomfortable in crowded spaces because their culturally attuned sense of appropriate interpersonal distance is much greater than in some other cultures. Body-space researchers see personal space as, 'effectively an

extension of the self's presence in space, and violation of this space by another is felt to be like the violation of the body itself' (Rodaway 1994: 59).

A combination of crowded and small shops and differing ideas of intimate body space often makes Ashfield's intercultural encounters fraught with discomfort and unease. Uncomfortable encounters between Chinese and Anglo-Celtic residents were commonly present in queuing behaviour (where the 'appropriate' distance between people in the queue differs), among pedestrians walking along the footpath on the high street, and behaviour on public transport.

> I don't know whether it is that they've never learned to queue. We came from a country where we learned to queue. But even down at the bus stop, they will get on the bus irrespective of whether you've got on the bus or not (Ruby, Anglo-Celtic, late 70s).

> And also the pushiness and the abruptness . . . I'm not being racist. Yes, there's this real abruptness and pushy habits. And, and there is no excuse. And they will push you out of the way. And if you were standing there and you were next to be served and suddenly you get 'whoop' and somebody else's in front of you in the line. . . . So I don't go to the shops anymore, I try not to go into them. I prefer to shop at Coles [a supermarket chain] (Asha, Indian, late 60s, resident 30 years).

A number of times I witnessed a Chinese shopper 'push' into a queue thinking that the wideness of the space between two queuers was actually the end of the line. In some cultures, body contact in shopping spaces is simply par for the course. However many of the Anglo-Celtic seniors in my study come from a generation where intimate space is even wider than for many Anglos of a younger generation today.

For the Anglo seniors, bodily control, comportment, and the maintenance of a relatively distant intimate bodily space are extraordinarily important aspects of bodily homeliness. What is interesting in the above extracts, however, is that a number of the longer-term migrants in my study seemed to have re-tooled their bodies toward more Anglo forms of habitus. For both groups, nonetheless, certain forms of body contact are considered important in establishing a sense of trust and acceptance. Consider the role, for example, of Sunil and his expectation that shopkeepers should place his change directly in his hand, or the gentle guiding hand on the back to welcome a new stranger into the room at a social event.

Smell and Urban Difference: Disgust and Matter out of Place

Smell, disgust, pollution, purity and defilement have long been topics of interest to anthropologists and sociologists, from Mary Douglas' 'matter out of place' (Douglas 2002) to Norbert Elias's *Civilizing Process* (Elias 2000). Stimulated by this literature, a chief concern emerging from my ethnography is what happens when groups with different schemas of purity and defilement encounter one another in an urban dwelling place.

> The bus stop opposite the mall, there are two shops there, two restaurants and a fish shop. They bring their slops, *their swill*, in buckets and empty it on the footpath

> into the grating right where the seat is where people sit waiting for the bus. Now that was filthy. And the smell! They do it regularly, two or three times a day. I told them it was wrong and they more or less told me to go and mind my own business (Sunil, South African Indian man, resident since 1975).

I heard various versions of this fish-shop story from a number of the Anglo and European seniors I spoke with, all of whom use the bus-stop that Sunil refers to. It is often used as an example of how Ashfield has changed for the worse. As Douglas (2002) has argued, purity and pollution are complementary and self-reinforcing categories concerned with classification and order—differing, as we know, between cultures. Conceptions of dirt, and particularly smelly dirt, are so deeply enculturated that our experience of such matter out of place becomes epidermalised, felt on the skin and inside the body, able to evoke the most palpable emotions of revulsion. Kroker and Kroker (in Lupton 1999: 128–9) use the term 'panic bodies' to describe 'the emotions that people feel about their bodies and the threat of penetration' by malign phenomena. The modern European autonomous, individuated body is closed off from other bodies (see Lupton 1999: 125–6). It emerged through a history of bodily self-discipline, management and regulation of what 'went in and out of the body and how the body was deported' (Elias 1978; Lupton 1999). The closed body is counter-posed to the pre-modern 'open' body, which can be characterised as a porous, volatile, sensuous body, open to all manner of contagion, material and spiritual. The modern body—concerned to close off from and eject such invasions—is racked with anxieties around hygiene, body boundaries, 'fluids that flow in and out of the body, the ways in which others touch one's body' (Elias 1978: 126–7; Lupton 1999).

The boundaries of the modern body extend to modern urban forms where distinctions between purity and defilement are encoded into the built environment and the regulatory framework of the city (Sibley 2001: 244). For Anglo-Celtic Ashfield seniors, fish swill belongs behind the scenes at the shop. It may be washed away at the back door, but never on the footpath at the front door. Worse still, not at the feet of those waiting at the bus-stop for it may permeate their bodies. Chewing gum, spit and rubbish belong in the bin, not on the footpath, and smells should be cleansed away or at least confined to certain kinds of space.

Obviously one of the reasons the Chinese fish shop story was raised by a number of my research participants has to do with the smelliness of fish and fishy waste. In Lefebvre's view, the sense of smell is intricately intertwined with experiences of Otherness. He argues that if ever 'an intimacy occurs between "subject" and "object" it must surely be the world of smells and the places where they reside' (Lefebvre 1991: 197). Smell is a very direct encounter with the world, it is a sense that cannot be turned on and off (Urry 2000: 96). As Simmel (1997) has argued, smell is more often associated with revulsion and disgust than anything neutral (see also Low 2005; Miller 2005; Urry 2000). Smells permeate our bodies in ways the other senses do not. They represent an involuntary *involvement* in the environment; as Rodaway argues, we 'feel' the 'taste of a strong odour as much as we smell it' (1994: 67). Not surprisingly, 'foreign' aromas recur as common points of intercultural discomfort in my study, most often among those

living in blocks of flats, and in stories about shops such as the butcher and the fish shop selling raw food. A typical interview extract:

> You go into a block of units, their cooking is different, so people don't like, necessarily, the aromas all the time. They don't mind it when they go to a restaurant, but that's only a one-off. It's not something that they've been used to. When you get groups together then you're going to have those strong aromas around. If you're in your block of flats, and you were the only couple of Anglo-Saxons in there, and they're all Asians, and you'd think 'Oh God, the smell of this place'. It's something you're not used to. I think once integration gets more then it's dispersed more, so you don't have these other things around, that maybe you don't like, they just sort of gradually disappear. It becomes less intense, it dissipates (Angela, Anglo-Celtic woman, 70).

Perhaps more so than matter, smells are hard to keep in place. However hard you try to contain them, aromas waft and weave their way around corners, through space, into the noses of anybody who happens by. In Angela's experience, smell out of place is particularly significant in the close confines of unit accommodation where cooking smells permeate the ambiguously defined spaces of shared hallways. The cooking aroma story came up several times and always by residents in flats. It is almost as if the smell wafting under the door threatens to colonise them. But just as interesting are Angela's comments on how 'with integration the smells dissipate', as if somehow the smells magically disappear or mesh with other more familiar smells as the new residents blend in over time. Although she might not be aware of it, this is more likely to be a function of Angela's nose and its pleasurable integration over many years of new food aromas (pasta, garlic, tomatoes, I'm sure no longer smell to her) than it is of her migrant neighbours 'integrating'. Another quote:

> You walk past the Asian butcher, I wouldn't go in there either, because I don't like the smell of the meat. That really turns you off (Ernest, Anglo-Celtic man, 78).

Malodorous smells also have the uncanny ability to magically appear when they are associated with something foreign. Olfactory system at the ready, I visited the butcher Ernest refers to and sniffed my way around it. For the life of me, it smells just like an average Australian butcher. I stood at the window for a bit and then it struck me. The meat was just meat, but it was all labelled in Chinese, and, curiously, I realised the whole shop was lit in red tinted lights, casting a pinkish red wash across the meat in the window. I suspect the combination of the red light, the differently displayed meat and the Chinese labels created a mental picture of foreignness for Ernest which makes present to him certain meaty smells that would remain invisible to him in an Anglo butcher's shop washed with 'clean' white fluorescent light which 'de-meats' the meat.

Windows, Lighting and Space

Some of the most passionate emotions had to do, not with abstract otherness, but with body-in-space feelings in relation to the materiality of shops along Ashfield's

shopping strip. Ashfield's Chinese shops, particularly the numerous small Asian grocery stores, are very different to the shops familiar to most Anglo-Celtic seniors. The Chinese-run stores are typically small, and often have boxes of goods clustered in and around the single entrance door (see Figure 2). Typically the windows are covered in posters, often advertising international telephone cards. Interiors are typically much more crowded, with aisles close together and many more items for sale crammed onto the shelves. The haptic experience of Ashfield's Chinese shops among my non-Chinese research participants is one of discomfort, primarily to do with the size of shops, the dim light, the closeness of objects, their height around the body, the narrowness of the aisles, and the availability of windows. The following extracts give a sense of some of the bodily responses reported:

> You go into these shops and they've built the aisles where you can barely walk a shoulder square. You can't walk straight, you've got to sidle along sideways. It's dark, it's gloomy, the front doors and windows are plastered with posters. You cannot see in, and you cannot see out. Inside the light is never bright, it is dark. Stuff is stacked in such a way that it is difficult to move. And boxes protrude onto the pavement (Brian).

> If you go to some of the shops down in Ashfield now, and you'll also find out in their windows, their windows are completely blocked off . . . . There's not even a view into the shop. It's totally blocked off (Margaret).

> It makes me feel isolated. I came here to live like an Australian, to have a free life. Free, free moving, free, the freedom seems to have gone. It's changing completely and utterly. . . . I never felt like that with the Italians or Greeks (Bill).

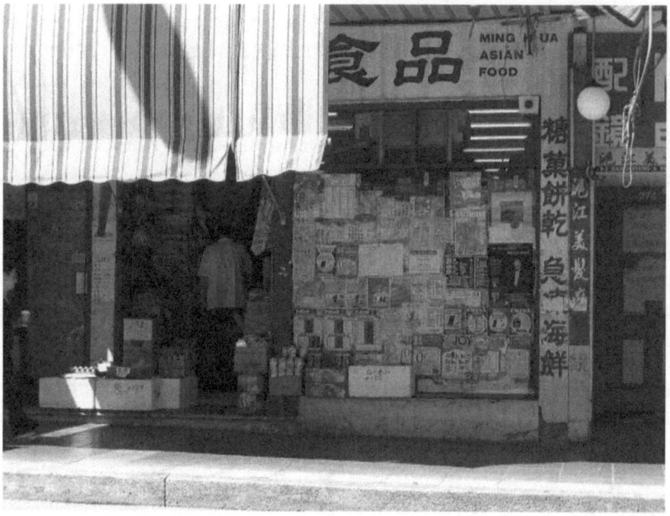

Figure 2. Another Chinese grocery store on Liverpool Road, showing narrow doorway and aisles, Chinese signage and papered windows. Photo by A. Wise (2005).

> Here in Ashfield, people miss the old kind of shopping. The shops now, you find pokey little rooms where you don't have enough room to swing a cat. You walk in and it's a very unfriendly atmosphere (Ron).

As Rodaway (1994), Tuan (2001) and others have pointed out, we become habituated to certain tactile worlds from early childhood, through touching, sucking, tasting, smelling, banging, hearing, turning around, exploring. Haptic habituation also occurs through 'the movement of body parts (arms and legs, hands and fingers) and the locomotion of the whole body through an environment', and in this way we learn to discern the thousand-fold 'tactile properties of [our] surroundings, surface texture, the solidity of objects, relative size and form, and moving through space using a kind of haptic map of the most familiar places' (Rodaway 1994: 51). Most importantly, Rodaway points out that, because of the participatory and reciprocal quality of haptic geography, each space or place discerned or mapped is in a sense *our* space and in this way we come to belong to it (1994: 54). Haptic habituation, by its very nature, is at once rooted in memory and expectation. Thus a radical disruption of familiar haptic environments can cause a deep-seated sense of rupture between past and future because familiarity has the capacity to kind of propel our bodies along. There is a sense that there are certain things we can (in our subconscious muscle memory) expect around the corner, up the road, in there, that propel our bodies on to the next moment, while at the same time drawing on past experiences to do so. Unfamiliarity with the material environment, on the other hand, pulls us back into the conscious realm of rational thought, stalling, or placing a crease in the unfolding of durational time.

It is interesting to note some of the bodily expressions my research participants used in describing their experiences. As Brian says, 'aisles where you can barely walk a shoulder square'; or (Ron) 'you don't have enough room to swing a cat'. And Margaret: 'Doors are just slots in the wall', connoting a sense of squeezing through into a dark unknown space. And importantly ideas about being able to see through and past objects, and about light, seem, for those habituated to 'Western' spaces, to articulate with feelings of freedom and movement. I was struck by Bill's comments that the posters and covered windows create for him a sense of isolation which he feels contrasts with the sense of 'freedom to move'. For many, the lack of light and of see-throughness of the new shops gives them a distinct bodily sense of confinement, of a barrier to entering the space.

Paths Well Trod: Embodiment, Orientation and Muscular Memory

Together, the issues raised above contribute to what I call body maps, which are the ways in which our bodily habitus orientates or disorientates us in urban space. These are deeply embodied routes carved out through paths well trodden over years, punctuated by familiar landmarks. According to Bachelard, the contours of landscape enter into what he calls our 'muscular consciousness'. In an especially evocative turn

of phrase, he suggests that 'it is as though the road itself ha[s] muscles, or rather, counter-muscles' (Bachelard 1994: 11). Long-time residents in Ashfield have made paths through the suburb, along regularly trod routes, past familiar shops with familiar faces, sedimented into the very muscular fleshy memory of the body and marked out into segments through familiar landmarks.

Spatial research has shown that our muscles, indeed our whole proprioceptive, haptic system, our body's twists and turns, its movement and rhythm through and upon the contours of space are fundamental to our spatial experience and orientation (Massumi 2002: 180). Landmarks also orient us, but not so much as in a visual map. Instead, as Massumi argues, in the actual course of orientation, they are what we habitually head to or away from. And importantly, they 'trigger *headings*. Vectors that allow us to "habitually flow". . . . giving the space of orientation a *qualitative* dimension' (Massumi 2002: 180–1). Because of this vectoral quality, the erasure of such landmarks can cause a distinct sense of disorientation.

Place for the not-so-mobile is also important in the apprehension of 'thick' memory. As Bachelard argues, the more memories are 'fixed in space, the sounder they are' (1994: 9) And our bodies and senses and their interaction with the environment play an enormous part in this rendering of place memories.

For many of the very elderly in Ashfield, the radical erasure of Ashfield's old urban landscape removes all those material and bodily markers, or 'evocateurs of memory' (Nora 1989), that we all lay down throughout our lifetimes. It is here that the significance of their length of residence, their very localised lives and their health-induced inability to travel far offers some clues as to why the Anglo and other long-term elderly of Ashfield feel such a sense of homely dissonance in the new Ashfield. The intensity of their discomfort with Ashfield derives from the fact that it is not just the erasure of memories at the level of words. The disappearance of an environment which functioned as a kind of bodily mnemonic system for place-based memories ruptures memories that have been laid down through real, physical, bodily, interactions with a place.

The bodily, muscular, visceral quality of place relations can, under conditions of radical change, produce affective counter-responses that are all the more emotionally intense, filled with bodily revulsion and neurotic bitterness. Because the sensusous geography of Ashfield has changed so profoundly, the muscles, noses, eyes, ears and skin of the longer-term residents are now quite out of synch with the counter-senses Ashfield's environment offers today. One of the magical functions of habitus, in Bourdieu's conceptualisation, is that the encounter between habitus, field and incorporated history allows us to anticipate the future in a near-perfect fashion. The fit, if you like, propels us forward, gives us a sense of past and what the near future might hold. The dis-synchronisation of memory and habitus, as described here, ruptures or kinks time. It is this quality-of-place relationship, I believe, that creates among Ashfield's elderly such neurotic emotions associated with nostalgia, change and the presence of otherness.

Emotions

In closing, I would like to return to the theme of emotions, the topic of this *JEMS* special issue. There are several intersecting domains in which emotions figure in this paper.

Emotional Grammars

Svašek and Skrbiš (2007: 379) pose the question 'To what extent can alternative discourses of emotivity co-exist in particular socio-historical settings?'. They go on to ask how it '[*feels* to be] confronted with unfamiliar routines, landscapes, or ideas' when confronted with another's mobility. This is indeed a key question in situations of intense interaction in multicultural urban settings such as Ashfield, where it is clear that different emotional grammars underpin many of the 'failed encounters' related in this article. Group mismatches in emotional style, which Middleton (1989: 189) describes as 'emotional dissonance', are now the focus of a robust literature in anthropology, cognitive psychology and other disciplines which underlines the extent to which emotional experience and display are culturally framed. Our emotions 'bear . . . the stamp of time and place' (Middleton 1989: 188). The face and body are primary sites for communicating emotions—pleasure, welcome, care, dislike, disinterest, for example (Adolphs 2002; Carroll and Russell 1996; Damasio 2000; Leavitt 1996)—yet there are differences in where, when and how emotions are displayed. Emotional dissonance was what the European women were experiencing in the foyer of the Town Hall at International Women's Day; it underpins much of the confusion and insult expressed by participants surrounding shopping-related interactions. This feeling of emotional dissonance is further compounded by the rupture of familiar rituals.

Encultured Senses and Alienation

The second area where emotion stands out involves what has been termed 'emotional geographies'. Humans are socialised to associate particular emotions with different kinds of spaces, for example feeling trapped and claustrophobic by dark and crowded spaces, or feeling free and happy in open and light spaces (Davidson and Milligan 2004). As I have argued, our senses are the means by which we apprehend our environment and these senses are habituated, linking our bodies to experiences, sensations and emotions, and in this way, places evoke *structures of feeling* (Williams 1965).

Depression and Ageing

There is a good deal of evidence now that the elderly are more susceptible to depression. Feelings of loss, sadness and loneliness are not uncommon, and typically tend to be more prevalent among the elderly when health and physical mobility decline. With the decline in mobility and physical ability, the geographical life-world tends to contract

(Rowles 1978). There is also evidence that reduced social networks are positively correlated with feelings of loneliness and depression (Lee 1987). Clearly, then, emotions play a key part in the experience of place among elderly people. Rowles (1978) has described how elderly people come to rely more and more on memories and pleasurable nostalgia to make up for the contraction of their geographical life-world. Positive memories become important in replacing this loss. However, I suggest that where the place itself has changed, and this change is experienced by elderly people as negative, then these fantasies can take on a more acute and neurotic nostalgic form.

Environmental change is an inevitable part of life, and most people manage to adjust to new urban spaces. As Yi Fu Tuan points out, we do become familiar with new places in time. In time a 'new house ceases to make little demands on our attention; it is as comfortable as an old pair of slippers' (Tuan 2001: 184). Memories are more deeply embedded when experienced with emotions; however, ageing makes it ever-more-difficult to lay down new place memories with positive emotional associations. Positive emotions associated with places and times past are then re-remembered in contrast to emotions of loss and alienation associated with age and change.

Emotions, Affect, Memory and Representations

Perhaps the most important thing we can say about emotions is that they are the medium through which the body (affect), memory, and the representational sphere intersect. Emotions are the socially mediated reflective interpretive filters through which we experience our embodied affects (Conradson 2007: 236–7; Damasio 2000; Lyon and Barbalet 1994).

It will be obvious by now that many of the senior citizens in the study contrast their negative emotions surrounding the 'new Ashfield' with memories of a more pleasant Ashfield that supposedly existed in years gone by. However memory is not simply an unmediated recollection of the past. What we see among Ashfield residents is a complex juxtaposition between memory, emotion, body and place,; between what is now and what was there before; the discursive environment that allows us to apprehend this past and present; and a mixture of first-hand and borrowed nostalgic sentiment, brought on as much by present absence as by past presence.

While younger residents are more capable of adapting to new environs, the elderly are less able to re-tool their bodies. The level of attention (rather than embodied flow) required to navigate the new place can produce a sense of exhaustion among them. It is harder for them to lay down positive new place memories and their experience of the place becomes imbued with negative affects, and tends to end up in nostalgic longing for a past, now remembered through the present. The Chinese community became the *object* of their negative affects, despite the fact that the causes are more complex. In making meaning of these experiences, seniors inevitably draw on available representations and discourses, and oftentimes these can be exclusionary and racist.

Conclusions

The problem in a lot of the literature on racism is that it assumes the challenge is simply to change the discursive environment. While that is important, it ignores the extent to which the representational regimes 'out there' become, over time, deeply embodied, habituated and sedimented into the very fleshly fibres of our beings (Svašek and Skrbiš 2007). What has emerged through this study is that little recognition has been given to the fact that sharing real places contact zones, if you like is not always an easy thing to do. It is something we learn to do through practice and everyday negotiation, and it is more difficult for some groups—particularly the elderly—than others.

All this is not an argument to succumb to nostalgia and return to the Ashfield of years past. This would amount to inscribing an exclusionary form of belonging in recognising the right of one group, white Australians, to manage the local and national space (Hage 1998). Instead, it suggests that we need to develop more imaginative and inclusive modes of managing 'togetherness-in-difference' (Ang 2001: 193; see also Wise 2005; Wise and Velayutham 2009). It is perhaps counter-intuitive, but tackling localised racism needs to include and be empathetic to *both* those who are displaced when neighbourhoods change due to migration, *and* the newcomers, who have an equal right to belong and to create a sense of homeliness for themselves.

What possibilities are there for commensality across difference? Arab Australian writer Abbas el-Zein (2003: 239)[6] says that, in a sense, migrants 'survive by growing new body parts'. This echoes Bourdieu's notion that our arms and legs are full of numb imperatives. What is clear, however, is that it is not just migrants who need to grow new limbs, but all of us who inhabit diverse contact zones. We need to grow new bodies, new sensory responses, and emotional, affective grammars; in short, nothing less than new bodily ways of being in multicultural suburbia.

Notes

[1] The title of this paper obviously references Paul Stoller (1997), who gave me some important feedback at a previous conference presentation of this paper in 2004.

[2] 'Anglo-Celtic' is used in the Australian context to denote the dominant white majority community. Anglo-Celtic signals the broadly intermeshed culture of white descendants of English, Irish and Scottish immigrants to Australia, who made up the majority population in Australia until the 1970s. It should be noted that this is a somewhat contested term as it elides the fact that there were significant hostilities between English and Irish (Protestant and Catholic) descended Australians up until as late as the 1960s. However the term 'white' is somewhat of a misnomer to refer to the dominant majority as, in the Australian context, immigrants from Southern Europe were, until the 1980s, not considered 'white'.

[3] This needs to be seen in the context of 1960s Australia where speaking a 'foreign' language in public was frowned upon. This woman is drawing her picture of the 'good migrant' from this era.

[4] As a female researcher I had built up a good relationship with this women's group over time which meant that these women felt comfortable talking to me about their lives in the area. However as an Anglo-Celtic Australian I was also perceived to be an outsider—hence the

women's discomfort at revealing their feelings to me when the discussion took the turn it did.

[5] There is actually quite a bit of science to support this proposition. Studies in social psychology and cognitive neuroscience tend to support the idea of collectively shared facial responses to a set range of expressions (Adolphs 2002; Carroll and Russell 1996; Dimberg *et al.* 2000).

[6] Thanks to Ghassan Hage for pointing me to el-Zein's work.

References

Abu-Lughod, L. and Lutz, C.A. (1990) *Language and the Politics of Emotion*. Cambridge: Cambridge University Press.

Adolphs, R. (2002) 'Neural systems for recognizing emotion', *Current Opinion in Neurobiology*, *12*(2): 169–77.

Ang, I. (2001) *On Not Speaking Chinese: Living Between Asia and the West*. London: Routledge.

Archer, M. (2000) *Being Human: The Problem of Agency*. Cambridge: Cambridge University Press.

Bachelard, G. (1994) *The Poetics of Space*. Boston: Beacon Press.

Bourdieu, P. (1990) *The Logic of Practice*. London: Blackwell.

Carroll, J.M. and Russell, J.A. (1996) 'Do facial expressions signal specific emotions?: judging emotions from the face in context', *Journal of Personality and Social Psychology*, *70*(2): 205–18.

Conradson, D. (2007) 'The affective possibilities of London: Antipodean transnationals and the overseas experience', *Mobilities*, *2*(2): 231–54.

Csordas, T. (1994) *Embodiment and Experience: The Existential Ground of Culture and Self*. Cambridge: Cambridge University Press.

Damasio, A. (2000) *The Feeling of What Happens: Body, Emotion and the Making of Consciousness*. London: Vintage.

Davidson, J. and Milligan, C. (2004) 'Editorial: embodying emotion, sensing space: introducing emotional geographies', *Social & Cultural Geography*, *5*(4): 523–32.

Dimberg, U., Thunberg, M. and Elmehed, K. (2000) 'Unconscious facial reactions to emotional facial expressions', *Psychological Science*, *11*(1): 86–9.

Douglas, M. (2002) *Purity and Danger*. London: Routledge.

el-Zein, A. (2003) 'Being elsewhere: on longing and belonging', in Hage, G. (ed.) *Arab Australians Today: Citizenship and Belonging*. Sydney: Pluto Press, 225–40.

Elias, N. (1978) *The Civilising Process*. Oxford: Blackwell.

Elias, N. (2000) *The Civilizing Process*. London: Blackwell.

Fisher, J. (1997) 'Relational aesthetics: towards a haptic aesthetic', *Parachute*, *87*: 4–11.

Forrest, J. and Dunn, K.M. (2007) 'Constructing racism in Sydney, Australia's largest ethnicity', *Urban Studies*, *44*(4): 699–721.

Goffman, E. (2005) *Interaction Ritual: Essays in Face-to-Face Behavior*. Edison, NJ: Aldine Transaction.

Hage, G. (1997) 'At home in the entrails of the West', in Grace, H. (ed.) *Home/World*. Sydney: Pluto Press, 99–153.

Hage, G. (1998) *White Nation*. Sydney: Pluto Press.

Leavitt, J. (1996) 'Meaning and feeling in the anthropology of emotions', *American Ethnologist*, *23*(3): 514–39.

Lee, G. (1987) 'Social interaction, loneliness, and emotional well-being among the elderly', *Research on Aging*, *9*(4): 459–82.

Lefebvre, H. (1991) *The Production of Space*. Oxford: Blackwell.

Low, K.E. (2005) 'Ruminations on smell as a sociocultural phenomenon', *Current Sociology*, *53*(3): 397–417.

Lupton, D. (1999) *Risk*. London: Routledge.

Lyon, M.L. and Barbalet, J.M. (1994) 'Society's body: emotion and the "somatization" of social theory', in Csordas, T. (ed.) *Embodiment and Experience: The Existential Ground of Culture and Self.* Cambridge: Cambridge University Press, 48–66.

Massumi, B. (2002) *Parables of the Virtual: Movement, Affect, Sensation.* Durham: Duke University Press.

Middleton, D.R. (1989) 'Emotional style: the cultural ordering of emotions', *Ethos, 17*(2): 187–201.

Miller, W.I. (2005) 'Darwin's disgust', in Howes, D. (ed.) *Empire of the Senses: The Sensual Culture Reader.* Oxford: Berg, 335–54.

Noble, G. (2005) 'The discomfort of strangers: racism, incivility and ontological security in a relaxed and comfortable nation', *Journal of Intercultural Studies, 26*(1): 107–20.

Noble, G. and Watkins, M. (2003) 'So, how did Bourdieu learn to play tennis? Habitus, consciousness and habituation', *Cultural Studies, 17*(3/4): 520–38.

Nora, P. (1989) 'Between memory and history: les lieux de mémoire', *Representations, 26*(Spring): 7–25.

Pratt, M.L. (1992) *Imperial Eyes.* London: Routledge.

Rodaway, P. (1994) *Sensuous Geographies: Body, Sense, and Place.* London and New York: Routledge.

Rowles, G.D. (1978) *Prisoners of Space? Exploring the Geographical Experiences of Older People.* Boulder: Westview Press.

Sedgwick, E.K. and Frank, A. (1995) *Shame and Its Sisters: A Silvan Tomkins Reader.* Durham and London: Duke University Press.

Sibley, D. (2001) 'The binary city', *Urban Studies, 38*(2): 239–50.

Simmel, G. (1997) 'Sociology of the senses', in Frisby, D. and Featherstone, M. (eds) *Simmel on Culture: Selected Writings.* London: Sage, 109–20.

Stoller, P. (1997) *Sensuous Scholarship.* Philadelphia: University of Pennsylvania Press.

Svašek, M. and Skrbiš, Z. (2007) 'Passions and powers: emotions and globalisation', *Identities: Global Studies in Culture and Power, 14*(4): 367–83.

Tuan, Y.-F. (2001) *Space and Place: The Perspective of Experience.* Minneapolis: University of Minnesota Press.

Urry, J. (2000) *Sociology Beyond Societies: Mobilities for the Twenty-First Century.* London: Routledge.

Williams, R. (1965) *The Long Revolution.* Harmondsworth: Penguin.

Wise, A. (2005) 'Hope and belonging in a multicultural suburb', *Journal of Intercultural Studies, 26*(1): 171–86.

Wise, A. and Velayutham, S. (eds) (2009) *Everyday Multiculturism.* London: Palgrave.

Gossiping in the Polish Club: An Emotional Coexistence of 'Old' and 'New' Migrants

Aleksandra Galasińska

This paper explores the emotional coexistence of three groups of Polish migrants in the UK. In particular it focuses on how this coexistence is reflected in narratives-in-interaction produced by members of Polish communities. Methodologically the paper is anchored in a constructivist view of emotions, when they are seen as discursive practice, as way of speaking, rather than as some internal states associated with physiological conditions of our bodies. Consequently, discourse and narrative analysis is my chosen way to analyse emotions in a given research area of Polish migration. The data come from my current project on leisure activities as well as cultural consumption among Polish migrants and were collected in established Polish 'centres' in the UK. My informants belong to three different groups of immigrants: 1) post-World War Two immigration; 2) post-1989/pre-enlargement immigration; and 3) post-enlargement immigration.

Introduction

Poland is a country with a long and distinctive history of emigration (see Cyrus 2006; Iglicka 2001; Iglicka-Okólska 1997; Slany 1997) which resulted in two main outflows of people. The first strand of political emigration, associated with a romantic narrative of exile and loss of homeland, is highly contextualised in a political history of nineteenth- and twentieth-century Europe and in particular in the Polish struggle for independence, as well as changes in the political system after World War Two (see Burrell 2006; Hładkiewicz 1997; Iglicka 2000; Sword 1996). In 1831, after defeat of the November Uprising (a military rebellion against the Russian Empire occupying the

country after the 'Partitions of Poland'), a large wave of intelligentsia fled to France. The incident is known in Polish history as the 'Grand Emigration' and it set certain standards and expectations, which stayed in the Polish mentality, with regard to the question of who Polish migrants are. They were mainly highly educated patriots, who fought for Polish independence and were forced to flee to avoid persecution for their actions. The second strand of Polish migrants was the one associated with economic outflow which began at the end of the nineteenth and the beginning of the twentieth century (Morawska 1989), mainly to the USA but also to Germany, Belgium, Holland and France. This wave's 'grand narrative' is one of success of the penniless Poles who succeeded in the West and is contextualised in the economic development of modern Western societies as opposed to Central and Eastern Europe's 'backwardness'.

Having such a strong and vivid tradition of migration, it is not a surprise then that consecutive waves of Poles had to deal emotionally not only with local host-country communities, but also with existing Polish communities in the country of destination. In this study I concentrate on how Polish migrants in the UK talk about other waves of newcomers from Poland. In particular I focus on how their narratives are used as forms of emotional evaluation of other groups of Poles as well as a 'boundary making' process between these groups. In doing so I hope to shed light on conflictual discourses of Polish migration in the context of social and economic transformation and EU expansion after 2004.

Aims and Assumptions

This article's aim is to discuss an emotional coexistence of different groups of Polish migrants to the UK, and in particular how this coexistence is reflected in *narratives-in-interaction* (Georgakopoulou 2006) produced by members of Polish communities. I shall focus on discursive stances and stories about migrants that are formed by migrants during encounters in places which are associated with migrants' life, such as the Polish club, Polish shops and a Polish restaurant. By doing so I follow Georgakopoulou's (2006) postulate on stretching narrative research in linguistics by analysing less-often-researched stories told outside a research interview. Such choice of data avoids co-authoring and co-construction of stories elicited by the researcher during research interviews and shuns asymmetrical power relations during an interview process. Moreover, it allows us to look at stories' 'embeddedness in discourse surroundings' and 'the way in which stories transposed, (re)shaped and recycled across time and space' (2006: 252). Georgakopoulou's dynamic and dialogical approach to narrative has demonstrated that interactional data become a rich source of *narratives-in-interaction.* Focusing on this type of story in my research, I present the role of personal narrative in argumentative discussion (Ochs and Capps 2001) on migration and its experience.

Blommaert *et al.* have explained how migrant places such as the ones I mentioned above are ruled by *interactional regimes* understood as 'a set of behavioural expectations regarding physical conduct, including language' (2005: 212). Although

'Polish' places are multifunctional they are regarded by Poles mainly as places to meet and exchange news and gossip, including gossip about the Polish community. Most of the data I collected took the form of gossip defined by Svašek as 'evaluating and speculating about people's public and private behaviour' (1997: 102). Moreover, collected stories were emotionally charged by their narrators. For the purpose of this article I adopt a constructivist view of emotions, where they are seen as discursive practice, 'as a way of speaking, rather than as some internal states associated with physiological conditions of our bodies' (see Galasiński 2004: 6). As Lutz and Abu-Lughod (1990) have argued, emotions are linked to social life and as such they are contextually bounded (see also Lutz 1988; Milton and Svašek 2005). Stressing its similarity to Foucault's concept of discourse and its embeddedness in social, cultural as well as political contexts, such authors see emotion as social practice, thus closely related to issues of power and domination within communities (see also Reddy 2001). There is a common claim within discourse analysis research to regard discourse as historical, based on and shaped by earlier discourses disseminated and distributed in the past within society (Fairclough 1992, 1996, 2003; Reisigl and Wodak 2001; Wodak 1996, 2001, 2006). By the same token there is a view of emotions as being closely associated with history and past events (see Svašek 2000; Zeldin 1998), as well as being used in politics of everyday life (see Ahmed 2004; also in contributions to Svašek 2006). In the latter case, emotions are formulated and displayed in the form of judgements and moral evaluations (see for example Lacoff 1996), which 'can be regarded as reactions to past and present social events' (Leutloff-Grandis 2006: 118). In the context of Polish migration it is precisely its history which influences the discourse within and about a Polish community in the UK. Discursive practices such as telling stories, gossiping and passing judgmental comments, often strongly influenced by past experiences of groups or individuals, help members of the Polish community to build their identity in contrast to other groups of Poles abroad.

The narrative turn in discourse analysis shows that narratives are an important part of our constructions of the self (see Bamberg 2000; Brockmeier and Carbaugh 2001; Bruner 1991; Linde 1993; Thornborrow and Coates 2005; Wortham 2001), but it is precisely within the case of migrants that their narratives are particularly rich in elements of their social and cultural identity (Baynham and De Fina 2005; De Fina 2003). Moreover, narrative is not an autonomous event but one interwoven with the socio-cultural, political-historical and spatio-temporal contexts. Different groups of Polish migrants developed different models of their respective grand narratives by repeating individual stories in the same or a similar canonical form. Those stories are closely linked to and enacted in migrants' places, where individual subjects give shape to them through interactions underpinning different social practices, such as socialising, celebrating, praying, or shopping. In what follows I outline characteristics of various groups of Polish migrants, elaborating on who they are, what constitutes the narratives they identify with, as well as on what the places and interactions they usually engage in are.

Poles in the UK: People and/in their Places

I collected my data in the English Midlands in dedicated 'Polish' places such as the Polish club (or centre) attached to the Polish Catholic Church, a few grocery shops recently established by Poles selling Polish products mostly, but not exclusively, to Polish customers, as well as a Polish restaurant operating on the same principles. I interacted mainly with three different groups of migrants: postwar, post-1989/pre-enlargement, and post-enlargement.

Postwar Migration

This group of migrants was established from former soldiers and officers (and also their families) who fought during the Second World War. The group's history is firmly associated with the history of Poland during and immediately after the war, including the change to a communist regime in 1944. They were prevented from returning to Poland after the War, or decided not to, escaping imprisonment, torture and even death in communist Poland. They settled down, built churches and clubs/cultural centres, organised themselves (i.e. the government-in-exile in London), opened Polish shops, established the Polish education society and mainly carried 'the torch of Polishness' for generations to come.

Analysing these migrants' life stories, Burrell (2006) identified several elements which construct a grand narrative of the postwar migration. These elements are: 1) a long story about getting to the UK (i.e. narratives of walking from Siberia); 2) views of the nation as the most treasured possession, mythologisation of the state, history, and their own personal histories (i.e. the myth of no return); 3) knowledge of Polish history—'without exception, every Polish person interviewed exhibited an intricate, and for the most part factually accurate, knowledge of Poland's modern history and an emotional empathy with the historical fate of the Polish nation' (Burrell 2006: 77); 4) active participation in church and religious ceremonies; 5) recognition of the importance of the Polish language as a mother tongue of future generations; 6) a sense of community. Creation of such a narrative was achieved by repeated patterns of a community-bounded dialectical production and consumption of their cultural needs, usually taking place in a Polish church and a Polish cultural centre. Premises were not only properties of the migrants' community but also, more importantly, locations with symbolic capital attached to them. They were 'our' sites, where a community's life evolved, and where people experienced their community's cohesion. In that sense, a Polish centre had a similar notion to that of home, 'inhabited' and 'guarded' by members of the postwar Polish migrant community. No wonder, then, that a main characteristic of this group of people is one of a closed community, suspicious of newcomers trying to enter, despite the fact that newcomers have also been Polish. However, when it comes to practical desire for material needs in the form of ethnic food, this group is happy to visit new Polish grocery shops, recently opened by newcomers.

Post-1989/Pre-Enlargement Migration

The second migration has to be contextualised with reference not only to post-communist transformation and EU enlargement, but also to pre-1989 Central and Eastern European countries' historical reality of closed borders. Up until 1989 passports to leave the Eastern bloc were strictly rationed, with people going to extremes to leave the country. Getting to the mythologised West was an achievement in its own right. At the same time, visas and work permit restrictions in the West for Eastern-bloc citizens from CEEC were strictly implemented, 'symmetrically' making borders difficult to penetrate. Democratic reforms in the late 1980s enabled ordinary people in the East to get their passports and presented the possibility of unrestricted travel. However these restrictions were waived from one side of the border only, leaving landing in the Promised Land still often dependent upon pure luck. Fortress Europe did not like visitors from behind the former Iron Curtain. These migrants left Poland in the early 1990s when the Polish borders were open but one still had to have an invitation from either a private person or a public subject in Britain to enter the United Kingdom. Still, the decision whether to let the person in or not was up to the British immigration official. There were also restrictions that made getting legal work a difficult task.

Having this context in mind, it is not difficult to understand why the general narrative of post-1989/pre-enlargement migrants is based on a construction of space as fixed and closed. The post-1989 group of migrants narrated their experience of moving as an extremely hard and critical moment in their lives—a rite of passage. Despite having a passport and the possibility of going back and forth, a journey to the United Kingdom was constructed as a final step into leaving one space and moving into another. Two elements of this group narrative are important: firstly, the overwhelming feeling of an extraordinary experience, struggle and final decision. Secondly, it is presented as an individual and not a group experience. Thus this group of migrants is not 'attached' to any specific 'Polish' locations. Indeed, they usually had problems being accepted in centres 'ruled' by the postwar group. In consequence they use both the church and the club pragmatically for *ad hoc* and superficial socialising but are usually not involved emotionally in these places. On the other hand, these people did not have enough power or capital to organise new migrant sites such as shops or restaurants.

Post-Enlargement Migration

The situation for migrating Poles changed dramatically almost overnight, when eight Central and Eastern European countries—Poland being the largest among them—entered the EU in May 2004, followed by Bulgaria and Romania in January 2007. The United Kingdom was one of the first countries from 'Europe 15' to open its labour market for 'new' Europeans since that date. As the post-1989 migrants usually repeated historically grounded patterns of the clandestine character of economic

migration from Poland, based on existing networks of fellow Poles (Morawska 2001; Triandafyllidou 2006), post-2004 arrivals gradually changed these patterns, moving, travelling and looking for jobs more independently. As Garapich argues, 'temporary, circular, unpredictable, open-ended, strategically adaptive migration activities have flourished after full liberalization of the migration regime' (2006: 15). Suddenly Polish migrants became 'well-adapted transnational actors, using—or at least trying to—the best of both worlds, keeping feet in both places and building their class identities in both settings with stronger emphasis on individual achievement, human agency, self-determination and flexibility' (2006: 4).

Not surprisingly, the post-enlargement group discursively constructed themselves in opposition to other waves of Polish migrants and also constructed their migration as a temporary or open-ended period in their lives. However, I would argue that they have achieved some degree of generational identity. Amongst other things, this is due to the mediated character of personal narratives, both in the British and the Polish press, an omnipresent use of new communication methods and networks fortified by the newest technology. It is their generation story. They could use it in the construction and legitimisation of their migrant status (see Galasińska 2009).

An unproblematic movement of thousands of Poles, their ideas, their way of life and their capital has significant material evidence on the ground in the UK. In the area of my fieldwork, several Polish shops and a restaurant have been established during the last two years. Although a primary role of these sites (at least for the owners) is the creation of business, for many members of the post-enlargement group these are multifunctional Polish spaces catering to the other needs of newcomers, including socialising and the exchange of information. In that sense these are the post-enlargement group's places, just as the club is the postwar group's space.

Gossiping

In this article I am interested in how elements of an emotional evaluation about different groups of migrants are (dis)played explicitly and implicitly in narratives produced, performed and circulated within the Polish migrants' community. In what follows, I focus on what narrators *do* while narrating (Bamberg 2007), and in particular how narrators are engaging in the activity of narrating as evaluating. While identifying certain content-related arguments (see Reisigl and Wodak 2001; Wagner and Wodak 2006) and their textual realisation in analysed narratives, I offer, at the same time, a broader macro-interpretation of bottom-up discourses of migration in the era of transition.

I identified as my collected data, with regard to the mutual evaluation of fellow Poles in the UK, items of gossip which were passed to other members of the group during semi-formal and mostly informal meetings in the 'Polish' places under investigation. People were employing characteristic *framing devices* while gossiping, such as the use of constructions *pronoun+noun*: '*You know, **those Poles** …*' or '*… but in **this club** …*'. The other linguistic feature I recognised was a frequent use of

pronouns instead of nouns for description of the other group, i.e. *they, those*, or (a very difficult case to translate as pronoun in English) *what comes here* ... (Polish—***To** co tutaj przyjeżdża*).

In the case of the **postwar group**, I collected my 'gossiping' data in the club. Here people were in the position of hosts and held power by virtue of their control over the place. Over several months club officials held a number of meetings to discuss, resolve and overcome financial difficulties the club came into, due to a falling number of members. The ageing population of the postwar group, coupled with a lack of interest from the younger generation in maintaining the same level of participation in the club's activities, resulted in economic problems. A significant influx of post-enlargement migrants, who participate in Sunday masses in the Polish church next door and who started to use the club's premises afterwards, became an important aspect of 'healing' the club's finances. Administrators decided to organise more social events, in which newcomers could participate, cashing in for tickets. After one open evening in the club, when live music was performed and people were dancing, I was engaged in a conversation about the event. A woman I talked to summed up the entire night as follows:

> It ended in blows, of course.
> *Oczywiście się pobili.*

This short utterance reveals several interesting points. There is its shortness, to begin with, which could be evidence of a lack of interest in the topic or the group/subject the woman was telling me about; hence a distancing strategy of a short form was used. On the other hand, she may have decided to demonstrate the most important part of that evening, the part which involved conflict and was a tale worth telling. Making an impact on the listener is crucial for storytelling activity (Holmes and Marra 2005), and my interlocutor presented evidence of an extraordinary event whose real subjects are actually hidden (Polish grammar allows the speaker to build sentences with a hidden/implicit subject). But not mentioning who those implicit *they* are is also another distancing figure employed in this utterance. *They* are clearly not part of 'us', moreover *they* are not even spoken of. Finally, there is an extreme case formulation *of course,* which here is an indication for foreseeing the bad (or undignified) behaviour of *them.*

Another episode: recently I was talking to a woman who is a volunteer helping newcomers to deal with matters to do with the city council. She reported some cases as illustrations of her work and then she added:

> [W]hat comes here is trash, it is a catastrophe.
> *[T]o co tutaj przyjeżdża to jest dno, to jest katastrofa.*

My interlocutor speaks of newcomers using an even more explicit (and depersonalised) pronoun *it,* confirming that distancing strategies from the other group of migrants are common and that they are constructed in a similar way to the previous

example. Her choice of descriptive vocabulary (*trash, catastrophe*) is an explicit way of passing an emotionally negative judgment on newly arriving Poles.

One very important feature of the club's life is a series of children's performances in connection to national and church festivals. Up until the post-enlargement-migrants' children joined the Saturday language school attached to the club, these performances were far from perfection, mainly due to a limited knowledge of Polish by the second and third generations of club members. Since 2004, performances improved significantly and it is visibly clear to an observer that the older members of the audience enjoy these occasions very much. During one such performance my neighbour from the audience told me:

> [Y]ou know, they were communists and since they came here they are learning how to be Poles
> *[W]ie pani, to byli komuniści i jak tu przyjechali to uczą się jak być Polakami.*

Here again we hear evidence of how 'old' migrants implicitly distanced themselves from a group of newcomers by naming them using emotionally charged labels such as *communists* (a synonym of all evils for them). An interesting aspect of this statement is the fact that this woman talked about children who were born long after communism in Poland collapsed in 1989. Nevertheless she decided to anchor her narrative in a familiar context of Europe divided by rival political systems. Thus her quote illustrates how the postwar group narratives became historically static and not developmental in time and how emotional judgement is influenced by a community's previous experiences.

Interestingly, once they hit national labels, my interlocutors immediately changed their discourses. Witness the following example when one club member is talking about newcomers as a group of Poles:

> [T]hose Poles are doing very well, they are happy, all have good jobs and accommodation.
> *[C]i Polacy sobie bardzo dobrze radzą, są zadowoleni, wszyscy maja dobrą pracę, mieszkania.*

This example presents an unequivocally positive view of Poles and Polishness with only a hint of reservation revealed by the distancing pronoun *those.* For my informants it was impossible to talk in a bad way about such a huge group of Poles in Britain. Even the ideological dilemmas (Billig *et al.* 1988) introduced by references to the newer migration groups are smoothed out and incorporated within the monolithic (and nationalist) view of Polish migration. It is an interesting observation mainly because earlier waves of migration were less likely to get such a good reception in the Polish club. As I mentioned before, these were closed and quite hostile places, at least in my other interlocutors' stories.

In contrast, the **post-enlargement group** (I interacted with them in various 'Polish' places) was straight away dismissive of the old migration and usually uninterested in the other waves. In relation to post-WWII migrants they compared them to living

museums. Patronising comments were often reinforced by open criticism. Witness both examples below:

> [T]here are nice grandads there, like from the insurrection.
> *[T]am są fajne dziadki, jak z powstania.*

> [T]hey don't even speak English well after all those years.
> *[O]ni nawet po angielsku dobrze nie mówią po tylu latach.*

Judgmental statements are clearly constructed here along historic (*insurrection*), generation (*grandads*) and education/adaptive (*proper English*) lines. A mirrored use of the distancing *they*, known already from the old group's discourse, alongside a new and interesting spatial mode of distancing *there*, shapes gossip about older Poles in opposition to 'us'.

The fact of not belonging on an emotional level to the Polish places associated with the postwar group is evident most vividly in the religious field. Post-enlargement migrants are often looking for alternative means of catering for their spiritual needs, choosing English Catholic churches (interestingly sometimes also staffed by priests from Poland). In the example below a young couple implicitly evaluated a Polish church as not normal:

> [W]e don't go there, we go to a normal English church.
> *[M]y tam nie chodzimy, chodzimy do normalnego Angielskiego kościoła.*

During collection of the data in shops and the restaurant, I was told by owners and employees about all groups of customers visiting those places. Although these premises serve mainly Poles, people who worked there stressed that the place welcomes members of all communities in the vicinity. Consider how post-WWII migrants are differently positioned from other Polish or English visitors in the following example:

> [All] people come here, Englishmen, Poles, even these old Poles.
> *[T]u przychodzą wszyscy, Anglicy, Polacy, nawet ci starzy Polacy.*

I would argue that there are specific post-enlargement-group stories, or indeed counter-stories (Andrews 2004), and lived experiences of an unproblematic translocation, which helped them to achieve a negative discourse about postwar migrants and to discursively distance themselves from the old migration. Implicitly members of this group positioned themselves as modern, open, mobile, egalitarian, highly skilful and well-educated, in striking contrast to postwar migrants, who are living in the past and not able to move with the spirit of the time. Interestingly, issues of class as such do not come to the fore here, as indeed they did not in other cases. All my interlocutors seem to be 'class-blind'.

The most surprising result of my research concerns **post-1989/pre-enlargement migrants.** This is the most ambiguous group in my opinion. They are balancing

between looking for approval from, and being critical of, both postwar and post-enlargement groups. Consider the next example whereby one woman, describing her early years in the UK, juxtaposed her experience with the situation of newcomers:

> [W]hen I came here I had to sort everything out all by myself and nobody helped me, while these new Poles want everything, all should be theirs, accommodations, benefits.
> *[J]ak ja tu przyjechałam to wszystko musiałam sama załatwiać i nikt mi nie pomógł a ci nowi Polacy to chcą wszystko mieć, wszystko im się należy, mieszkania, zasiłki.*

In this short passage she distances herself from both groups: the old migrants who did not help her when she started a new life in Britain, and the post-enlargement group whom she 'accuses' of overusing the benefits system. This fact did not prevent her from articulating, a little later in her narrative, her joy over the establishment of new Polish grocery shops:

> [N]ow one can buy everything [Polish food, etc.] and it is not as it was before.
> *[T]eraz to można wszystko kupić a nie tak jak dawniej.*

My interlocutor this time explicitly praises the entrepreneurship of energetic newcomers while at the same time implicitly criticising the stagnation of the old migrants. Here is another example of how the post-1989 group's discourses of both postwar and post-enlargement migrants are subject to change, and are thus less stable than narratives produced by the other groups. It is probably as a result of the fact that these narratives are embedded in the context of both communist ideologies and discourses of post-communist transformations. As gossiping involves a power struggle I would argue that this is the least powerful group. Their grand narrative of struggle (see *all by myself and nobody helped me*) is less powerful than that of the postwar veterans. On the other hand, they do not hold strong arguments about their entrepreneurship in comparison with the post-enlargement group, often officially praised by the British media for their commitment to work and their contribution to the country's budget. By contrast to the newcomers, post-1989 migrants were rejected by the old Polish diaspora ('They were not Polish enough'; 'How you could leave a free motherland?'), rejected by the UK as a new home country (permanent residence and work permit struggles) and not appreciated or else ignored by the 'new Europeans'. This in turn fuels even more gossiping.

Conclusions

Analysing my data for this special issue of *JEMS* devoted to the theme of emotions and human mobility, I have tried to show how stories which popped out in a given context of a multilayered Polish migration could be seen as a specific way of discursively addressing the problem of emotional coexistence amongst different waves of Polish migrants in the UK. For different groups of my Polish interlocutors, emotions are demonstrated in different ways in their stories. Some of them are quick

to evaluate or even judge those who came to the UK at a different time. Others are more careful in their opinions, but knowing their group's narratives which underpinned their sense of making meaning of migration and also their lived experience of migration, one could perhaps decode an implicit emotional display interwoven in the discourses they produce.

The utterances analysed here are free of vocabulary usually associated with emotions. My interlocutors avoid naming their feelings toward other groups of Poles; hence labels such as disrespect, dislike, contempt, resentment, antipathy or scoff are not in use, even though the overall emotional evaluation is clear to interpret. As Galasiński observes, 'Other lexico-grammatical resources of language can also construct emotional experience without labelling it, without even implying it by certain (...) vocabulary' and these are based on 'our abilities as social actors to interpret the world' (2004: 126). He mentions, *inter alia*, metaphors, idioms, emotional verbs, stylisations (see also Fiehler 2002; Foolen 1997), and also recalls Greenwood's (1994) language of moral commentary on actions and social relations. In the case of Polish migrants, a negative critique is made along historic, generation, adaptation and spatial lines. It is worth repeating here that a national affiliation with Poland is out of the question when it comes to an emotional judgement. In other words, one can disapprove of and resist a particular embodiment of Polishness (see in the data: *new, old, those, they*) but Polishness itself as a general category is not contested at all (see also Galasińska 2006).

One aspect of the collected data is apparent—all groups are emotionally involved in inter-group relations, they negotiate their way of dealing with other Poles and sometimes struggle to cope with different version of Polishness abroad. For all of them, a particular group of challenging 'others' is, first of all, not a local community of the country of destination but, what is more important, their fellow-countrymen in the UK. Frequent gossiping becomes a handy way to express negative feelings against other groups and, at the same time, to form and build an attachment to 'our' group. Discursive analysis of gossip helps to understand how group formation is performed and shaped through this unique genre, and how emotions play a central and essential role in it.

Finally, conflicting discourses of the Polish migration in the context of a social and economic transformation in Europe show how historical processes shape and are shaped by the language we use in everyday encounters. It is indeed the micro level of personal experience which (discursively) reflects broader historical, political and social global issues.

References

Ahmed, S. (2004) *The Cultural Politics of Emotion.* Edinburgh: Edinburgh University Press.

Andrews, M. (2004) 'Counter-narratives and the power to oppose', in Bamberg, M. and Andrews, M. (eds) *Considering Counter-Narratives. Narrating, Resisting, Making Sense.* Amsterdam/Philadelphia: John Benjamins, 1–6.

Bamberg, M. (ed.) (2000) Theme issue on narrative identity, *Narrative Inquiry, 10*(1).

Bamberg, M. (2007) 'Stories: big or small—why do we care?', in Bamberg, M. (ed.) *Narrative: State of the Art.* Amsterdam/Philadelphia: John Benjamins, 165–74.

Baynham, M. and De Fina, A. (eds) (2005) *Dislocation/Relocation. Narratives of Displacement.* Manchester: St. Jerome Publishing.

Billig, M., Condor, S., Edwards, D., Cane, M., Middleton, D. and Radley, A. (1988) *Ideological Dilemma. A Social Psychology of Everyday.* London: Sage.

Blommaert, J., Collins, J. and Slembrouck, S. (2005) 'Polycentricity and interactional regimes in "global neighborhoods"', *Ethnography, 6*(2): 205–36.

Brockmeier, J. and Carbaugh, D. (eds) (2001) *Narrative and Identity: Studies in Autobiography, Self and Culture.* Amsterdam: John Benjamins.

Bruner, J. (1991) 'The narrative construction of reality', *Critical Inquiry, 18*: 1–21.

Burrell, K. (2006) *Moving Lives.* Aldershot: Ashgate.

Cyrus, N. (2006) 'Polish emigration: permanent and temporary patterns', in Triandafyllidou, A. (ed.) *Contemporary Polish Migration in Europe. Complex Patterns of Movements and Settlement.* Lewinston: Edwin Mellen Press, 25–46.

De Fina, A. (2003) *Identity in Narrative: A Study of Immigrant Discourse.* Amsterdam: John Benjamins.

Fairclough, N. (1992) *Discourse and Social Change.* Cambridge: Polity Press.

Fairclough, N. (1996) 'Technologisation of discourse', in Caldas-Coulthard, C.-R. and Coulthard, M. (eds) *Texts and Practices: Readings in Critical Discourse Analysis.* London: Routledge, 92–106.

Fairclough, N. (2003) *Analysing Discourse: Textual Analysis for Social Research.* London: Routledge.

Fiehler, R. (2002) 'How to do emotions with words: emotionality in conversations', in Fussel, S.R. (ed.) *The Verbal Communication of Emotions.* Mahwah: Lawrence Erlbaum Associates, 79–106.

Foolen, A. (1997) 'The expressive function of language: towards a cognitive semantic approach', in Niemeier, S. and Dirven, R. (eds) *The Language of Emotions. Conceptualization, Expression, and Theoretical Foundation.* Amsterdam/Philadelphia: John Benjamins, 15–32.

Galasińska, A. (2006) 'Border ethnography and post-communist discourses of nationality in Poland', *Discourse and Society, 17*(5): 609–28.

Galasińska, A. (2009) 'Small stories fight back: narratives of Polish economic migration on an internet forum', in Galasińska, A. and Krzyżanowski, M. (eds) *Discourse and Transformation in Central and Eastern Europe.* Basingstoke: Palgrave Macmillan, 188–203.

Galasiński, D. (2004) *Men and the Language of Emotions.* Basingstoke: Palgrave Macmillan.

Garapich, M. (2006) 'De-localizing class and transnationalizing super-diversity: Polish migrants in London'. Bristol: paper presented to the 9th EASA Biennial Conference, 18–21 September.

Georgakopoulou, A. (2006) 'The other side of the story: towards a narrative analysis of narrative-in-interaction', *Discourse Studies, 8*(2): 235–57.

Greenwood, J.D. (1994) *Realism, Identity and Emotion.* London: Sage.

Hładkiewicz, W. (1997) 'Bilans i Perspektywy Emigracji Polskiej w Wielkiej Brytanii', *Przegląd Polonijny, 23*(2): 53–64.

Holmes, J. and Marra, M. (2005) 'Narrative and the construction of professional identity in the workplace', in Thornborrow, J. and Coates, J. (eds) *The Sociolinguistics of Narrative: Theory, Context and Culture in Oral Story-Telling.* Amsterdam/Philadelphia: John Benjamins, 193–213.

Iglicka, K. (2000) 'Mechanisms of migration from Poland before and during the transition period', *Journal of Ethnic and Migration Studies, 26*(1): 61–73.

Iglicka, K. (2001) *Poland's Post-War Dynamic of Migration.* Aldershot: Ashgate.

Iglicka-Okólska, K. (1997) 'Społeczne, Ekonomiczne i Polityczne Uwarunkowania Emigracji z Polski w Latach 1945–1995', in Zamojski, J.E. (ed.) *Migracje i Społeczeństwo.* Warsaw: Instytut Historii PAN, 97–112.

Lacoff, G. (1996) *Moral Politics. What Conservatives Know that Liberals Don't.* Chicago/London: University of Chicago Press.

Leutloff-Grandis, C. (2006) 'Claiming ownership in postwar Croatia: the emotional dynamics of possession and repossession in Knin', in Svašek, M. (ed.) *Postsocialism. Politics and Emotions in Central and Eastern Europe.* New York/Oxford: Berghahn, 115–37.

Linde, C. (1993) *Life Stories: The Creation of Coherence.* Oxford: Oxford University Press.

Lutz, C.A. (1988) *Unnatural Emotions.* Chicago/London: University of Chicago Press.

Lutz, C.A. and Abu-Lughod, L. (eds) (1990) *Language and the Politics of Emotion.* Cambridge: Cambridge University Press.

Milton, K. and Svašek, M. (eds) (2005) *Mixed Emotions. Anthropological Studies of Feeling.* Oxford: Berg.

Morawska, E. (1989) 'Labour migration of Poles in the Atlantic world economy, 1880–1914', *Comparative Studies in Society and History, 3*(2): 237–72.

Morawska, E. (2001) 'Structuring migration: the case of Polish income-seeking travellers to the West', *Theory and Society, 30*(1): 47–80.

Ochs, E. and Capps, L. (2001) *Living Narrative: Creating Lives in Everyday Storytelling.* Cambridge, MA: Harvard University Press.

Reddy, W.M. (2001) *Navigation of Feeling. A Framework for the History of Emotion.* Cambridge: Cambridge University Press.

Reisigl, M. and Wodak, R. (2001) *Discourse and Discrimination.* London: Routledge.

Slany, K. (ed.) (1997) *Orientacje Emigracyjne Polaków.* Kraków: Uniwersytet Jagielloński, Instytut Socjologii.

Svašek, M. (1997) 'Gossip and power struggle in the post-communist art world', *Focaal. Journal of Anthropology, 29*: 101–22.

Svašek, M. (2000) 'Borders and emotions: hope and fear in the Bohemian–Bavarian frontier zone', *Ethnologia Europaea, 30*(2): 111–26.

Svašek, M. (ed.) (2006) *Postsocialism. Politics and Emotions in Central and Eastern Europe.* New York/Oxford: Berghahn.

Sword, K. (1996) *Identity in Flux. Polish Community in Britain.* London: University of London, School of Slavonic and East European Studies, occasional papers.

Triandafyllidou, A. (ed.) (2006) *Contemporary Polish Migration in Europe. Complex Patterns of Movements and Settlement.* Lewinston: Edwin Mellen Press.

Thornborrow, J. and Coates, J. (eds) (2005) *The Sociolinguistics of Narrative: Theory, Context and Culture in Oral Story-Telling.* Amsterdam/Philadelphia: John Benjamins.

Wagner, I. and Wodak, R. (2006) 'Performing success: identifying strategies of self-representation in women's biographical narratives', *Discourse & Society, 17*(3): 385–411.

Wodak, R. (1996) *Disorders of Discourse.* London: Longman.

Wodak, R. (2001) 'The discourse-historical approach', in Wodak, R. and Meyer, M. (eds) *Methods of Critical Discourse Analysis.* London: Sage, 63–94.

Wodak, R. (2006) 'Mediation between discourse and society: assessing cognitive approaches', *Discourse Studies, 8*(1): 179–90.

Wortham, S. (2001) *Narratives in Action.* New York: Teachers College Columbia Press.

Zeldin, T. (1998) *An Intimate History of Humanity.* London: Vintage.

Emotional Ambiguity: Japanese Migrant Women in Mixed Families and their Life Transition

Naoko Maehara

Through the narratives of Japanese migrant women in Ireland, this paper focuses on their perceptions of 'home' and their emotional processes in the context of their life transition. In order to explore the interactive and relational nature of their emotional processes, three questions are examined. How do migrant women manage their emotions in the process of constructing motherhood as their main social identity? How do their emotional orientations complement or conflict other emotion rules? In changing social and familial settings, how are their feelings navigated? The narratives of two Japanese mothers illustrate their contradictory, inconsistent and ambiguous emotional experiences which are created through physical mobility and transnational family relationships. Through changing social roles, obligations and expectations, they participate in different 'feeling rules' to frame the lived experiences in which their relationships with their new country and home place are renewed. Through changing their life course, they also experience 'emotional resonance' or 'dissonance' with others, which affects their sense of belonging/non-belonging in different places. The context of motherhood provides examples of such dynamics of multiple, interdependent processes in which subjectivities and feelings emerge.

The Japanese migrant women featured in this study live in Northern Ireland and the Irish Republic.[1] Their migration backgrounds are various. Some of them migrated for career or study prospects and eventually settled down with local husbands and/or children. Others met Irish or Northern Irish husbands in Japan or in other countries, and eventually migrated to their husband's home place. Since settling in Ireland, they

have all developed relationships with their in-laws and new friends, while often maintaining important ties with their places of origin. For many of them, migration was not meant to be permanent. One woman in her early 40s, who migrated from Japan to her husband's home in Derry in 1993, said 'I was curious to see . . . but if life went wrong, and if I didn't like it here, I thought we could always go back to Japan'. Fifteen years later, she still lives in Northern Ireland, noting that 'It must be a good place'. Another woman in her mid-30s, who migrated to Portrush to marry a man who was originally her pen-friend in 1995, reflects:

> I didn't think so carefully about my future, whether I wanted to go back to Japan some time or not . . . You know, I was in my early twenties, I didn't think about my old age . . . which is different from now . . . I was thinking only about myself then . . . not about the future at all . . . I just thought I could survive here somehow . . .

Her husband died of a heart attack two years ago. She now intends to stay in Northern Ireland with her two daughters, describing her adopted town like this:

> Here (Portrush) has become like 'my home' . . . although there're not so many things here . . . how can I describe it? . . . Portrush is . . . very peaceful somehow . . . I used to have my family-in-law nearby . . . and you know, everybody is like my relatives. They know each other well. So, I already knew everybody in the first few months after I came . . .

In this paper, I focus on migrants' perceptions of 'home' and their emotional processes in the context of their life transition. In recent years, a growing number of scholars have been concerned with the emotional dimensions of human mobility (Conradson and McKay 2007; Svašek 2008; Svašek and Skrbiš 2007). The life-course perspective is useful to develop their studies, allowing us to consider how migrants' social roles, obligations and expectations are largely dependent upon what stage they have reached in the life cycle (Gardner 2002). Each migrant thus creates a sense of belonging or 'feeling at home' in a new country differently, and these experiences are often ambiguous (Rapport and Dawson 1998: 9). At a different point in their life course, they experience transitions in their relationships with the new and home places. Through marriage, having children, having elderly parents or parents-in-law, losing their parents or husbands, they change their priorities, concerns, expectations, goals and plans, all of which affect, and are affected by, emotional processes.

Motherhood and Emotional Adjustment

Pregnancy and childrearing are two of the most significant aspects of the life transition for many Japanese migrant women. As mothers of half-Irish and half-Japanese children, they participate in the socially constructed set of activities and relationships involved in child-nurturing and caring. New social fields are created: for example, by being involved in children's play groups, and later parents' groups. Their

extended family relationships, neighbourhood and friendship relationships are also renewed through the arrival of new family members. For example, receiving hands-on assistance and emotional support with childcare, they may cultivate new relationships with in-laws in Ireland. Through establishing meaningful social fields and a sense of responsibility, they create a new sense of belonging in the present surroundings.

Their relationships with the homeland also change when migrant women become mothers and have to cope with young children. Ryan (2008) describes, in the case of Irish nurses in Britain, how migrant new mothers express feelings of loneliness and homesickness for their own families, as this is often a time of intense emotion for the women and family support becomes more important than it had been during their care-free years. Likewise, many Japanese new mothers whom I interviewed talk about how they miss, particularly, their own mothers who would be very helpful in terms of childcare, and who would also love to see their grandchild. Many of them are also eager to introduce Japanese language and other cultural aspects (diet, manner, life style, etc.) to their children. Through such childrearing practices, they may relive memories of their own childhoods which bring them to re-evaluate their past experiences.

In order to explore the dynamic relationships that Japanese migrant women create between their new country and home place, this paper focuses on the interactive and relational nature of their emotional processes. In past decades, scholars from different disciplines have sought broader understandings of emotion without assimilating it either to pure sensation or to pure cultural cognition, to feeling or meaning (Svašek 2005). An increasing number of studies now acknowledge that emotion should not be seen in the realm of pure individuality but in an interactive world lived by mind and bodies. As Leavitt (1996: 527) wrote:

> Affective or felt associations, like semantic ones, are collective as well as individual; they operate through common or similar experience among members of a group living in similar circumstances, through cultural stereotyping of experience, and through shared expectations, memories, and fantasies.

This paper mainly outlines the concept of 'emotion work' to examine how mothering and motherhood shape relationships, and emotional involvements, with places and families 'here' and 'there'. According to Hochschild (1979, 1983), emotion is subject to acts of management in which how we want to feel is directed by a set of socially shared 'feeling rules' (1979: 563). Through the emotion work socio-culturally defined, we are accepted as part of a specific social group to which we belong. In the contemporary globalising world, however, individuals are increasingly confronted with the feeling rules from different communities in which they participate (Hermans and Dimaggio 2007: 46). Unexceptionally, Japanese migrant mothers in this study talk about their struggles to manage often different, inconsistent 'feeling rules' in new and old places. Their narratives also reflect how, through a different stage in their life course, they change 'the official frame' of the lived experience, which guides

'appropriate' feelings (Hochschild 1979: 567). This study thus examines how Japanese migrant mothers manage their often contradictory, inconsistent and ambiguous emotional experiences which are created through movement over time and space.

The concepts of 'emotion work' and 'emotional labour' have been influential, being used in various forms such as organisations and occupational roles (Hochschild 1983), mothering and motherhood (Erickson 1993), and also transnational family relationships (Baldassar 2007a, 2007b; Ryan 2008). This paper focuses on the processes of 'emotion work' in the contexts of motherhood and migration. As Erickson (1993) notes, mothering carries a heavy moral connotation and entails extensive, ongoing emotion work in which feelings must be managed and directed. The context of migration and intermarriage adds unique dimensions to such emotion work, since migrants are often required to manage their feelings in a conscious effort to establish relationships with significant others in multiple places. How do migrant women navigate their emotions in the process of constructing motherhood as their main social identity? Also, how do their emotional orientations complement or conflict with other emotion rules?

To consider these questions, it is also important to consider that emotions are not only consciously and cognitively managed (or unmanaged), but also unconsciously shaped through interactive relationships with others (Anderson and Keltner 2004; Hatfield and Rapson 2004; Theodosius 2006). For example, Hatfield and Rapson define emotional contagion as three propositions: '(1) that people tend to mimic others; (2) that emotional experience is affected by such feedback; and (3) that people therefore tend to "catch" others' emotions' (2004: 140). In this case, emotions are shaped less consciously and more automatically through interaction with others. Similarly, Anderson and Keltner argue that emotional convergence occurs in close relationships: '[r]elationship partners became more similar in their emotional reactions to events, and this similarity was exhibited even in the contexts in which they were not in each other's company' (2004: 154). Borrowing insights from these studies, this paper is also concerned with how transnational family relationships shape and reshape emotional orientations of the individuals involved. In changing social and familial settings, how are their feelings navigated?

Life Narratives of Two Japanese Migrant Mothers: Reflexive and Empathetic Approaches

The questions of implicit, unconscious emotions are particularly challenging, because it is empirically impossible to access what is subjectively felt within individual minds.[2] What needs to be examined here, however, is not a completely 'objective' understanding, but a less distorted view of their psycho-cultural processes. To minimise my own presumptions and preoccupations, reflexive and empathetic approaches are applied in the life-narrative method.[3]

As the Japanese wife of an Irish spouse and mother of two children, I have shared not only language but also many similar experiences with the interviewees. In the

research process, such a shared understanding has helped to create 'empathy sentiments' and 'resonance' between the researcher and the researched, which contributed to convey not only the meanings of emotions, but the feeling-tones as well, in my translation of emotions (Leavitt 1996: 530). I also acknowledge that self-narration is part of a multifaceted process: the cultural, the hermeneutic, the psychosocial and the psycho-cultural (e.g. Davies 1999; Driessen 1992; Peacock and Holland 1993). Peacock and Holland see life stories themselves as both developed in, and the outcomes of, the course of story-telling and other life events (1993: 371). In this regard, my study pays attention to how life stories are situated in different processes crucial to human life: collective meaning systems and their dynamics, self–other communication and discovery, social relations and the formation of sociality, or self-formation (1993: 377).

This study draws upon the narratives of two Japanese migrant mothers. I conducted the interviews as part of my ethnographic research among Japanese migrants in mixed marriages who live in Northern Ireland and the Republic. The actual number of Japanese residents in these regions is unknown. However, over 40 Japanese nationals in Northern Ireland, and 400 in the Republic, are currently estimated to hold permanent residency visas.[4] To my knowledge, an increasing number of young Japanese have recently migrated to these regions and married Irish or Northern Irish spouses. At an early stage of my research, I also found that many more Japanese women than men migrated and these women are involved in various organisations and informal networks. Through participant observation within these groups, and also personal friendship, I have tried to grasp the background of their narrative contexts.

The two interviewees in this paper represent different stages in the family cycle and the migration cycle. As a new mother of a young son, and a relatively new migrant, Hiroko, in her mid-30s, talks about how her views on life in Ireland have changed since her son was born. She also talks about her uneasiness and confusion over cultural expectations in Ireland. Kaori, in her late 40s, who has lived in Northern Ireland for 16 years, talks about her struggles with feelings of guilt about her inability to provide more support to her own parents in Japan. Although their stories represent their unique psycho-cultural processes, their contradictory, inconsistent and ambiguous experiences show the dynamic complexities of subjectivities and feelings that emerge through physical mobility and the social relations of transnational migrants.

Creating a Sense of Belonging through 'Feeling Up'

Hiroko lives in a small town in Co. Donegal. In the summer of 2007, I visited her for the first time for an interview. We had known each other through a social networking website, of which she was the group organiser and I was one of the members. The interview was conducted in her detached house. It was an exceptionally nice day. In her sunny kitchen, we were talking about the flowers and vegetables she was growing

in her garden. I started the interview by asking about her migration process. She initially came to Dublin to learn English in 1996. Like some of the other Japanese women, she didn't intend to stay in Ireland before she met her future husband, Thomas. In 2003, she decided to marry him and moved to Co. Donegal, where he was from, and got a new job. Settling down in Ireland was never her wish:

> I couldn't get rid of Thomas. We broke up a couple of times because I wanted to live in Japan. But we couldn't do really. We had a long-distance relationship for a long time. I wanted to have a normal life. I was tired. I thought I could enjoy my work if I lived in Japan. Here, in Ireland, I would only be a person who speaks poor English. But in Japan, I would be a person who can speak English ... which would also help me to get a job. But because of Thomas ... I was really not sure whether I should come back to Ireland or I should settle down in Japan. I was thinking too much and was tired. In such a way, marriage was a very difficult option.

She used to work as an administrator in Japan and Dublin, and wanted to work in a trading company in the future. In Donegal, there were almost no job opportunities for her. To settle down there meant that she had to give up such a future career. In her mid-twenties, she thought it was time to develop her work career. She saw her migration as a negative move: 'I didn't love this country. Because I had lived here for a long time, it wasn't an attractive place for me any more'.

Two years after marriage and migration, her son was born. At the time of the interview, he was two years old. I also had my small children including a new-born baby with me during the interview. As new mothers, we talked about how our lives had changed since we had children. For Hiroko, having previously been concerned with work possibilities in Donegal, other concerns now came to the fore in terms of the education system, healthcare, social surroundings, natural environment, and family relationships:

> My way of thinking changed, so did my pace, everything has changed ... my way of thinking ... I sometimes think Ireland is a better place to raise children. At the same time, I sometimes think the Japanese education system is better than here ... I think especially early education is better in Japan. The school facilities also aren't good here. And, children here don't learn how to clean, you know. They don't treat public things well, either. Things like that ...

Transitions from singlehood to marriage, to motherhood, require a good deal of 'emotion work' to re-orient 'appropriate' feelings in situations as wives and mothers. A sense of new 'rights' and 'duties' is applied to feelings, and in Hiroko's case she seemed to have modified previous 'feeling rules' for her career-oriented life. A new set of rules for framing the work and family life is assumed, and accordingly she has attempted to change images, ideas or thoughts of new surroundings and the home place. The subsequent extract shows a process of such cognitive emotion work, as she said:

> Irish families are tight, which is good, isn't it? The best thing in Ireland I thought was that people prioritise their families. I used to wonder whether Japanese men are

> better or which nationalities are better. But after all, Thomas was a good person, and there is no doubt that he treats his family members, including me, very well. So, I thought I could live here calmly, mentally, and also there's no materialism here ... which really contrasts with Japan.

Since she eventually decided to marry Thomas and settle down in Ireland, these images of idealised Irish family life and problematic Japanese life may have played a significant role in managing her emotions. However, the work of 'feeling up' is often a struggle for a new mother and a new migrant like her, whose sense of self is not fulfilled only with gender-ascribed roles as a wife and a mother. Her inconsistent concerns and desires in terms of work prospects and family life bring a lack of clarity about what the rule actually is, causing conflicts and contradictions between contending sets of rules (Hochschild 1979: 567–8). Such emotional ambiguity was expressed when she talked about her future prospects. When I asked her if she intends to stay in Ireland in the future, she replied uncertainly: 'I'm trying not to think about the future'. Towards the end of the interview, however, she talked of 'her dream' of having a Japanese-style guesthouse which is eco-friendly:

> Thomas' parents have a farm. They are too old to work it. So, if possible, I want to have an eco-friendly guesthouse there in the future. I would start with a normal guesthouse and, if it goes OK, it would have great potential, you know. As I love flowers, I want to grow lots of clematis, and make a clematis nursery garden .... Because it is farm land, I could have animals too ... I'm just dreaming ... And if possible, I want to have a Japanese bath and *tatami* rooms. I want many Japanese people to come to my guesthouse. Especially Japanese people who live in Europe ... when they feel like having a Japanese bath, for example. I would make some Japanese food for them. I want to develop a market for Japanese corporate families in Europe. Ireland is not exploited yet, you know ... When I'm thinking about such things, I feel excited ... life would be enjoyable, if it goes well ...

In this narrative, reminding me of the fact that she always liked working with soil, and had studied agriculture in college in Tokyo, she weaved a sense of continuity into her future prospects. She temporarily manages to 'feel up', bringing 'exciting' and 'enjoyable' images of her future life in Ireland. Through re-evaluating positive future perspectives, she orients her identifications with the present over the past, and creates a new sense of belonging in Ireland.

Emotional Dissonance in a New 'Home'

One of Hiroko's concerns in relation to life in Ireland was Catholicism. Thomas' parents are devout Catholics, and even sent him to a special school to become a priest when he was young. Because of that experience, she explained, he developed a 'Catholic allergy' (i.e. he became anti-Catholic). Thomas wanted to have a secular marriage (he even wanted to get married on Good Friday, which is taboo for Catholics), and in the end they had a wedding at a Shinto shrine in Japan. Because of

strong opposition from her husband's parents, nobody came to their wedding from Ireland, and there were only Hiroko's family and friends. Even after marriage, Thomas' parents asked them to have a blessing in a Catholic church but they refused. She expressed frustration towards her in-laws:

> They (my parents-in-law) are always telling him (my husband) such things. I feel like they don't accept our marriage, although they've never told me that directly.

Nevertheless, since marriage she has tried to build a good relationship with her parents-in-law who live nearby, for example through sometimes inviting them for dinner. When her son became four months old, she even accepted their expectations that he would be christened, although she didn't like the idea of her son becoming a Catholic. Even Thomas, who had a 'Catholic allergy', accepted their son's christening, seeing it as 'just an event'. However, she didn't like the idea that her son would become a Catholic long before he was able to decide such things for himself. She had a dilemma. Should she keep her stance on religion, or should she accept her parents-in-law's expectations? She was also concerned with the local primary school where her son would be expected to take religious classes and prepare for first communion:

> But there is Thomas' mother. I don't want to destroy our relationship. But I don't want to do something against my will. Thomas thinks first communion is just like an event, rather than religion. So, he thinks why not. He thinks it would be a pity for our son to be different from the other kids. But in my view I want him to have his own will. I know he would be sad at the beginning ... it would be difficult ... but he would understand it when he grows up ... But also I don't want to make a crack in the family relationship. If my mother-in-law gets very angry and says to us she doesn't want to see us any more, what could we do ...?

Her conflict is not unusual, as studies on intermarriages have described how migrant wives often experience conflict over various differences in everyday rituals (Breger and Hill 1998). To be sure, not only Hiroko but some of the other Japanese mothers I met expressed uneasy feelings about Irish in-laws' expectations over their children's religion. This conflict may reflect certain differences over 'emotion cultures' for framing religious beliefs and customs in Ireland and in Japan. In the following quote she reflects on Japanese people's attitudes towards religion (including her parents'), which, she emphasised, were very different from those of her parents-in-law. However, she was also aware of the multiplicity of 'emotion cultures' within the societies, and the fact that their attitudes are not so different from her husband and many other Irish people:

> (My parents are ...) Buddhist, but they also seem to believe in Shinto gods. My mother goes to the Shinto shrine. In Japan you don't care about such things, do you? While you are Buddhist, you celebrate Christmas, go to the Shinto shrine to celebrate a baby's first one hundred days etc. (They) are not sticklers for details. I know I contradict myself. I wanted to visit a shrine when my son was one hundred days old. I wanted to put a kimono on him, go to a shrine in Japan, and take a

> photo of him. If Thomas sees first communion in the same light, well . . . I would be better not to keep my ground. I know, people here too, they would have first communion just because they want to dress up their children . . . But because it (Catholicism) is so rigid, I feel like opposing first communion . . .

She tried to accept the idea of first communion, like her husband did, seeing its cultural and social aspects, although this was not successful. Analysing the reasons why she feels so opposed to her son's first communion, she talked about why she regarded Christianity negatively, linking it to racism:

> Another thing I was always concerned about is . . . racial discrimination . . . in some way . . . which may be not so related to religion, though . . . Not everyone, but many Irish people, I feel, have a sense of superiority over non-white people. I feel such a thing when I am talking to various people, such as neighbours, or people I meet for the first time. I know it's bad to think in this way, but I can't stop connecting this feeling of superiority with Christianity and white Westerners.

In this next narrative, she talks about how emotional detachment with many other Irish people restricted her ability to 'catch' the emotions of her husband and in-laws. A sense of marginalisation in Ireland and 'emotional dissonance' were not something that she expected before she settled down in this country:

> It's a bit disappointing for me to have such a feeling. At the beginning (when I came to Ireland), I was forgetting I was Japanese . . . Although my English was bad, I tried my best to mix with local people. But as I got used to life here, I gradually felt some distance from them. But I don't know where this impression came from . . . whether my understanding of local people has got better or just my attitudes towards them have changed . . .

In the process of constructing motherhood as a main social identity, I assume that she needed to find the way in which she could feel 'at home' in the new place. Creating 'emotional convergence' (Anderson and Keltner 2004) in relationships is important to developing such a sense of belonging in Ireland. Since there were no other Japanese people living around her town, she had organised an online community for those who have settled in Ireland with their Irish spouses, noting: 'I was like grasping at straws. We need to express our thoughts and hear other people's thoughts, don't we?' Through the website, members have discussions, exchange information, or chat, about various topics—including children's religion, education, bilingualism, Japanese school experience, how to get Japanese ingredients, recipes, getting visas, visiting home, husbands' Japanese language skills, etc. Through the involvement in the community, she has got to know many Japanese migrants living in Ireland. Regarding children's religion, she has also found that some of the women do not mind about it at all, while others feel uncomfortable with devout Catholics' expectations. Through interacting with other Japanese women, it seems that she has loosened her negative feelings towards Catholicism:

> I usually don't like things which I can't accept ... But these days I really don't know ... Since I got to know many other Japanese people through that community, I've been able to express my feelings little by little ... and feel I don't care so much about it (my son's christening). So, my way of thinking has changed a lot since I set up that community ...

Conflicting Loyalties Towards Families 'Here' and 'There'

Kaori lives in Belfast. We met for the first time for an interview in the spring of 2007. We were at a café in a shopping centre, and talking about our ageing parents in Japan. The café was a bit crowded but, since we were talking in Japanese, and nobody would understand what we were talking about, it was as if we were in a private space. She started by asking me 'How do other people cope with this problem? I really want some advice ...'. What I was able to tell her was only the fact that many other migrant women have similar problems when their parents begin to require old-age support; there are Japanese organisations which support care across distance; this is a big issue for me too. She talked about her parents who were in their late seventies. Her father was in hospital, while her mother went to see him every day. Her younger brother appeared not to be so dependable, and she seemed to struggle with feelings of guilt about her inability to provide more support to her parents because of the distance.

> My father had a stroke when I was just over 20 years old. He was very lucky. All the other patients in his room in the hospital died, only he survived. But since then, his brain, his memory and his body have little by little got worse ... About two years ago, he finally became bedridden. He can't eat, talk, or get up, he can only open and close his hand ... apart from that, he has no way of communicating ... Since June, two years ago, my mother goes to the hospital every day. Fortunately, she is a positive person. But even for a very positive person, it must be very depressing ...

She said she usually phones her mother three times a week. Apart from that, she also uses e-mail and mobile text messages. As is typical of her generation, her mother cannot use the Internet; instead she sends messages from her mobile to Kaori's e-mail address. They exchange simple messages every day, such as 'he has got a temperature today' or 'it dropped now'. For Kaori, this was the only way to know about her father's condition. She thus seems to bear out Baldassar's view that the advantage of contemporary technologies appears to bring heightened levels of obligation in their transnational care-giving practices (2007a: 294).

Kaori and her husband met and married in Tokyo, and migrated to Northern Ireland in 1991. Their three children are now teenagers. Like other mothers of school-age children, her life is filled with responsibilities towards her husband and children. For example, she has to give her children daily lifts to school and after-school activities. She also works as a part-time Japanese teacher in local schools. She also has

a sense of responsibility towards her parents-in-law who live nearby, who have helped her to establish her life in Northern Ireland. Since her oldest sister-in-law died, she has played the main role in family gatherings, hosting Christmas dinner and Sunday lunch:

> I cook Christmas dinner for everybody. My husband's aunt, uncle and the children of his older sister who died, all of them come together in my house. They wouldn't gather unless I played a role like their mother. This makes it all the more difficult for me to leave here.

Her worries about her parents and sense of guilt coexist with her feelings of obligation towards her family (husband and children) and in-laws in Ireland. Struggling with conflicting loyalties, it seems that she has tried to suppress a strong sense of guilt towards her parents, and to orient her feelings through the fulfilment of roles as a wife, a mother, and a daughter-in-law:

> In my case, it seems that my sense of obligation, responsibility and guilt are being dealt with by doing things like inviting my parents-in-law for dinner and chatting with them. They don't need any nursing care yet. They are in their early eighties. My mother-in-law had a heart bypass operation 13 years ago, and she is not so well. My father-in-law is fine. They live in Bangor. Every Sunday, I ask them to come for Sunday lunch. Because he likes driving and she likes to get out of the house . . .

Hochschild (1983) noted that suppressing one's feelings over an extended period can lead to feelings of alienation, self-estrangement and emotional exhaustion. Kaori's 'emotional stamina' was strained and this caused her to suffer from depression. She could not orient her feelings towards life in Northern Ireland any more, and her incompatible roles as a mother and daughter led to emotional disorientation:

> I'm physically very fine. So, I always thought I would be all right. But I started suffering from depression, I became very unstable . . . That's why I kept away from friends and the Japan Society . . . I hated myself, I felt I couldn't forgive myself . . . and became depressed . . . After I got tablets, I became OK . . . I can talk about this with a smile now, but at that time I would have refused to meet you as soon as I saw your notes . . . It was about a year ago . . . about a year after my father went into hospital. I couldn't accept that I couldn't be in two places at the same time. It was tough at that time . . . although my pain is nothing compared to my mother's. I knew my mother would have kept herself going, tried not to complain, not showing her pain even to me on the phone . . . It was very painful . . .

The image of her mother who is always 'positive' and 'tries not to complain' reflects on the image of Kaori herself who mainly presents relational and role-oriented selfhood. Her mother may have been one of her salient 'rule reminders', navigating her 'fulfilled' feelings regarding care for her new family members in Ireland. But, at the same time, 'emotional contagion' or 'convergence' could have occurred in

the transnational mother–daughter relationship. In this case, she might have 'caught' her mother's distress as well. She talked about the journey home from Japan last year:

> I hated the airport. My mother came to see me off. My feeling was getting oriented toward my family here, wondering how are they, they must be waiting for me, etc . . . But at the same time I imagined my mother's feeling . . . after my plane took off, she would be left alone in the airport, going back to her house on her own . . .

Svašek and Skrbiš indicate that 'migrants are prone to experience emotional destabilization as their emotional dispositions, learned "back home," may not be acceptable in their new locations' (2007: 374). In Kaori's case, conflicting expectations and concerns bring emotions tearing apart between families 'here' and 'there'. She said that she couldn't go to Japan this year, because her son was taking his GCSE exams: 'Well, I know I couldn't do much even if I was there. It's very heavy . . .' Her voice was monotonous, but her strong distress communicated itself to me. At the end of the interview, she also commented on positive aspects of her mother's life. Through bringing the image of her mother as a happy person, it seemed that she tried to 'feel up' temporarily and to reassure herself that her life is here and her mother's there:

> My mother says it's her job to be healthy. She grows vegetables in the garden and cares about what she eats . . . She also plays table tennis with young people in a club. They are very good to her. They often give her a ring or an e-mail. That's why when I asked my mother to come to live in Ireland, she always said she couldn't because of her friends. Her neighbours are also good to her. In this sense, I feel she is blessed.

Conclusion

This paper focused on the emotional processes of Japanese migrant mothers in the contexts of intermarriage and transnational family relationships. As Hiroko's first narrative showed, mothering and motherhood require a good deal of emotion work in which migrants must create a sense of belonging in a new place. One of the efficient techniques of her emotion work was a cognitive process: constructing images of idealised family life in Ireland and problematic Japanese life. Her future perspective was also re-evaluated through the process of emotion work. Her second narrative of Catholicism in Ireland described how emotional attachment/detachment is related to the achievement/failure of emotional management. Her emotional detachment from local Irish people other than her husband shaped her 'emotional dissonance', while emotional attachments with other Japanese migrant women contributed to losing her negative feelings towards Catholicism. Finally, Kaori's narrative described how transnational family relationships can shape inconsistent 'emotion cultures' and the complexity of 'emotional contagion'. In conflicting loyalties towards family in

Northern Ireland and ageing parents in Japan, her 'emotional stamina' was strained, although her emotion work was continued painfully.

The narratives of Japanese migrant mothers show how migrants' perceptions of 'home' are shaped and reshaped through their temporal and hierarchical constructions of the self and emotional orientations.[5] Through changing social roles, obligations and expectations, they participate in different 'feeling rules' to frame the lived experiences in which their relationships with the new country and the home place are renewed. Through changing their life courses, they also experience 'emotional resonance' or 'dissonance' with others, which affects their sense of belonging/non-belonging in different places. Motherhood, in this paper, provided the examples of such dynamics of multiple, interdependent processes in which subjectivities and feelings emerge.

Acknowledgements

I am grateful to the research participants for generously sharing their life experiences with me. I also thank Maruška Svašek for her encouragement and comments during the research and writing process, and the anonymous referees for their useful feedback on an earlier version of this article.

Notes

[1] All personal names and places used in this paper are fictitious.

[2] In the studies on emotions, many scholars have asked methodological questions regarding the complicated relationships between the expression and the experience of emotions.

[3] For the significance of reflexive and empathetic approaches, see Ryan (2008); Theodosius (2006); Throop (2003: 126–7).

[4] Based on information given by Japanese Embassies in the UK and the Republic of Ireland.

[5] In a constructivist model of mind, Hollan (2000) argues that subjectivities are actively constructed through intrapersonal processes of memory and symbol formation, and interpersonal, self–other configurations as organised and shaped through familial, social, historical processes. Accordingly, 'the self' is organised hierarchically, dynamically and temporally (2000: 539).

References

Anderson, C. and Keltner, D. (2004) 'The emotional convergence hypothesis: implications for individuals, relationships, and culture', in Tiedens, L.Z. and Leach, C.W. (eds) *The Social Life of Emotions*. Cambridge University Press, 144–63.

Baldassar, L.R. (2007a) 'Transnational families and aged care: the mobility of care and the migrancy of ageing', *Journal of Ethnic and Migration Studies*, *33*(2): 275–97.

Baldassar, L.R. (2007b) 'Transnational families and the provision of moral and emotional support: the relationship between truth and distance', *Identities: Global Studies in Culture and Power*, *14*(4): 385–409.

Breger, R. and Hill, R. (eds) (1998) *Cross-Cultural Marriages*. Oxford: Berg.

Conradson, D. and McKay, D. (2007) 'Translocal subjectivities: mobility, connection, emotion', *Mobilities*, *2*(2): 167–74.

Davies, A.C. (1999) *Reflexive Ethnography: A Guide to Researching Selves and Others.* London: Routledge.

Driessen, H. (1992) 'Introduction: trends, genres and cases in self-revelation', *Focaal*, *32*: 7–13.

Erickson, R.J. (1993) 'Reconceptualizing family work: the effect of emotion work on perceptions of marital quality', *Journal of Marriage and the Family*, *55*(4): 888–900.

Gardner, K. (2002) *Age, Narrative and Migration: The Life Course and Life Histories of Bengali Elders in London.* Oxford: Berg.

Hatfield, E. and Rapson, R.L. (2004) 'Emotional contagion: religious and ethnic hatreds and global terrorism', in Tiedens, L.Z. and Leach, C.W. (eds) *The Social Life of Emotions.* Cambridge: Cambridge University Press, 129–43.

Hermans, H.J.M. and Dimaggio, G. (2007) 'Self, identity, and globalization in times of uncertainty: a dialogical analysis', *Review of General Psychology*, *11*(1): 31–61.

Hochschild, A.R. (1979) 'Emotion work, feeling rules, and social structure', *American Journal of Sociology*, *85*(3): 551–75.

Hochschild, A.R. (1983) *The Managed Heart. Commercialization of Human Feeling.* Berkeley: University of California Press.

Hollan, D. (2000) 'Constructivist models of mind, contemporary psychoanalysis, and the development of culture theory', *American Anthropologist*, *102*(3): 538–50.

Leavitt, J. (1996) 'Meaning and feeling in the anthropology of emotions', *American Ethnologist*, *23*(3): 524–39.

Rapport, N. and Dawson, A. (eds) (1998) *Migrants of Identity: Perceptions of Home in a World of Movement.* Oxford: Berg.

Peacock, J.L. and Holland, D.C. (1993) 'The narrated self: life stories in process', *Ethos*, *21*(4): 367–83.

Ryan, L. (2008) 'Navigating the emotional terrain of families "here" and "there": women, migration and motherhood', *Journal of Intercultural Studies*, *29*(3): 299–313.

Svašek, M. (2005) 'Introduction', in Milton, K. and Svašek, M. (eds) *Mixed Emotions: Anthropological Studies of Feeling.* Oxford: Berg, 1–23.

Svašek, M. (2008) 'Who cares? Families and feelings in movement', *Journal of Intercultural Studies*, *29*(3): 213–30.

Svašek, M. and Skrbiš, Z. (2007) 'Passions and powers: emotions and globalisation', *Identities: Global Studies in Culture and Power*, *14*(4): 367–83.

Theodosius, C. (2006) 'Recovering emotion from emotion management', *Sociology*, *40*(5): 893–910.

Throop, C.J. (2003) 'On crafting a cultural mind: a comparative assessment of some recent theories of "internalization" in psychological anthropology', *Transcultural Psychiatry*, *40*(1): 109–39.

The Hindi Film's Romance and Tibetan Notions of Harmony: Emotional Attachments and Personal Identity in the Tibetan Diaspora in India

Timm Lau

In this article, Tibetans in the diaspora in India are shown to be engaged in emotional processes that connect very different themes of their lives. Their attachment to both Tibetan moral notions and Indian popular cultural representations is theorised with reference to emotional attachment as appropriation into the sense of what belongs with oneself. Both normative Tibetan moral notions and aspirational Indian popular-cultural representations are appropriated by Tibetans born and raised in India. On the one hand, Tibetan moral notions of harmonious relationships present generally salient norms for Tibetans, and are connected to polyandry and idealised representations of Tibet in older people's discourse. On the other hand, Indian popular film and television are ubiquitous in Tibetan everyday life. The ethnography presented demonstrates that Indian popular culture has helped to shape Tibetan diasporic aesthetics and historicity and provides an idiom for ideas and practices of love, romance and marriage for younger Tibetans in India.

In the anthropological literature on peoples in diaspora, attachment to the region or country of origin often takes a central place (e.g. Glick Schiller and Fouron 1999; Jing 1996; Kirsch 2001; Malkki 1995). This is reflected in the literature on Tibetans in exile: Tibet as a remote, lost 'homeland' has generally been attributed with continuing symbolic significance (Anand 2000; Diemberger 2002; Forbes 1989; Kolås 1996; Korom 1997; Nowak 1984; Ström 1994, 1997; von Fürer-Haimendorf 1990). Some

existing studies pay attention to questions of Tibetan adaptation, raising the issue of assimilation into the host country (see Grunfeld 1987: 202; Saklani 1984). However, they do so without presenting ethnographic descriptions of Indo-Tibetan relationships and the consequences for the Tibetan diaspora. The predominant tendency to focus on exclusively Tibetan social and cultural practices has served instead to minimise or obscure the importance of the Indian social environment for the Tibetans living there. In reality, social interaction across the lines of diasporic community and host society is common in India, as well as highly significant for the understanding Tibetans have developed of their own position in the Indian context.

In this paper I will demonstrate that Tibetans in India have appropriated notions and practices from both Tibetan and Indian cultural realms, and that the processes underlying these different appropriations can be conceptualised as emotional attachment. In this context, I will introduce emotional attachment as emotive appropriation into the subjective experience of what belongs with oneself. Both the moral notions of harmony discursively connected to an idealised notion of Tibet, and aesthetics and aspirations shaped through interaction with Indian popular culture represent such emotional attachments to Tibetans in India. My ethnography[1] shows that young Tibetans have appropriated elements from both of these seemingly disparate 'Tibetan' and 'Indian' realms. Both have been made 'their own' by them, and give them a sense of what belongs into their lives.

This article adds to the small but growing number of studies that explicitly integrate the study of emotions and globalisation (see Svašek and Skrbiš 2007). First, since having migrated in the last fifty years, Tibetans in India share the predicaments of diaspora with other mobile populations. Secondly, through Bollywood films shown on Indian television, they are engaging with popular-cultural representations associated with processes of globalisation. I will demonstrate below that Hindi film representations are appropriated by young Tibetans in India and provide an idiom for their ideal of love-marriage. The presence and negotiation of this romantic ideal also finds resonance in social changes within other societies, in which long-established marital practices are being contested (e.g. Larkin 1997; Mody Spencer 2000).

Emotions in Valuing Elements of the Social Environment

Generally speaking, the continuum of elements in our social environment is open in terms of attracting sustained interest and emotional engagement, while the construction of identity may be tightly circumscribed by notions of purity (cf. Malkki 1995). Therefore, it can be difficult for migrants to reconcile their social reality with the demands engendered by such notions. This is true especially where the co-presence of elements from different backgrounds causes anxiety, fear, or other antagonistic emotions (Lau 2009). Most younger Tibetans in the refugee settlements in Northern India in which I did fieldwork strongly identified with the goals of Tibetan cultural preservation, yet often said to me that a gulf existed between them

and their parents and grandparents. Actively reflecting on their own life in India, young informants often told me about their tastes and interests: their favourite music and films were mostly Indian (although some young men preferred American Hip Hop); their favourite clothes were those on display in modern Indian films; some young men told me that Indian women were the most beautiful; and, finally, they stressed that the food they ate was more often than not Indian, in spite of widespread discourse about the kinds of food eaten in Tibet. They spoke Hindi fluently and even preferred it on certain limited occasions such as joking, drinking and gambling, when it perhaps added to the subversive character of these activities. Some of my informants captured their sense of mixture and impurity by cogently referring to themselves as 'a *remix* of Tibetan, Indian and Western', using terminology borrowed from the Indian popular music with which they are so familiar.

Such circumstances can lead to a marked sense of ambivalence in young diasporic Tibetans, who may struggle to integrate the co-presence of both Tibetan and Indian elements in their lives. And yet, the fact that such mixing of elements happens brings home the point that the social environment engaged by Tibetans in India is in an important sense a *continuum* of elements, regardless of their label as 'Indian' or 'Tibetan' in the diaspora. In their social reality, Tibetans in India turn their attention to those elements which are most interesting or meaningful to them. To conceptualise this ascription of meaning or value in terms of emotions, let us first turn to a discussion of Kay Milton's recent work.

In her *Loving Nature*, Milton discusses the importance of emotions for the way in which people engage with and come to value specific elements in the environment. On a very general level, Milton asserts that 'all encounters with the external world involve emotion ... they must do so if we are to learn from such encounters' (2002: 86). She argues that emotions help us to learn about the environment, as well as about how to feel about the environment. The former aspect relates to the human capacity of direct learning through perception. Citing psychological approaches to perception, Milton maintains that emotions are central to this process as they guide our attention and interest, which are themselves both preceded and followed by perception. In discussing how emotions help us to learn how to *feel* about the environment, Milton refers to emotions in their social contexts as well as their social construction. Here, her argument is less extensive, essentially reiterating that we learn how to feel about specific elements of our environment by example, very prominently in childhood through parents or other influential figures.

Milton then emphasises emotions and their relation to personal identity to describe how individuals come to give value to specific elements of their social environment:

> What each individual comes to value most will depend on the context in which they learn about the world, the kinds of personal experiences they have, the ways in which they engage with their fellow human beings and with their non-human surroundings. The process of living, and learning to live, in particular contexts provides each individual with the *reference points for defining their own personal*

> *identity* ... The things that matter most to people are, self-evidently, the things that make their life most meaningful ... these are also, and inevitably, *the things that induce the strongest emotions and feelings* (2002: 108–9, emphasis added).

In sum, Milton's work establishes that emotions are central to both our learning about the world and our giving value to certain elements within it. She argues that, in doing so, emotions are crucially important for our personal identity. In Milton's words, this explains the 'fundamentally emotional character of all personal commitments' (2002: 109).

Emotional Attachment as Personal Appropriation

Kay Milton's approach to emotions helps us to understand their importance in the attribution of value to elements of the social environment. She explicitly highlights that emotions are central to our personal identity, and that this is why our personal commitments are fundamentally emotional in nature. However, this insightful line of her argument can be pushed further, through a closer examination of our relationship with the elements to which we experience such personal commitment. We also describe this relationship as having become emotionally attached. A now antiquated meaning of the word *attachment* carries significant insight into this type of relationship between self and environment. According to the Oxford English Dictionary, from the late sixteenth century onwards, 'attachment' had the meaning of 'taking of property into possession' (1971: 136). The act of 'taking into possession' can in other words be described as making something one's own. Following this meaning, we can describe emotional attachment as *the emotive appropriation of a thing, person, concept, or context into the subjective experience of what belongs with oneself.* This way of conceptualising emotional attachment importantly brings a sense of belonging ('with' or 'to') into relief, as well as a sense of self and identity. In a two-way process, emotional attachments tell us about our experience both of *what belongs* with us, and of *where we belong.* I will show that analysing emotional attachment as personal appropriation is fruitful for understanding young Tibetans' ambivalent senses of belonging in the diaspora in India.

Existing studies suggest that the value attached by Tibetans to elements of their diasporic social environment is often determined by the perceived Tibetanness of these elements. This is explained by the emphasis placed on cultural preservation by Tibetans in India generally, and the Dalai Lama's administration in particular. The often discussed central symbolic function and power of the Dalai Lama is perhaps the most predominant example of this dynamic (see e.g. Forbes 1989; Houston and Wright 2003; Michael 1985; Subba 1988: 54; 1990: 115; von Fürer-Haimendorf 1990). The Dalai Lama himself embodies the qualities associated with being Tibetan, as well as the hope of return to Tibet, for most Tibetans in the diaspora. An openly expressed and explicitly emotional commitment to the Dalai Lama is thus a very common feature among Tibetans in India. Other elements of Tibetan lives in the diaspora are also highly valued according to their perceived connection to 'Tibetan culture', e.g.

Tibetan Buddhist adepts, institutions and practices; Tibetan food and clothes; and the celebrations and demonstrations on 'Uprising Day' every 10 March. In the anthropological literature, these elements have often been analysed in terms of their symbolic value to Tibetans in relation to cultural preservation and political struggle (e.g. Klieger 2002; Kolås 1996; Nowak 1984). Following Milton, we may say that emotions help Tibetans in India to place these elements within their own lives. *Qua* emotional attachment, this placement entails a direct appropriation into the social self and enables its Tibetanness. Emotional attachment to symbols and practices therefore provides the crucial link between Tibetan cultural elements and personal identity. The emotional nature of this link is all the more significant for my following discussion of Tibetan notions of harmony, since they are essentially *emotional* concepts.

But emotions are also central in the development of interest in social elements not so closely connected to Tibetan culture. I will present ethnographic evidence for the assertion that the determination of value along the lines of Tibetan cultural identity is far from absolute. As briefly mentioned above, young Tibetans may refer to Indian influences when describing everyday preferences. The immense popularity of Indian television is crucial for the development of these tastes and interests. I will demonstrate Indian television's importance for Tibetan diasporic knowledge and historicity in detail below, as well as discussing another crucial aspect of Indian film in the context of emotions and value: its essentially melodramatic character, which means that it appeals to its audience by dealing with aspects of social change in *emotional* terms. Indian social and cultural elements, then, also give meaning to Tibetans in India. They may become reference points for Tibetan personalities in the diaspora, to paraphrase Milton, because they have been emotionally made their own by Tibetans in India.

This closeness of a sense of possession on the one hand and personal identity on the other, is reflected in Alfred Gell's notion of consumption as the incorporation of consumer goods into the definition of the social self (1986). In the local contexts of Tibetan diaspora, consumption of Indian goods as well as Indian cultural representations through television is ever-present. Gell observed consumption as an active and creative enterprise where it concerns the incorporation of new imaginations of oneself in the process. His argument is all the more pertinent for the consumption of images and representations, since they work directly on the imagination and extend the constant challenge of being invited to imagine oneself in connection to what is seen. Therefore, I will analyse Tibetan consumption of Indian popular culture in terms of incorporation into the social self, and specifically in terms of emotional attachment as personal appropriation.

In the following, I will first draw out Tibetan notions of harmony from discourse about familial relationships. I will demonstrate that the Tibetan concept of *'cham po* (literally, 'friendly'), and the notion of harmony inherent in it, are salient social norms for Tibetans. In local discourse, polyandry is represented as centrally based on *'cham po* relationships, and as the ultimate form of marriage. Tibet is thought of as

the locus of continuous polyandrous marriage and therefore of unabated harmonious relationships. My older informants' emotional conviction towards *'cham po* ways of being thus ties into an emotional attachment to Tibet as a mythologised 'homeland'. As I will show, normative notions of familial harmony are also salient for younger Tibetans in India. However, they are co-present with other influences born of the diasporic context. I will discuss the aesthetic and aspirational impact of Hindi film and Indian television programmes on younger Tibetans in India. A moral-aesthetic understanding influenced by these media has become part of the taken-for-granted, everyday knowledge of Tibetans in India, and of their historicity as a social group in the diaspora. Furthermore, Hindi films provide highly significant aspirations and idioms for romance and marriage, which are appropriated by younger Tibetans in the diaspora. The latter aspirations, then, are co-present with Tibetan moral notions such as *'cham po*. I will argue that the value and meaning younger Tibetans ascribe to both are crucially related to an appropriation, through emotional attachment, into a sense of personal identity.

The Importance of Familial Harmony

To be friendly and not to hurt others or their feelings was generally valued very highly by my Tibetan informants and listed as one of the essential qualities of a 'good person'. There is, of course, a religious underpinning of this, as it is not only sin (*sdig pa*) in Tibetan Buddhist representations to hurt physically or to kill, but also to hurt emotionally. Thus, *'cham po* and *'cham po byed* (harmonious action) stand at the very base of the moral and ethical and in contrast to negative emotional states. Naturally, my informants were also aware that conflict and disharmony may lead to violence. But even more immediate than this, conflictual relationships and disharmony are understood to attract misfortune. Discord amongst relatives is considered especially bad as it is thought to bring 'bad luck' into the family. The misfortune thus incurred could become evident in economic terms, or in terms of disarray and even illness in the family. Sometimes, I was told that such misfortunes were caused by disharmony and conflict because they were displeasing to the Three Precious Jewels of Buddha, Dharma and Sangha (*dkon mchog gsum*). The concept of *dkon mchog gsum* was commonly used in a way analogous to the English-language concept of 'God' or 'the gods', for example when I was told that '*dkon mchog gsum* are always watching us'. The gods, then, are pleased by harmony and loving relationships, and, as it were, displeased by disharmony and conflict. The consequences of each were seen as the rewards for one's own attitude and behaviour, the latter two really being aspects of the mind (*sems*), whose all-important role was stressed to me very often: it was explained to be of prime importance to have a 'sharp' (*sems sangs po*) and 'good mind' (*sems yag po*). This reaction to harmony or disharmony by the divine realm and the consequential effects, benign or otherwise, in the realm of humanity, were clearly represented both in daily discourse and in more explicit and didactic explanations of matters to me. The consequences of familial harmony/disharmony

were also related as closely connected to protection through divine agents or principles in local popular religious understandings. The fact that familial disharmony incurs problems because it displeases the gods was as self-evident for my informants as the fact that we need their protection. Acting in harmonious ways within the family is, for Tibetans in India, an obvious prerequisite of divine protection for the household.

Additionally, conflict and disharmony in the domestic realm are thought of as causing neighbourly gossip and bringing the household into disrepute, something of which my Tibetan informants were extremely wary at all times. Thus, they are keen to avoid conflict within the household, and within the circle of relatives more generally. This contributed to the expectation of solidarity between kin: Tibetans expect relationships between relatives (*spun kyag*) to be more likely to be *'cham po*. Avoiding conflict and *'cham po byed* are indeed thought of as the moral default position, and thus represent a social norm for behaviour. They are also understood to be at the base of the social relationships that are the most intimate and sustaining for the community: *'cham po* is highly significant in everyday discourse about marital relations, and particularly salient in discourse about polyandry.

Harmony and Marriage

In the settlements where I did fieldwork, prospective marriage partners for one's children are best sought from families with whom one has a long-standing and *'cham po* relationship; the married couple is thought to carry on such a harmonious relationship in their marriage. Ideally, relationships forged in marriage are an extension of, or at least positively imprinted by, *'cham po* relationships between the families and individuals involved. But marriage holds ambivalent aspects for Tibetans, who say that disharmonious marital unions could disintegrate easily. Elder Tibetan informants perceived bringing a person from the 'outside' into the family through marriage as carrying the potential for disruption. This corresponds to Nancy Levine's description of Tibetans in general as assuming more cooperation between kin than between kin and outsiders. She describes a 'low valuation of marriage and distrust in in-laws' for Tibetans in Purang, and writes that 'in-marrying daughters-in-law were regarded as outsiders and distrusted' (1994: 476). For the Tibetan Nyinba in Nepal, 'kinship is seen as providing the most reliable basis for trust, and this notion has effects on the patterning of interpersonal relations in households and in marriages' (Levine 1988: 278). My Tibetan informants also shared the widespread notion that in-laws did not always get on, and that there was thus a significant risk in acquiring them. While the Nyinba use the ideal of kinship-based trust to explain their practice of cross-cousin marriage, strict exogamous marriage rules in my fieldsite marked that type of union as highly incestuous. These rules pertain to marriage between people within the same clan (signified by *rus*, 'bone') and those with common kin as distant as seven or more generations back, and make for a different context of possible marriage arrangements from that of the Nyinba. Yet, as we shall

see shortly, my informants would certainly agree with the statements about polyandry's advantages which Levine derived from Nyinba cultural representations. She writes that siblings 'are thought to have less trouble as co-spouses' and that 'the kin relationship mitigates rivalries and lessens hardships' for siblings involved in marriage (1988: 149).

Polyandry and Harmony

In terms of Tibetan kinship bonds, the bond between brothers is especially culturally elaborated. Harmony between siblings was often described to me as *spun kyag brtse ba*, in literal translation 'love between relatives'. However, this was often translated to me as 'brotherly love' or 'real brotherhood'. This betrays the tendency to think of the kinship bond between brothers as the most salient type: solidarity between brothers was often stressed in explicit expectations or reports of sibling solidarity. Elder brothers are expected to 'look after' their younger siblings, in the sense that the latter's interests are ideally equated by the elder brother to his own (see also Levine 1988: 120–1). Fraternal solidarity, then, is a core value pertaining to Tibetan kinship ties (e.g. Levine 1988: 84, 159; 1994: 470). This is reflected in the Tibetan marital practice of fraternal polyandry: as Levine puts it, fraternal solidarity is accompanied by 'a deep sense of obligation to brothers in polyandry' for Tibetans (1988: 9).

My informants often connected the solidarity of brothers to polyandry. Indeed, polyandrous marriage (*bza 'gsum*) was held up as the ideal form of marriage by elder Tibetans. They understood polyandry to create a very harmonious unit, as the brothers' kinship bond is combined with the marriage bond they are jointly forming with their wife. Harmony was inevitably at the centre of the description of the relationship, as the distinctive feature of polyandry. As one informant put it, 'the meaning of polyandry is to make [the relationship] very friendly (*'cham po*)'; another told me that 'the biggest advantage [of polyandry] is this: that relatives want to give good harmony to one another.' The concept of polyandry (*bza 'gsum*) is very clearly related to the central notion of friendliness and harmony (*'cham po*), which implies being close to one another, and being friendly and loving.

My informants also raised economic factors in their discussions of polyandry. It was said to enable the household to deal with economic difficulties with more ease, as more than one husband is present to earn income. Furthermore, one husband would be able to stay at home and take care of the household, e.g. in case a member of the family fell ill at home, while the other(s) would go outside of the settlement 'for business'—which in the Tibetan diaspora in India mostly means itinerant trade in sweaters (cf. Lau 2007). This mirrors the economic element of Melvyn Goldstein's analysis of Tibetan polyandry, in which it appears as maximising economic utility and thus ensuring a better standard of life. However, Goldstein holds that Tibetans characterise polyandry as problematic, and 'more as the lesser of two evils than as the prized form of marriage' (1976: 233; also 1978: 328). His approach to polyandry is based on his Tibetan informants' own assessment, and my informants also offered the

kind of practical explanation Goldstein calls 'highly materialistic' (1976: 224) for their preference of polyandry. Yet, in their descriptions *'cham po* took centre stage and polyandry clearly appeared as a 'prized form of marriage' which older Tibetans aspired to for their own children. Thus, my ethnography suggests that some older Tibetans in India are in favour of polyandry for similar reasons to those noted by Levine (1988) and Levine and Silk (1997), who stress polyandry as a historically developed marriage-system embedded in cultural values, and integrated in political and kinship structures. However, in addition to the moral and cultural values connected to *'cham po*, the concept of *bza' gsum* elicited a rich description of an idealised Tibet, as well as a sense of contrast to the present in India.

Polyandry and Idealised Notions of Tibet

The often expressed conviction that 'in Tibet, all brothers marry one wife' connects the locally important representations of fraternal solidarity and *'cham po* with Tibet. The following excerpts from an interview with a Tibetan woman in her fifties, herself married to two brothers, present these elements very clearly:

> To stay in polyandry is very difficult. It is very good and very difficult. It is like a diamond. We don't get diamonds easily, right. In Tibet it is very good, in Tibet it is going on. But that didn't come here. Yes, it is difficult to come by. These days, it is very difficult to be good. But it is easy to be bad and mixed up. To get good things, to get work is very difficult. It's like that [now]. In Tibet, it is very good, brothers all agree with each other, are together.

In these statements, there prominently appears the feature of a mythical, idealised notion of an unchanged Tibet, which is generally salient in local discourse about polyandry. This notion of Tibet is contrasted to the present in India and younger Tibetans living there:

> *Q: Why won't [your children] stay in polyandry?*
> They are looking to the foreign countries; it's just because they are looking. Before, when we were in Tibet, we didn't have anywhere to look, to foreign countries. We have freedom at that time, and that's why we are independent, we don't have to look at anyone. Then we were all very close... When we got to India, then we saw different things. Then people take different outlooks. And they don't take better outlooks, they take the worse. So, like that, it doesn't happen [polyandry is not practised].

Here, my informant stresses that the Tibetan children's outlook changed because they were 'looking' to 'foreign countries', and that attitudes changed 'just by looking'. The emphasis on looking will become centrally important in the following sections on the influence of Indian film and television. The outlooks resulting from the influences of the diaspora, the un-free and post-independent state of Tibetans in India,[2] are characterised as 'worse', and as the reason for the demise of polyandry:

> ... times have changed, for the worse. People think they can't be together, they are afraid of each other, that's why they don't want to stay together (in polyandry). It is considered to be bad. Before in Tibet, all stayed together... In Tibet, all are like that. It is good in Tibet, the bad times haven't come in Tibet. No one is like that, and you don't have doubt in your mind. Being *'cham po*, being put together (in arranged polyandry), they don't think that something bad will happen. ... Since we came here, it's all bad times, bad people, everything got bad. This country and foreign countries will not keep this (good thing), they will all look after that (other thing), and that's why I said polyandry is difficult. That's why it's difficult to put (young people) into polyandry. It is easy in Tibet. Our country was like that from the beginning. Everything is good. There is nothing bad.

The predominantly negative evaluation of present circumstances in India is explained in the temporal terms of living in 'the bad times'. This relates to the Buddhist cosmological notion that the present age or *kalpa* is one of moral decline. My informants' evaluation of time does not conform to the Buddhist scriptural knowledge of cyclical cosmological time, where a Buddhist *kalpa* can be 15,998,000 years long (Sadakata 1997: 96–7). The multitude of named *kalpas* and aeons stretch across massive periods of time, rather than the span of two generations or so which my informants are evaluating. Yet, it is important to note that their notions of moral decline, which are instantiated by the decline in polyandrous marriages and by the change in attitude among younger Tibetans toward family and marriage, are connected to Buddhist cosmology, adapted by my informants to talk about their present circumstances. By contrast, Tibet as a place is connected to and fused with the superior moral conditions of earlier times—its essential quality of 'goodness' is de-temporalised in discourse. Polyandry clearly belongs in this context: it is described as quintessentially good, and emphasised as rare in the present in India (precisely because of its goodness). In this context, the 'good practice' of polyandry is also explicitly perceived as *Tibetan* practice. Most of my informants hold the notion that Tibetans have practised polyandry in the past and do so continuously in Tibet, and that times have changed in India and elsewhere. The concept of polyandry is thus firmly *located* in a mythical Tibet, the process encompassing both time and space.

My informant's discourse on polyandry and the importance of *'cham po* and 'staying together' illustrates understandings that are widespread among older Tibetan refugees. The majority of young Tibetans, however, do not share their elders' enthusiasm for polyandry, and aspire towards love-marriage. They are at times confronted by the kind of discourse which is damning of their new, and 'worse', perspective on marriage, and call this type of discourse (and those who dispense it) '*orthodox*' (from English) or 'hard' (*mkhregs po*) amongst themselves. But they usually do not argue openly with their elders. On the one hand, young Tibetans share the positive notion of *'cham po* as a moral default position. Emotional commitment to *'cham po* ways of being is equally present and important for them; and although they may question some of their parents' other concepts, many do not disagree with the conception that harmony is important because disharmony can cause misfortune. On the other hand, their own muted behaviour in such situations avoids transgression of

the moral default of *'cham po* which would result from open conflict, as well as the shame such a transgression would entail. Yet, it is generally understood that the 'silent majority' of young Tibetans cannot be kept from pursuing their romantic interests. The next section will illustrate that Indian television and its popular cultural representations have been important influences for Tibetan diasporic historicity, and the ideas and practices of romance and marriage among young Tibetans in India.

Indian Television and Tibetan Diasporic Aesthetics and Historicity

Hindi film, television and popular music are ubiquitous and well-loved in the Tibetan diaspora in India. The television sets in Tibetan houses are nearly constantly showing Hindi films: colourful, impassioned, violent and romantic spectacles. The TV sets are rarely turned off; if this seems to be the case, it is more likely than not the temporary outcome of a power failure (see also Abu-Lughod 1995: 202). Since the economic opening of India's markets in the 1990s, up to two dozen cable TV channels are beamed into Tibetan households. These images often represent for my informants what, for want of a better term, we may describe along with them as 'modernity'. This is very often a specific Indian modernity transported through images and objects in tandem, such as advertisement for and presence of the same consumer goods (from shampoo to motorcycles), and the representations of modern India inherent in recent Hindi cinema. The Tibetan viewers of Indian television are of course not passive, but choose, deconstruct and reconstruct elements of their consumption (cf. Abu-Lughod 1995; Das 1995).

To provide a conceptualisation of Tibetans' consumption of Indian popular cultural images, I turn to Alfred Gell's description of consumption as 'the appropriation of objects as part of one's *personalia*' (1986: 112). Ingeniously, Gell portrayed the 'incorporation of consumer goods into the definition of the social self' as a process that may display boldness and vitality in taking on new objects of consumption, involving a 'leap of the imagination' (1986: 115). Indian television has had a highly significant and continuing impact on Tibetan socio-history in Indian settlements, involving new imaginations of themselves for Tibetans. This is clearly reflected in the following interview with another Tibetan woman, taken together with my Tibetan research assistant (KT):

> I was ten [when I saw my first movie]. Yes. *Parwarish* [title of the 1977 film]. I went to see it in Palampur. We... there is the monastery, right ... the Nyingma monastery, we were carpet weaving there. During a party, we went for a movie, on a tractor. (laughs) That makes me laugh. We were really like villagers (*gaon gaon*) back then, Lord Buddha! (laughs) The police caught us. So many people are not allowed to go on a tractor! We went inside to see the movie, and the police caught the driver. We came back from the movie, and the driver had given money to the police so they let us go. We didn't know the law. Even the adults didn't know. We asked them to take us, so they took us on the tractor. ... [To KT:] Our story is more funny than yours! We were really like villagers. It was really funny, Lord Buddha.

Q: How is the difference between now and then?
I don't know. But the channels on TV at home make a huge difference. Times have changed, now. Earlier, our perspective (*lta ba*) was like in Tibet. We stayed together with our grandparents, so our perspective was like in Tibet. To watch TV, we had to pay 25 *paise*, at the school. There was only one TV for all of the people then.

Q: You used not to have a TV at home. Now that you have a lot of channels it brought a lot of change ...
The TV channels, yes. Star TV and many others are there. Since they have come there is a lot of change. Before that, there was a little change. But not a lot of change like that.

(KT adds:) At that time we had no TV. We would go to the one family who had a TV to watch.

Q: Since all the TV channels have arrived, what are the changes?
The way to dress. And cleanliness. The cleanliness has become better. The clothes... and keeping the children clean. And then as they get older, just by watching TV some things get better and some things get worse.

Q: What got better?
The cleanliness has become better. The cleanliness has become better and that is the positive change.

Q: How is the cleanliness... like cleaning up, or ... ?
Yeah, like to clean up, and putting things into place (points around the living room). Like we saw it in the movies. We don't have any education, right? We know a few words of English, here and there.

Q: And other things?
Like, the way to talk to people. Not to shout, but to talk slowly. If you do bad things, bad will come to you. To think that. That it is good character to do better and better things, to think that this is good. To talk to elders, to think that it is good, like doing these things; whatever it is, it is a bit better now. To talk to people... like this, many small things. When we watch a film, we are not only watching the bad things—really, we don't have an education. If we watch bad things, it's not ok. If you have got a good education, you have good understanding about what to do and what not to do. We don't have that. We know a little bit from the TV.

Q: What has become worse?
What has become worse? How to say, like, one's own culture... it's like style, the children are put in fashion clothes by their parents; in reality, we should put them in Tibetan dress according to our culture. In the films, we see children wearing beautiful clothes, for the children; so we put those clothes onto our children. We lose our way of dressing. The children themselves don't think of this. We see something beautiful over there, see beautiful children, then we think I want to make my children beautiful like that. Parents might think and feel that way. Then Tibetan culture gets lost.

> *Q: What are other changes since TV has come?*
> For example, before when we were going on a tractor, and we were caught. This will not happen. . . the point of view (*lta ba*) comes from watching movies. What is beautiful (*snying rje mo*) and what is smart (*'dzig po*), we catch it there (*'jus ba*). That thinking has changed now. Before, we didn't know. We're going on a tractor, breaking the law.

My informant's reminiscing about being taken on the back of a tractor to watch a film provides a revealing characterisation of the Tibetans' way of life at her time as a child. She effectively describes them as backward, and significantly used the Hindi expression *gaon gaon* (literally, village village) to express this backwardness of the earlier Tibetan population of the settlement. In returning to this image of backward village people when explaining the changes that have come with the advent of television, she states that knowing 'what is beautiful and what is smart'—the perspective of a 'changed thinking'—'comes from watching movies'. The image of a bunch of villagers careening into town on the back of a tractor, and being 'fined' for it by police, provides the contrast of ignorance ruling during the time before television came: 'Before, we didn't know'.

It is important to take this evaluation of earlier times in context with other narratives, which were often characterised by tales of how 'rough' the early Tibetan refugees were. Immediately after fleeing Tibet, many early Tibetan refugees led an existence as extremely impoverished, homeless road labourers (see Kharat 2003: 288). Even for the time after settlements had been established, the appearance of early Tibetan refugees was often recounted to me as unkempt, ragged and violent. The heroic undercurrent of the fierce Tibetan warrior figure notwithstanding, these early Tibetan refugees that were 'a bit wild' now appear, in an important sense, as backward. I was, for example, told a story that Tibetans died soon after arrival because they had drunk large amounts of cheap Indian vegetable oil. The morale of these types of story about early Tibetan refugees was uniformly that they did *not know*: they did not know what to eat, how to live in India, or how to live peacefully with each other. It is important to note that Tibetans in India today make these judgments from a perspective that has already incorporated many aspects of their way of life as obvious knowledge, and as valued, taken-for-granted qualities such as (largely) non-violent behaviour. For Tibetans born and raised in India, the earliest Tibetan refugees have become something of an *other* that yet represents the earliest incarnation of *us* in India. As in the earlier interview excerpts on polyandry, recent diasporic changes are often conceptualised as changes in perspective (*lta ba*) which are dependent upon 'looking' (*lta*)—the major difference being that these changes were seen as negative in the former context.

Along with its difference in connotation, the second interview cited illustrates the emergence of a reflexive judgment about the recent Tibetan past in India. The main characteristics of the new perspective learned from television described here are elements such as fashion, cleanliness, arranging the domestic scene and ideas about 'what is beautiful and smart'. The general 'style' of the scenery alluded to by my

informant contains what we may call aesthetic elements, in the sense that they are concerned with cleanliness, order and beauty. Yet, they clearly appear as moral elements in her discussion. A point to consider here is that the interviewee's introduction of ethical elements alongside her statements about cleanliness and beauty demonstrates that she emphasises their *moral nature*: the things talked about have a moral element that is congruous with familiar ethical concerns, e.g. those expressed in 'If you do bad things, bad will come to you'. What is being 'learned' from television, then, is essentially of a *moral-aesthetic* nature. Importantly, this learning happens through emotions: the emotions of joy at beauty, for example, and of aspiration. The knowledge thus gained differentiates the early times of the settlement and the television-informed present. The overall message conveyed is that the aesthetic of Tibetan diasporic modernity, influenced by Indian television, is of moral importance and at the core of knowing how to act appropriately in the present. It represents the significantly emotional 'change in thinking' that defines the Tibetan diaspora in India now—and that at the same time represents the threat of losing authenticity: 'Parents might *think and feel* that way. Then Tibetan culture gets lost.' Moreover, the aesthetic and aspirational processes connected to the consumption of Indian television are important in Tibetans' historicity of themselves as a social group in the diaspora. This historicity, and the advent of television as an avenue of emotional learning within it, form part of the background to the reception of Hindi films by Tibetans in India.

Hindi Films: Contexts of Origination and Consumption

Analysts of consumerism in Europe and the United States have argued that commodity images provide a crucial idiom of public agency and expression for individuals and groups marginalised by mainstream forms of public discourse, the common factor being the way in which commodity images add a dimension of sensuous embodiment to an otherwise abstract ideal of citizenship—promising a 'reconciliation between embodiment and self-abstraction' (Warner 1992: 39; cf. Mazzarella 2003: 100). Another way of putting my argument in this section is to say that, if the romantic imagery and narratives of Indian popular culture can be read as kinds of 'commodity images', their consumption and related romantic practices represent forms of 'sensuous embodiment' to young Tibetans, who are themselves a marginal group in two ways: first, in relationship to India as a place they at the same time understand to be a foreign place and their home; and secondly, in their relationship to the abstraction of Tibetan identity which they (in their own perception) sometimes fail to embody completely. The fact that the commodity images that provide such embodiment to young Tibetans originate from the Indian social context from which they experience themselves as marginalised in other ways, reflects the ambiguity of the Tibetan diasporic experience in India.

In *All You Want Is Money, All You Need Is Love*, Rachel Dwyer argues that Hindi commercial cinema is the cultural expression of an emerging middle class in India

(2000). Dwyer's main achievement is to suggest that this new middle class's attitudes towards love, romance and kinship are reflected in the cinematic representations of Bollywood movies. She points at an association between the kind of romantic relationships portrayed in Hindi films and the shared desires and ambitions of their consumers. This is reflected in the film industry's output, breaking box office records with 'big-budget, plushy, romantic films, which ... mark the dominance of the values of the new middle classes as they find their audience across social categories' (2000: 100). However, Dwyer also suggests an important relationship between erotic romance in popular media and what she calls 'wider frameworks of kinship', especially parental control over arranged marriage, which do not comply with the implications of this imagery (2000: 50). She argues that Hindi films attempt to resolve the romantic import of love matches and eroticism with a perception of being rooted in Indian family values. Young Tibetans in India face a similar contradiction in their negotiation of romantic experience and social norms, and Hindi cinema presents them with a means to imaginatively explore possibilities of social change because it deals with a situation of perceived conflict between the 'old' and the 'new'.

Hindi cinema's often discussed emphasis on emotions has led most of its scholars to classify it as melodramatic (see e.g. Dwyer 2000; Mishra 2002; Nandy 1998; Thomas 1985, 1995; Vasudevan 1989). The consensus of the literature on melodramatic film is that it achieves the 'pleasure of being touched and giving way to tears' (cf. Neale 1986: 6). Following Ien Ang's work on soap opera (1985), Dwyer writes of melodramatic cinema that its emphasis on 'being true to emotions rather than any other aspect of life' motivates viewers to watch (Dwyer 2000: 107, 170). Stressing the relationship of these aspects to social tension, film theorist Christine Gledhill argues that the genre of melodrama indicates that social change is worked through in private contexts and emotional terms (1991: 208). Hindi cinema, then, may be seen as dealing in emotional terms with aspects of social change which the audience relate to in their own lives. Often, Hindi films were remarkable for Tibetan viewers because of their emotional effects. As one informant told me after a movie theatre visit with her friend: 'That film made me cry, and her too. We sat there like this [blinking as if fighting back tears] all the way through the end of the film!' What is really significant here is emotive power or emotional movement—often expressed to me as 'that film made me cry'.

There are striking similarities between Tibetans in India and Hausa in Nigeria described by Larkin (1997). In his ethnographic account of Hindi films' immense popularity in Nigeria, he contends that, through their narratives in which characters struggle over 'whether they should marry the person they love or wed the person their parents choose', Indian films 'raise, consider and resolve minor and major anxieties within contemporary Indian society, anxieties that are relevant to Hausa viewers' (1997: 410). In spite of cultural differences, young Hausa in Nigeria and young Tibetans in India appropriate the romantic representations of melodramatic Hindi films, because they are relevant to their own lives amidst social changes, and because they induce strong emotions in them. As Milton (2002) demonstrates, those things

that induce the strongest emotions and feelings make our lives most meaningful, and may become reference points for social action and personal identity. The emotional content of Hindi film representations is therefore all the more important for their appropriation.

In sum, Hindi film and television's avenues of influencing their Tibetan audience are mainly emotional and aesthetic, and both of these work through emotional attachment in the sense of appropriation into personal identity. The romantic practices of young Tibetans, described in the next section, reveal this: they are seeking the 'perfect love match' for marriage according to their individual emotional perspective, and engage in romantic relationships in ways that include the fusion of romantic experience and consumption.

Romance and Marriage for Young Tibetans

Young Tibetans in my fieldsite were very much concerned with finding the right person to marry. Romantic marriage as a goal was very clearly present in their minds, and informed both the way they chose their partners and the ways of engaging in such relationships. A situated desire for romantic relationships is thus expressed in terms of finding a long-term partner, ultimately for marriage, based on compatibility and love. The emotions young Tibetans talk about differ from those emphasised by their elders when talking about ideal marriage and family relations. The most important emotion mentioned by younger informants in relation to marriage is the notion of 'love' (*brtse ba*)—used alone and not as *spun kyag brtse ba*, the love between relatives or brothers. In relation to girlfriend/boyfriend relationships or marriage, *brtse ba* clearly signifies romantic love between two individuals, stressing the emotions of attraction binding a couple together. The main difference between *brtse ba* and the concept of *'cham po* ('friendly') as used by older Tibetan informants in talking about how marriage is best to come about, is that the former is focused on individual emotional concerns for a relationship, while the latter is used in relation to the families involved in a marriage as well as in relation to the individual couple. Speaking about marriage was for older informants not separate from speaking about the interrelations of families and about forms of sociality that favour harmony in the group. For this reason, there is a close connection in elder Tibetans' complaints about the disappearance of arranged marriages and polyandry—proper marriages, so to speak—and the disappearance of the communal sense of sociality inherent in the concept of 'staying together'.

In pursuing romance, young Tibetans emulate the kind of consumption portrayed in films which connotes the fusion of consumption and romantic experience. The middle-class lifestyle portrayed in films includes romantic activities such as couples going out for dinner to restaurants, going to the movies, vacationing in exotic and European places, or at the very least walks on the beach or in the park as part of their narrative development of romance. In the development of romantic relationships by my Tibetan informants, these types of activity played a very important role. As one of

my young male informants in a sweater market in Rajasthan told me: 'When you meet a nice girl here that you like, and you get to know her well, then you take her out to dinner, go to the movies with her ... then you really get to know her better.' Another young informant of mine told me about trips he had made on the motorcycle he owned, taking his girlfriend to 'nice places' in the forests close to his settlement in Northern India. For him, as for many other Tibetan youths, the kind of consumption of leisure activities that were part and parcel of Hindi films' description of romantic relationships were very important for his own romantic experience. Importantly, Dwyer notes that the two main elements of her description, consumption and romance, are not separate realms of desire, but are instead combined through mass media, including cinema and advertising (Illouz 1997; cf. Dwyer 2000: 13). Dwyer writes that this fusion of consumption and romance is expressed in the middle class's celebration of erotic love and romance through Hindi film: 'For them the commodity is where they base their aesthetics; their sentiments are expressed in spectacle. Hence commodities and consumption are not opposed to romance but form a key part of it' (2000: 13). Through the extensive exposure of young Tibetans to Hindi films, the portrayed fusion of romantic and consumption practices has become influential on their aspirations and attitudes toward romantic experience. Consumption, in the sense suggested by Gell of incorporation into the social self, must be understood as having become an intrinsic part of young Tibetans' romantic experience.

However, while the attitudes of young Tibetans who are seeking the perfect love match stand in contrast to their elders' ideals of marriage and sociality, this contrast is not a total contradiction. Be it in arranged marriages that are accepted, attempts at arranged marriages that are rejected, or love marriages entered, the family and its interests (followed or fretted over) do remain a central concern of younger Tibetans in their practices. While sometimes rejecting arranged marriages outright, young Tibetans are emotionally attached to Tibetan notions of harmony in familial relations. Two sibling informants and friends of mine, brother and sister and both in their twenties, present a clear example of this. Both were as much part of the romantic economy of their Tibetan settlement, and Bollywood enthusiasts, as any other Tibetan youth I came to know during my fieldwork. Yet, my friend told me that his sister would remark to him in the strongest tones that, whatever he chose to do with himself, he could under no circumstances upset his parents. He himself stressed the importance of being 'good' to his parents, and of living together with them to support them. The fact that they fully embraced the glamour of Bollywood's motorbikes and romances, yet still reminded each other of the highly important moral aspects of Tibetan notions of familial harmony, illustrates that they are emotionally attached to notions and convictions from both realms. They had appropriated both romantic elements from Hindi film and Tibetan moral notions into their sense of personal identity; both are therefore simultaneously present and effective in their lives.

Young Tibetans in India, then, have not abandoned familial interests and norms of harmonious social relations, because they are attached to notions such as *'cham po* that support these interests. It is an outcome of this emotional commitment that they negotiate their strong concern over romance and marriage with an equally strong socially normative context. Such negotiation between romantic love and social norms has been pointed out for the urban Indian context in Perveez Mody Spencer's work about love-marriage in Delhi (2000). In the context of British Pakistani transnational marriages, Shaw and Charsley note that it may be 'misleading to draw too sharp an analytical distinction between cultural expectations on the one hand and individual choice and action on the other, because conformity to social and cultural expectation can be an important element of individual motivation in marriage choice' (2006: 407). Similarly, convictions and social conventions held by older Tibetans are not discarded by younger Tibetans in India, but are instead shared to some extent and thus hold considerable sway over them as they engage with new realities and practices.

Conclusion

At the beginning, I suggested that senses of belonging can be conflicting for Tibetans in the diaspora in India, leading young Tibetans to characterise themselves as a 'remix'. In the course of my argument, I have laid out some of the elements involved in this perception. I have illustrated diasporic Tibetans' idealised representations of their 'homeland' in my discussion of elder informants' discourse about polyandry. The local construction of this idealised Tibet is connected to the affective state of *'cham po*, since it supposes that, in Tibet, 'brothers all agree with each other, are together'. My ethnography importantly demonstrates the centrality of *'cham po* for not just older, but also younger Tibetans in India, who are emotionally bound to it. But I have shown that, especially for younger diasporic Tibetans, emotional processes are also highly relevant to their engagement with Indian popular culture. Hindi films present them with imagery and narratives that deal with familiar social tensions between 'old' and 'new' ways in relation to romance and marriage. Very importantly, these representations link up with and work through their own imagination and emotions, and provide them with an idiom for their own romantic aspirations. Both the ideals of familial harmony and of romantic love are thus emotionally salient for younger Tibetans in India, and have been appropriated into a sense of their personal identity.

The fact that emotional attachments arise in such different and in some senses even opposed contexts of the Tibetan diaspora is significant for understanding the ambivalent self-perception of young Tibetans in India. However, such ambivalence is certainly not limited to them, to diasporic peoples, or even the 'age of globalisation'. Perhaps personal identities are generally so complex and multi-dimensional because the different things we are emotionally attached to are not unidirectional, but may instead pull our subjectivities in different directions at the same time.

Acknowledgements

This article developed out of a paper first presented to the panel 'Emotional attachments in a world of movement' at the annual EASA conference, 19 September 2006, in Bristol, England. I would like to thank King's College and the Department of Social Anthropology, Cambridge University, for their financial assistance in attending the conference, Maruška Svašek for comments and support, and an anonymous *JEMS* reviewer for comments on a later draft of the paper

Notes

[1] The fieldwork on which this article is based was carried out from March 2004 until July 2005 in Tibetan settlements in Himachal Pradesh, Northern India, and during the Tibetan itinerant trading season from October 2004 to February 2005 in Rajasthan. Research was supported by a Dissertation Research Grant of the Wenner-Gren Foundation, a Research Studentship of the Economic and Social Research Council, a Reginad Smith Studentship of King's College Cambridge, a Cambridge European Trust Bursary, a Wyse Trust Grant of Trinity College Cambridge, and a Ling Roth Scholarship of the Department of Social Anthropology, Cambridge University.

[2] It is interesting to note that the 'freedom' enjoyed in Tibet in the past is here connected to isolation from outside influences, when Tibetans 'didn't have anywhere to look, for foreign countries'—which is quite a different conceptualisation to the idea of freedom as implying the widest possible range of information and thus sources of potential influence.

References

Abu-Lughod, L. (1995) 'The objects of soap opera: Egyptian television and the cultural politics of modernity', in Miller, D. (ed.) *Worlds Apart: Modernity Through the Prism of the Local.* London and New York: Routledge, 190–210.

Anand, D. (2000) '(Re)imagining nationalism, identity and representation in the Tibetan diaspora of South Asia', *Contemporary South Asia*, 9(3): 271–87.

Ang, I. (1985) *Watching Dallas: Soap Opera and the Melodramatic Imagination.* London: Routledge.

Arakeri, A.V. (1998) *Tibetans in India. The Uprooted People and their Cultural Transplantation.* New Delhi: Reliance Publishing House.

Das, V. (1995) 'On soap opera: What kind of anthropological object is it?', in Miller, D. (ed.) *Worlds Apart: Modernity Through the Prism of the Local.* London and New York: Routledge, 169–89.

Diemberger, H. (2002) 'The people of Porong and concepts of territory', in Buffetrille, K. and Diemberger, H. (eds) *Territory and Identity in Tibet and the Himalayas. Proceedings of the Ninth Seminar of the International Association for Tibetan Studies.* Leiden: Brill, 33–55.

Dwyer, R. (2000) *All You Want Is Money, All You Need Is Love. Sex and Romance in Modern India.* London and New York: Cassell.

Forbes, A.A. (1989) *Settlements of Hope: An Account of Tibetan Refugees in Nepal.* Cambridge, Mass: Cultural Survival.

Gell, A. (1986) 'Newcomers to the world of goods: the Muria Gonds', in Appadurai, A. (ed.) *The Social Life of Things: Commodities in Cultural Perspective.* Cambridge: Cambridge University Press, 110–40.

Gledhill, C. (1991) 'Signs of melodrama', in Gledhill, C. (ed.) *Stardom: Industry of Desire.* London and New York: Routledge, 207–29.

Glick Schiller, N. and Fouron, G.E. (1999) 'Terrains of blood and nation: Haitian transnational social fields', *Ethnic and Racial Studies, 22*(2): 340–66.

Goldstein, M.C. (1976) 'Fraternal polyandry and fertility in a high Himalayan valley', *Human Ecology, 4*(3): 223–33.

Goldstein, M.C. (1978) 'Pahari and Tibetan polyandry revisited', *Ethnology, 17*(3): 325–37.

Grunfeld, T. (1987) *The Making of Modern Tibet.* London: Zed Books.

Houston, S. and Wright, R. (2003) 'Making and remaking Tibetan diasporic identities', *Social & Cultural Geography, 4*(2): 217–32.

Illouz, E. (1997) *Consuming the Romantic Utopia: Love and the Cultural Contradictions of Capitalism.* Berkeley: University of California Press.

Jing, J. (1996) *The Temple of Memories: History, Power, and Morality in a Chinese Village.* Stanford, Ca: Stanford University Press.

Kharat, R. (2003) 'Gainers of a stalemate: the Tibetans in India', in Samaddar, R. (ed.) *Refugees and the State. Practices of Asylum and Care in India 1947–2000.* New Delhi: Sage, 281–320.

Kirsch, S. (2001) 'Environmental disaster, "culture loss," and the law', *Current Anthropology, 42*(2): 167–98.

Klieger, P.C. (2002) 'Engendering Tibet: power, self, and change in the diaspora', in Klieger, P.C. (ed.) *Tibet, Self, and the Tibetan Diaspora. Voices of Difference. Proceedings of the Ninth Seminar of the International Association for Tibetan Studies.* Leiden: Brill, 139–54.

Kolås, Å. (1996) 'Tibetan nationalism: the politics of religion', *Journal of Peace Research, 35*(1): 51–66.

Korom, F.J. (1997) 'Introduction: place, space and identity: the cultural, economic and aesthetic politics of Tibetan diaspora', in Korom, F.J. (ed.) *Tibetan Culture in the Diaspora. Proceedings of the Seventh Seminar of the International Association for Tibetan Studies.* Vienna: Verlag der Österreichischen Akademie der Wissenschaften, 1–8.

Larkin, B. (1997) 'Indian films and Nigerian lovers: media and the creation of parallel modernities', *Africa, 67*(3): 406–40.

Lau, T. (2007) The Tibetan Diaspora in India: Approaching Itinerant Trade, Popular Cultural Consumption and Diasporic Sociality. Cambridge: University of Cambridge, unpublished PhD thesis.

Lau, T. (2008) 'Understanding Tibetan shame and hierarchy through emotional experience in fieldwork', in Chua, L., High, C. and Lau, T. (eds) *How Do We Know? Evidence, Ethnography and the Making of Anthropological Knowledge.* Cambridge: Cambridge Scholars Publishing, 157–78.

Lau, T. (2009) 'Tibetan fears and Indian foes: fears of cultural extinction and antagonism as discursive strategy', *vis-à-vis: Explorations in Anthropology, 9*(1): 81–90.

Levine, N.E. (1988) *The Dynamics of Polyandry.* Chicago: University of Chicago Press.

Levine, N.E. (1994) 'The demise of marriage in Purang, Tibet 1959–1990', in Kvaerne, P. (ed.) *Tibetan Studies. Proceedings of the Sixth Seminar of the International Association for Tibetan Studies. Vol. 1.* Oslo: Institute for Comparative Research in Human Culture, 468–80.

Levine, N.E. and Silk, J.B. (1997) 'Why polyandry fails: sources of instability in polyandrous marriages', *Current Anthropology, 38*(3): 375–98.

Malkki, L.H. (1995) *Purity and Exile: Violence, Memory, and National Cosmology among Hutu Refugees in Tanzania.* Chicago: University of Chicago Press.

Mazzarella, W. (2003) *Shoveling Smoke: Advertising and Globalization in Contemporary India.* Durham and London: Duke University Press.

Michael, F. (1985) 'Survival of a culture: Tibetan refugees in India', *Asian Survey, 25*(7): 737–44.

Milton, K. (2002) *Loving Nature. Towards an Ecology of Emotion.* London and New York: Routledge.

Mishra, V. (2002) *Bollywood Cinema: Temples of Desire.* London and New York: Routledge.

Mody Spencer, P. (2000) Love-Marriage in Delhi. Cambridge: University of Cambridge, unpublished PhD thesis.

Nandy, A. (1998) *The Secret Politics of Our Desires: Innocence, Culpability and Popular Cinema.* London: Zed Books.

Neale, S. (1986) 'Melodrama and tears', *Screen, 27*(6): 6–22.

Nowak, M. (1984) *Tibetan Refugees: Youth and the New Generation of Meaning.* New Brunswick, NJ: Rutgers University Press.

Oxford English Dictionary (1971) *Oxford English Dictionary.* Oxford: Clarendon Press.

Sadakata, A. (1997) *Buddhist Cosmology: Philosophy and Origins.* Tokyo: Kosei.

Saklani, G. (1984) *The Uprooted Tibetans in India: A Sociological Study of Continuity and Change.* New Delhi: Cosmo Publications.

Shaw, A. and Charsley, K. (2006) 'Rishtas: adding emotion to strategy in understanding British Pakistani transnational marriages', *Global Networks*, 6(4): 405–21.

Ström, A.K. (1994) 'Tibetan Refugees in India: aspects of socio-cultural change', in Kvaerne, P. (ed.) *Tibetan Studies. Proceedings of the 6th Seminar of the International Association for Tibetan Studies.* Oslo: Institute for Comparative Research in Human Culture, 837–47.

Ström, A.K. (1997) 'Between Tibet and the West: on traditionality, modernity and the development of monastic institutions in the Tibetan diaspora', in Korom, F.J. (ed.) *Tibetan Culture in the Diaspora. Proceedings of the Seventh Seminar of the International Association for Tibetan Studies.* Vienna: Verlag der Österreichischen Akademie der Wissenschaften, 33–50.

Subba, T.B. (1988) 'Social adaptation of the Tibetan refugees in the Darjeeling-Sikkim Himalayas', *The Tibet Journal, 13*(3): 49–57.

Subba, T.B. (1990) *Flight and Adaptation. Tibetan Refugees in the Darjeeling-Sikkim Himalaya.* Dharamsala: Library of Tibetan Works and Archives.

Svašek, M. and Skrbiš, Z. (2007) 'Passions and powers: emotions and globalisation', *Identities: Global Studies in Culture and Power, 14*(3): 367–83.

Thomas, R. (1985) 'Indian cinema: pleasures and popularity', *Screen, 2*(3–4): 116–31.

Thomas, R. (1995) 'Melodrama and the negotiation of morality in mainstream Hindi film', in Beckenridge, C. (ed.) *Consuming Modernity: Public Culture in a South Asian World.* Minneapolis and London: University of Minnesota Press, 157–82.

Vasudevan, R. (1989) 'The melodramatic mode and commercial Hindi cinema', *Screen, 30*(3): 29–50.

von Fürer-Haimendorf, C. (1990) *The Renaissance of Tibetan Civilization.* Oracle, Arizona: Synergetic Press.

Warner, M. (1992) *The Letters of the Republic. Publication and the Public Sphere in Eighteenth Century America.* Cambridge, Mass: Harvard University Press.

The Politics of Hope and Disappointment: Ambivalence in the Post-1989 Homeland-Related Discourses among Hungarians in Australia

Petra Andits

In this article, I look at the ways in which the homeland-related discourses among Hungarians in Australia have shifted as a result of the political and social transformations in Hungary around and after 1989. In order to disentangle this question, I place a specific emphasis on the dynamics between identification, emotions and politics. I demonstrate that the aftermath of regime change produced a sense of ambivalence in discourses about Australian-Hungarians' relationship with the homeland. The desire for inclusion into the new democracy became dialogically intertwined with the simultaneous feelings of distrust and disappointment, producing what Bakhtin calls 'double voiced' homeland-related discourses. I examine how these contradictory emotions are evoked and expressed in the post-1989 Australian-Hungarian discourses. I argue that they became powerful moral forces which affect diaspora members' understanding of their selves and enable and constrain the diaspora's political actions towards the homeland.

Introduction

While the construction of 'new cultural landscapes' (Berdahl 2000: 1) in Eastern Europe following the *annus mirabilis* of 1989 has gained plenty of scholarly attention (see

Lemon 2000; Ries 1997; Verdery and Burawoy 1999; Wanner 1998), the impact of the collapse of communism on Eastern European *émigré* communities has been much less documented. The political and social transformation of the region, the possibility for transnational mobility, and the renewed 'discourses of the national' (Niedermüller 1999) in the newly born democracies have opened up new avenues for new forms of subjectivities, emotions and diaspora politics to emerge within these diasporas. In this paper, I look at the ways in which the tumultuous events in Hungary around and after 1989 influenced the ways in which Australian-Hungarians feel about their sense of self and their connection to the new–old homeland. In order to comprehend this transformation, I analyse the post-1989 diasporic homeland-related discourses and the thresholds and tensions of the newly emerged relationship between the Hungarian authorities and the Australian-Hungarian community. The analysis is focused primary at the meso and macro levels of community and state politics but the article also addresses micro-level accounts of personal return visits of Australian-Hungarians and the experiences of belonging at the level of individuals.

In examining the subjectivities that emerge through such dynamic changes, my starting-point is the understanding of the self as a relational achievement (see Conradson and McKay 2007). From this perspective, subjectivities are the results of the complex interplay between various influences and encounters. While the social, political and geographic factors need to be considered, these factors alone cannot explain the issues associated with the transformation of Australian-Hungarians' sense of self and belonging. I argue that a specific emphasis on emotions can shed light on previously neglected aspects of identity, identification and belonging. An increasing amount of research shows that emotions play a major role in the construction of post-socialist Europe (see, for instance, Golanska-Ryan 2006; Leutloff-Grandits 2006; Mihaylova 2006; Muller 2006; Skrbiš 2006; Svašek 2002, 2006). These works document how the tumultuous political and economic transformations have generated strong emotional responses, ranging from hope and euphoria to disappointment, envy and nostalgia (Svašek 2006: 9). By investigating the dialectics of emotions and politics in Post-Cold-War Eastern Europe, these studies demonstrate that emotions, politics and identity construction are closely intertwined phenomena. The emotional landscape which developed in the Eastern European diasporas after 1989, however, has remained an unexplored field in the literature.

In this paper, I examine how emotions are evoked and expressed in the post-1989 homeland-related diasporic discourses and the ways in which these emotional discourses are implicated in the negotiation of diaspora members' sense of self and connection to the homeland. My particular focus is the dynamics between structural transformations, emotions, identity construction and political actions, and the ways in which they mutually condition one another (see Bourdieu 1985; Emirbayer and Goldberg 2005). I consider the relation between these factors as 'dynamic, ongoing, dialogic processes-in-relations' (Emirbayer and Goldberg 2005: 507).

While the diaspora's symbolic return to the nation after 1989 has been a way to reconcile, reintegrate and heal the scars of the past, it has also given rise to new tensions

and boundaries (see Long and Oxfeld 2004). The aftermath of the regime change produced a sense of ambivalence in discourses about Australian-Hungarians' relationship with the homeland. After decades of structural segregation and exclusion, the regime change opened up a strong discourse of belonging, inclusion and connectedness in the diaspora. This sense of desire for inclusion proved to be a powerful moral force, which strongly affected and motivated the diaspora's political actions towards the homeland (see Lyons 1980: 52; Rosaldo 1984). After the early negotiations between homeland and diaspora, the initial desire for inclusion was overshadowed by the feelings of disappointment. As a result, a powerful discourse of 'not belonging'—of abandonment, distrust and anxiety—also developed. Later on the sense of belonging and not belonging became dialogically intertwined, producing what Bakhtin (1981: 324) calls 'double voiced' homeland-related discourses. These 'double voiced' discourses of 'belonging and not belonging' to the homeland in turn, enabled and constrained possibilities of action and thought. They affect diaspora members' understanding of themselves, inform their actions and impact upon the processes of negotiating the relationship with Hungary.

Australian-Hungarians Pre-1989

Emotions are constructed in particular cultural, social, historical and political contexts (Lutz and White 1986: 408, 415, 420; Reddy 1997: 329, 331; Svašek 2006). They are informed by norms which developed in a long process of socialisation (Reddy 1997: 335). When analysing the emotional dynamics and identification processes of the Australian-Hungarian diaspora, it is important to consider the structural position of the diaspora and its culturally and historically specific discourses, pre-1989 (Lutz and Abu-Lughod 1990; Svašek 2006).

There are approximately 62,000 Hungarians in Australia. The vast majority of the first generation arrived during the communist dictatorship in Hungary. The first large wave of Hungarian immigration (about 15,000 people) arrived in Australia as Displaced Persons between 1948 and 1954. The second large wave occurred after the 1956 Revolution. Roughly 250,000 'fifty-sixers' fled Hungary after the Revolution (Huseby-Darvas 2004: 77); and around 15,000 arrived in Australia. After the Revolution, no other clearly defined waves of Hungarian refugees migrated to Australia. Between 1958 and 1980, around 100 so-called 'defectors' arrived each year in Australia (Kunz 1985: 538). Individuals in each of these immigrant waves were officially labelled 'political refugees'.

Over a period of over 40 years, while Soviet-style communism dominated Eastern Europe, the Hungarian community in Australia enjoyed little formal or institutional links with Hungary. During the 1950s and early 1960s, communist propaganda in Hungary labelled refugees as fascist criminals, class enemies and work-shy rabble (Kunz 1985: 102). After the amnesty in 1963, the Kadar regime officially differentiated between 'good' and 'harmful' émigrés (Borbandi 2006: 272). However, broad negative connotations still persisted. The only attempt by the Hungarian government to have connection with the expatriates abroad was the *Magyarok Vilagszovetsege* (World

Federation of Hungarians). The organisation was set up in Budapest after the 1963 amnesty and operated under close party control in order to monitor Hungarians and their organisations in exile (see Borbandi 2006).

Each of the emigrant waves was deprived of their Hungarian citizenship. Return visits for the 'good émigrés' to Hungary were possible, though not unproblematic. Travel to Hungary was only possible with a visa, which was granted by the Hungarian government only to those with 'excellent behaviour', which implied non-participation in exile-politics (Borbandi 2006: 273).

Most Hungarians in Australia maintained a conception of Hungary split by the dichotomy between their homeland on the one hand, and the regime on the other. This separation of national culture from the state was an important principle in exilic discourses (Slobin 2001: 516). While émigrés desired to return to the homeland, disconnection from communist Hungary was a focal constitutive element of the exilic condition. Maintaining the isolation for as long as the dictatorship remained in power in Hungary was propagated as a 'moral duty' of the émigrés. Hungarians in Australia during this period referred to their state as being in '*emigráció*' (exile). The term '*emigráció*' is heavily loaded with historical significance as it draws a link with prominent Hungarian émigré groups from the past (Andits 2007).

While being in exile is often described in the literature as an experience leading to fundamental *discontinuity* (Breytenbach 1991: 75; Said 1992: 360–1), the representatives of the *emigráció* did not entirely see their exile as an exclusion from history (Slobin 2001). While one had to bear banishment, many believed that being in exile was the only way to save both Hungary and Hungarianness from the 'complete devastation' of Communism.

Satzewich (2002; see also Hein 2004) documents that for many émigrés the urge for freedom from Communism and Soviet hegemony led to external political mobilisation against Soviet domination of their homelands. Further, Eastern European emigrant groups felt that in many ways their authentic language, culture and traditions were preserved only in exile. Similarly, Australian-Hungarian narratives from the pre-1989 period claimed that their mission was to fight Communism and to keep alive the 'purity' of Hungarian culture. Accordingly, exile politics and nation-preservation became key phrases in the pre-1989 period. A powerful element in the narratives was that the émigrés had the requisite knowledge and 'moral purity' to participate in the transformation of Hungary into a 'true nation'. This feeling prevailed despite the fact that their anti-communist political actions and attempts to institutionalise Hungarian culture in the *emigráció* were mainly symbolic and objectively largely weak (see Skrbiš 2002: 45).

Australian-Hungarians Post-1989

Structural Transformation

Revolutions swept across Eastern Europe in the autumn of 1989 and overthrew the Soviet-style dictatorships. The subsequent negotiated transitions were quick and

non-violent. In several Eastern European countries, including Hungary, liberal democracy ensued after the forty years of communist dictatorship. The legislation in 1989 transformed Hungary from a People's Republic into the Republic of Hungary, guaranteed human and civil rights, and created an institutional structure that ensured separation of powers among the judicial, legislative and executive branches of government. This transformation from dictatorship to democracy is popularly referred to in Hungarian as the *rendszerváltás* ('system change'). The *rendszerváltás* not only affected the citizens of the Hungarian Republic but also had repercussions for those Hungarians who live outside the country. The transformation in Hungary meant that the 'discourse of the national' (Niedermüller 1999) was revisited. The reorientation implied a new official policy towards Hungarians residing outside of the Republic. For example, in 1990 the first democratically elected Hungarian prime minister, Antall József (1990–93), declared himself to be Prime Minister 'in spirit' of 15 million Hungarians. The notion of '15 million Hungarians' embraced 10 million Hungarian citizens, 'minority-Hungarians' who are citizens of states which neighbour Hungary, and Hungarian émigrés all over the world. This reorientation entailed the granting of citizenship—the most important instrument of inclusion in a society (Kivisto 2001: 572)—to Hungarian émigrés and the reconfigured official relationship with the émigré organisations. Hungarian citizenship enabled émigrés to move back to Hungary or engage in frequent border-crossings. The reworked official relationship impacted on the opportunities for the diaspora to carry out transnational political, economic and cultural activities, and enabled unconstrained contact and cooperation between organisations in the Australian-Hungarian community and Hungary for the first time after forty years of official segregation.

Great Hopes: The Desire for Inclusion

'Uplifting' emotional processes after the fall of the communist dictatorships have been widely reported in Eastern Europe (see Svašek 2006). The euphoria was accompanied by widely shared expectations that the introduction of democracy and the market economy would result in the rapid improvement of peoples' lives. The *rendszerváltás* also evoked feelings of euphoria and hope within the Australian-Hungarian diaspora. A dichotomy which several Hungarians in Australia maintained until 1989, that is, a division between their homeland on the one hand, and the regime on the other, was finally broken down. After decades of being in exile, expatriates in Australia saw the moment of 1989 as a grand possibility, which would open up ways for their homecoming and reintegration. Building bridges between the community and the homeland became a major theme in diasporic discourses.

The desire for reintegration urged the Hungarian diaspora elite in Australia to call for a resurrection of national identity within the community and to mobilise members through different gatherings, programmes, speeches and plans. During this time national commemoration days and other community activities were used for mobilising the diaspora. For example, after the last Soviet troops left Hungary in

June 1991, more than 3,000 Hungarians gathered to celebrate the event with a mass in St Mary's Cathedral in Sydney. A passage of a speech on 15 March 1989 (Hungarian National Day) in the Sydney-based Hungarian Community House demonstrates how the desire for homecoming was used to motivate the community:

> We live in a never-to-be-repeated historical period. (...) Our homeland wants to climb out of the dark grave of 40-years-long communist dictatorship and claim its rightful place among the European nations. It is a difficult task and we, Hungarians, who live in the West should do everything we can to assist our country. (...) In order to rebuild the country we need to make enormous sacrifices.

On a different occasion in 1989 the president of the Hungarian Council of New South Wales, Béla Kardos, said the following:

> We have to wake up those who are sleeping, those who are tired, apathetic, and indifferent, and those who do not have any hope. As the free Hungary and the Hungarians in the Carpathian basin in the dismembered territories are looking at us with hope and the expectations of help from us.

Similarly, intense hope was experienced at the individual level in the diaspora. After the collapse of Communism, the previously unreachable Hungarian homeland 'of the mind' (Rushdie 1992: 10) became accessible again for Hungarian émigrés. Open borders enabled Hungarians—'haunted by some sense of loss [and] some urge to reclaim' (Rushdie 1992: 10)—to attempt to close the gap of 20, 30 and even 50 years, and to re-territorialise their identities in the newly rediscovered homeland. Several Australian-Hungarians visited Hungary for the first time in the hope of a rapid and complete reclamation of old relationships unaffected by the physical separation or the time that had elapsed.

The New Mission of the Emigráció: *'Diaspora Diplomacy'*

The strong sense of desire for symbolic homecoming and reintegration shaped the diaspora's political actions after 1989. The Hungarian community elite in Australia aimed to be reintegrated by portraying the diaspora as an important political body in the democratic transformations in Hungary. They intended to carry out political actions as a 'mobilised diaspora' while remaining in Australia, as illustrated in this quote from an optimistic speech on 15 March 1990—National Day—at the Hungarian Community Centre, Punchbowl, Sydney: 'We hope that the new democratic government together with us will start to rebuild the new Hungary'.

The Australian-Hungarian diaspora saw its own incorporation into nation-rebuilding as crucial in Hungary's transition to democracy. The *emigráció* envisaged itself as an 'ambassador' in the reconstruction of the homeland, a medium between the *fresh democracy* in Hungary and the *well-established democracy* in Australia (see also Huseby-Darvas 2004; Pomogats 1994; Shain 1995). This claim was based on the belief that the *emigráció* possessed 'double cultural competencies' (Vasta 1993: 220) or, as

Edward Said (1983: 172) calls it, 'plurality of vision'. By portraying themselves as both well-educated Western citizens, familiar with the system of democracy, and as 'authentic' Hungarians, the *emigráció* saw a facilitating role for themselves in the rebuilding of the Hungarian nation. This double identity was not seen as emerging in a space 'somewhere between the host land and the homeland' (Panossian 1998: 58), but claimed to be deeply rooted in both of them.

The representatives of the *emigráció* attempted to present themselves to the democratic homeland authorities as a professional and integrated group in the political system of the host country, capable of campaigning, networking and lobbying for Hungary's sake. As one of my participants, Endre Csapó, put it in a publication addressed to Géza Jeszenszky, Hungarian Foreign Minister:

> Hungary had never ever had so many potential ambassadors and foreign agencies as she has now. She has a diplomatic army.

The representatives of the *emigráció* stated that they had the ability to monitor foreign policies all over the world, based on their familiarity with another successful democratic country (e.g. Australia), its social and political circumstances, its trade, industry, language and other features. They claimed that this 'dead capital' could be channelled into the rejuvenation of Hungary (see also Huseby-Darvas 2004). A letter written by Endre Csapó, editor of *Magyar Élet* (Hungarian community newspaper in Australia) to Pordány László, Hungarian Ambassador, on 15 March 1991, emphasised the efficiency of the diaspora:

> I want to draw your attention to the fact that the Hungarian community enjoys a good reputation in the eyes of Australian authorities and governments. They [the Australian government representatives] are familiar with our institutions and media, we have official relationship and they consult us in Hungary-related issues.

Another prominent member of the elite, Béla Kardos, said:

> For the Hungarian Associations in Australia it always has been immensely important to put Hungary in a favourable light abroad. To this end, we have actively produced several publications in English drawn from trustworthy sources. We have continually emphasised our Europeanness, and the inequity of Trianon Treaties. We edited actual disclosing studies and booklets on regular basis in order to advocate for the rights of Hungarians living in dismembered territories and we sent them to every single member of the Australian Federal Parliament: to senators, ministers, public figures and so on. And we continuously furnish state and university libraries with books and documents which can raise Hungary's reputation.

The discourse also emphasised the lack of Hungary's intellectual resources, as Hungarians were unable to establish connections with the West, and were deprived of access to foreign media under Communism; therefore they lacked a sense of foreign politics. As one of my participants stated in *Magyar Elet* (25 September 1990):

'Hungary doesn't have ready intelligent diplomats who know how to deal with the West, how to behave'. This argument utilised the passionate *decommunisation* discourses, which emerged in Hungary (and throughout Eastern Europe) after 1989. While those promoting *decommunisation* argued that getting rid of the old *nomenklatura* who hold important positions is morally desirable, those opposing *decommunisation* argued that there would not be anybody in the country to replace them (see Rupnik 1995). Hungarian diaspora representatives in Australia attempted to solve the dilemma by advocating their own members for the new positions.

The other face of the ambassador figure was the 'true Hungarian'. While emphasising the community's 'Western' values at the same time, contemporary discourses in the diaspora underscored the view that the *emigráció* is not more disconnected from 'real Hungarianness' than people in Hungary. This argument was based on two claims. First, the representatives argued that the diaspora is only geographically separated from the homeland's territorial location. In fact, via 'nation-preservation' it managed to keep alive the 'real Hungarian spirit', while this was not possible in Hungary under communist rule. Second, the 'moral purity' of the émigrés was also highlighted. This was underpinned by the claim that, while in the homeland virtually every adult could be suspected of collaboration with the Communist regime, émigrés remained above suspicion. Further, representatives were eager to emphasise their rigorous engagement in anti-communist exile-politics and consequent benefits for Hungary. The *emigráció* representatives in Australia often made comparisons between themselves and other Hungarian *emigráció*s in the West and referred to themselves as the 'best of all *emigráció*s', as they rigorously isolated themselves from the 'damaging influences and resisted the siren songs of the Communist Hungarian government'. Such comparisons served further to underscore their anti-communist character, and thus their moral purity. In October 1990 the representatives of the first democratic Hungarian government were invited to the commemoration of the 1956 Revolution in the Sydney-based Hungarian Community House. The president of the New South Wales Hungarian Association, Béla Kardos, said the following:

> The Australian-Hungarian *emigráció* was the only one in the world which never acknowledged the dictatorial governments, not even during the *détente*. Accordingly, we never kept in touch with their embassies either.

The task the *emigráció* imagined for Hungary was to *activate* these 'diplomatic corps', to be the coordinator and to centralise the information and duties that would provide the institutional framework for their mission. The experiences of individual Hungarians show similar tendencies. Several returning or visiting Hungarians were eager to offer Western expertise, such as teaching English or volunteering for social and political organisations. Individual travel narratives reveal that Australian-Hungarians felt not only obligated but also entitled to participate in the reconstruction of Hungary.

Great Disappointments

As Milena Veenis (1999: 83) notes, in the post-socialist Eastern European context '[d]esire and disappointment go hand in hand'. It is widely documented that the euphoria that accompanied the fall of Communism was soon followed by disappointments in Eastern Europe (Rupnik 1995; Svašek 2002, 2006). As several scholars have pointed out, an important factor contributing to the widely shared disappointments in Eastern Europe was the rise of 'mythologized hopes' (Hochmann 2001: 281) and exaggerated expectations after 1989. Rightful hopes for quick solutions were often intermingled with misconceptions and false illusions. A negative emotional transformation also took place in the Hungarian *emigráció* in Australia, in which the unfulfilled ambitious expectations played a similar role. A general sense of bitterness and disillusionment followed the early initiatives of Australian-Hungarians, and has remained a powerful sentiment in the diaspora even 20 years after the change of regime. Satzewich (2002: 11) notes that, after decades of separation, the embrace between Eastern European diasporas and the homelands often had unintended and negative consequences, such as further feelings of alienation and estrangement instead of renewed connectivity.

One of the major sources of the disillusionment, in the case of Australian-Hungarians, was that their great hopes and desire for homecoming and reintegration were not realised. This sense of exclusion and abandonment was manifest in the perception that the establishment of the desired bridges between the diaspora and Hungary was not initiated by the Hungarian authorities. In particular, the expatriates felt that their offers of political help seemed not to be appreciated in Hungary and the Hungarian government failed to provide professional help to organise the diaspora for the 'new mission'.

The reason for the lack of the diaspora's inclusion into the political, social and cultural domain of the homeland are many. Émigré representatives saw, and presented, their activities during the exile period (nation-preservation and exile politics) as a sufficient basis on which equal belonging to Hungary could be claimed. Based on these activities, they saw their own reintegration into the nation as a necessary component of the democratisation of Hungary. These claims, however, turned out to hold uncertain promise. First, the homeland administrations regarded these competencies as non-imperative in Hungary's development. A small diaspora, which lacks substantial political or economic connections to influential allies in Australia, and which does not contribute to Hungary's GDP via remittances or investments, did not appeal to homeland governments. Magocsi (2005) also emphasises that those in exile had few concrete political plans, as they did not really expect that the collapse of the communist system in Eastern Europe would occur during their own lifetimes.

Second, the divergent discourses of 'rightful' belonging also fuelled miscommunication between the diaspora and the homeland authorities, and thus contributed to émigrés' sense of disappointment. Magocsi (2005: 175) argues that Eastern European political organisations in exile, after decades of hermetic separation, 'grew to be out of

touch with the political reality in Communist-ruled Central and Eastern Europe and, in particular, unaware of the changed civic, economic and moral values of those at home' (see also Cohen 1997; Panossian 1998, 2003). While the émigrés presented themselves as the last preserve of authentic Hungarianness, homeland authorities approached the émigrés' decades of being in exile as an absence of engagement with the temporal rhythms of life and the developments in Hungary. Through this prism, émigré representatives appeared outdated and idealistic. Again, what in the community context was an indicator of achievement and sacrifice turned out to be an insignificant factor in the context of *rendszerváltás* in Hungary (Stefansson 2004: 67). Hungarian authorities often argued against the incorporation of the diaspora into homeland politics by emphasising the great divide between the contemporary Hungarian society and the émigré community. The first post-1990 Foreign Minister, Géza Jeszenszky, is quoted as saying:

> Although every emigrant community was watching the course of events in Hungary [in the last 40 years], it caused problems for them to live through them as much as the ones who lived there during the decades of Communism. Accordingly, they couldn't take part in the struggle for liberation. Something has stopped inside them when crossing the borders [i.e. when emigrating]. [...] In a democracy with old traditions, internal political affairs are not brought outside the borders (*Új Magyarország*, 18 August 1991).

Árpád Göncz, the president of Hungary between 1990 and 2000, was even bolder in a speech delivered to the Melbourne-based Hungarian community; here he comments on the divide between the two communities:

> Everybody has that image of the country which he left. Time goes by, the country is changing. I would like you to know that I respect your loyalty to a country which doesn't exist in practice any longer. It's gone with the wind of the history... You got far away from your homeland. I repeat, I feel empathy with you and I am truly sorry for you. I owe that to 10 millions who are in Hungary... (*Demokrata*, September 1999).

After the President delivered his speech in Melbourne, several community members expressed disappointment at his comments, one of them publishing an article in the same Hungary-based journal in the same month:

> The latest speech of the President of the Hungarian Republic just confirms us in our concerns. We got to know on the best authority that the country to which we are so loyal vanished. Where it is now? What is there instead of it? Also those, who expected from the President a soul-stirring, optimistic speech, which would inspire us to act for our homeland, were disappointed.

Magocsi (2005) emphasises that Eastern European leaders in exile were politically out of step with the times. He suggests that émigrés held on to a more outdated vision of the nation-state as the ideal mode of political organisation, which characterised the political vocabulary of the past. The Hungarian context is similar. Even those

politicians and prominent figures who expected political help from the diaspora, for instance the famous Transylvanian bishop László Tőkés, found the political radicalism of certain segments of the *emigráció* objectionable. Tőkés warned of the nationalistic extremism of 'hero-Hungarians' and 'wild-Hungarians', who had been disconnected from reality in Hungary for 40 years. József Antall, the first democratically elected prime minister, who claimed to be the prime minister 'in spirit' of 15 million Hungarians, was accused of saying in an informal setting that the members of the '*emigráció*' are venomous, extreme-right-wing and impossible to talk to, and that time had passed over their heads.

Another component of the divergent discourses on belonging concerned Hungarians' 'moral purity' in the homeland and diaspora. While émigrés utilised the fact that they could not fall under suspicion of collaboration and complicity with the former regime, it is documented that stayees ascribed a guilt of desertion to the émigrés, emphasising that those who fled the country during hardship could not be regarded as 'real' Hungarians any more (Gefin 1997; Huseby-Darvas 2004). While President Göncz was delivering his Melbourne speech, reported above, several Hungarians in the crowd whistled, screamed and accused him of being a traitor, based on his activities as an informer in Kádár's prison after the 1956 Revolution and his current co-operation with the ex-Communists. As a reaction, the president turned the crowd's accusation against them: 'So who is the traitor here? The ones who stayed at home and endured the life-sentence? Or others . . . ? Each can judge for himself!' (*Demokrata*, September 1999). A disappointed community member reacted with: 'We received his words with scalding tears. So that would be the base of the loving relationship between the *emigráció* and the homeland?' (*Demokrata*, September 1999).

Beyond the resentment felt towards the newly elected governments for not including the diaspora in the democratic transformations, émigrés' utterances of disappointment also targeted the 'incomplete transformation'. It is widely documented that the 'unfinished transformation' to liberal democracy has created significant tensions, dissatisfaction and distrust in post-socialist Eastern European societies. In most Eastern European countries, a so-called 'thick line' was drawn under the communist past, strictly separating it from the present (Kalb *et al.* 1999: 16). It implied that the collapse of the Communist regime was not accompanied by expelling the 'nomenclature' from their positions; rather it enabled them to regain political power and to appropriate common public goods (Kalb *et al.* 1999: 16; see also Elster 1996). The consequences of the 'unfinished transformation' also resulted in great disappointment in the Australian-Hungarian diaspora. The diaspora representatives felt betrayed by the fact that the Hungarian government did not call to account the individuals who were responsible for political crimes during Communist rule. The incomplete transformation also entailed the proscription of irredentist voices regarding the Treaty of Trianon in the Hungarian political arena in the eyes of the diaspora. This became a particular resentment among many Australian-Hungarians, palpable in the passage below, which I draw from a 2002 resignation speech of one of my participants from his position in an Australian-Hungarian grassroots political organisation:

> In 1990 joint countries like Yugoslavia, Czechoslovakia are collapsing like house of cards... Aeroplanes getting off from Taszár [NATO station in Hungary during the Balkan War in the 1990s] are bombarding, interrogating Milosevic, Ceausescu are riddled, European borders are being shifted, every country becomes independent, everybody is privatising and scrounging ... only one is not taking part in the dog-fight. And as a gentleman gives again and again ... airports, back-supports, all that is needed without asking anything in change. Not even a tiny independence of Vajdaság [Hungarian populated region in Serbia, part of 'Historical Great Hungary'] ... nothing ... Stupid child of Europe. In the subject called 'Utilising great historical occasions' Antall József [first democratically elected prime minister in Hungary after 1989], Horn Gyula [prime minister between 1994 and 1998 in Hungary] and their governments absolutely failed.

What is more, the 'incomplete transformation' from dictatorship to democracy was also seen by the émigrés as the cause of the non-incorporation of the diaspora. It was seen as the reason why the government did not utilise the resources of the diaspora and continued to use the same labels, such as 'fascistic'. A community representative, Béla Kardos, who has been working on the building of the transnational bridge since 1989, confessed in one of his pessimistic writings:

> The current political elite in Hungary could still not get rid of the socialist reflexes and still doesn't realise that firstly, the Western *emigráció* is an incredible loss for the country, secondly, that after establishing its position in the West, it represents a fantastic diplomatic and economic opportunity for Hungary.

The *emigráció* representatives in Australia particularly resented that, while the new democratic government did not devote much attention to them, it showed greater interest in other Hungarian diaspora organisations in Canada and in the United States, such as the *ITT–OTT Kör* (Here and There Circle) and the *Magyar Baráti Közösség* (Hungarian Fellowship). These diaspora organisations demonstrated willingness in initiating connections with the Hungarian government before the fall of Communism. The fact that the government favoured these organisations after 1989 was again seen as a result of the 'unfinished transformation'. A resentful voice was published in *Magyar Élet* in 1991:

> The *Magyar Baráti Közösség* was one of those organisations, which approved of Kádár's dictatorship and regularly visited Hungary to co-operate under the cover of participating in the *Anyanyelvi Konferencia*. [...] I know their newspaper very well, [*Nyugati Magyarság* (Hungarians in the West)]. It has been eagerly attempting to propagate the Kádár government in the West. [...] I have no idea how the foreign minister can propagate this journal which represents a minority and actively attacks the national *emigráció* (cited in *Amerikai Magyar Ertesítö*, November, 27 November 1991).

These examples reveal that the negative or negatively perceived judgments of the Hungarian authorities were experienced as explicit signs of exclusion in the *emigráció*. Representatives of the diaspora felt that neither their 'great potential' or

'self-sacrificing' political efforts for the sake of the homeland, nor the hard work of the expatriate community to preserve Hungarianness were recognised in Hungary. Further, the well-known negative labels, such as 'extreme-right-wing' and 'fascistic', used by the communist propaganda to depict the *emigráció*, were still in usage by Hungarian authorities.

Individual community members' initial hopes similarly turned into disappointment when exilic dreaming of homeland and return gave place to practical homecomings. The imagined geographies of home often created high expectations for Australian-Hungarians, which were often not realised upon return. Several Hungarian returnees and visitors realised that the specific experiences they had during their return trips often contrasted with their memories from the past and dreams of return (Long and Oxfeld 2004). They painfully discovered that, in their period of absence, the homeland, their homes and communities had changed beyond recognition. In these cases, return was less about re-exploration and re-integration and more about rupture (see Huseby-Darvas 2004; Stefansson 2004; Tsuda 2004). Disappointments were particularly painful among those return migrants whose expectations were based on memories from childhood or youth. However, often not the transformations but the undesired legacy of the past hindered the visitors' feelings of reintegration and belonging. A great majority of returnees I talked to complained about the irrevocability of the 'Communist legacy' in Hungary. Returning expatriates conclude that Hungary and Hungarians could still not overcome the communist tradition of improper language, littering and negligence, and are still behind (Western) European standards. The other disillusioning aspect of homecomings was the cold welcome that Australian-Hungarian visitors often received. Several Hungarian returnees talked about being accused, either openly or covertly, of betraying Hungary by fleeing from the hardship to the rich West, where 'dollars are hanging on the trees, and all you have to do is to reach your hand to get them', as one of my participants formulated it. Returning Australian-Hungarians were often called 'Amerikás Magyar' in Hungary (see Andits 2008). The term implies that returnees cannot be regarded as real Hungarians any more, as they have lost connection with the present-day reality of the country and live in a dream-world of nostalgic memories.

The Discourse of Exclusion

The disappointments have generated a wide range of additional negative emotions within the diaspora which have undermined the community's sense of belonging to the new–old homeland and created a feeling of exclusion. First, the disappointments undermined the newly elected government's claim to be 'true democrats' in the eyes of the diaspora and created significant distrust towards Hungarian authorities. Several scholars have argued that distrust is one of the most widespread emotions in the Eastern European post-socialist political climate (Kalb *et al.* 1999; Mitszal 1996; Sevenhuijsen and Brinkgreve 2002; Sztompka 1999). I would argue that distrust also became a focal emotion within the Australian-Hungarian diaspora post-1989. A

community member stated, in a manuscript written for the Trianon Day commemoration in Melbourne in 1998:

> I am eliminating my ample archives and counting the number of the dead horses we were riding on with all of our energy and effort. [...] How many bitter disappointments we lived through during the last 10 years since the invader has got out of the country! [...] Our 'brothers in arms' *have stabbed us in the back several times*...[...] We are building brick by brick but somebody, often one of our allies, destroys everything. Our national leaders shrink away and subside into silence.

The collapse of trust between the *emigráció* and the new government proved to be a fertile ground in which a strong sense of anxiety was conceived. Even if community members were aware that communism was dead as a system of rule in Hungary, they nevertheless felt haunted by its encumbering legacy. A popular fear arose, fed by the climate of distrust towards the new authorities, that 'seemingly-democrats-but-in-reality-communist' forces would spy on the diaspora and try to destroy its homogeneity and power. Previous attempts on behalf of the Hungarian authorities during communist rule to 'manipulate' the expatriates abroad fuelled the exiles' sense of pride. Such attempts were ridiculed and reinforced the feeling of importance of the *emigráció*. However, after 1990 the suspicion that the 'new/old' political forces would try to monitor and destroy the overseas community distressed the diaspora elite and fed into their feelings of disappointment, distrust and sense of exclusion. This anxiety of connectedness however, does not completely overshadow the desire for inclusion in the diaspora. New organisations continue to emerge each year, trying for inclusion into the national body.

While we cannot talk about increased anxiety at the personal level, a discourse of exclusion and alienation has nevertheless developed among individual returnees. Instead of reconnection, return visits have often substantiated the longstanding separation from the old home (see Lomsky-Feder and Rapoport 2001). The experience of homecoming for many resulted in a 'second immigration'. After the taken-for-granted and long-cherished conceptions of home were shattered, in order to cope with the unpleasant and unexpected encounters, several Australian-Hungarians detached, for the second time, their cultural identity from the geographical homeland.

The Feeling of Ambivalence: Double-Voiced Discourses of Inclusion and Exclusion

The aftermath of the *rendszerváltás* produced a sense of *ambivalence* in the diasporic discourses in which the *hope* for dense connectedness to the homeland and the *anxiety* of such links are dialogically intertwined. This indicates a tension between the competing desires for connectivity and isolationism. These 'double-voiced' discourses index an ongoing negotiation attempting to come to terms with a 'new and yet paradoxically historic homeland' (Uhling 2004: 401), and also played an important part in the perception and shaping of homeland relations and the orientation of diaspora politics. The dilemma of whether or not to communicate with the

'democratically elected, but in reality non-democratic' governments has become a powerful and passionate debate within the *emigráció* community. However, the conflict did not create 'diasporic' and 'exilic' fractions within the community. Instead, exilic narratives often compete with diasporic dreams of connectedness.

After the loss of trust in the newly emerging state and due to the different anxieties the disappointments generated, certain voices in the diaspora called for the continuation of the comforting moral community of exile by regenerating the exilic narratives of separation. Several émigrés' insistence on using the old term *emigráció* to label the Hungarian community in Australia indicates a similar stance of exilic separation. Foreign Minister Géza Jeszenszky suggested in the Hungary-based newspaper *Új Magyarország* that the term '*emigráció*' had become old-fashioned and lost its validity; thus it should be replaced with the term 'Hungarian communities outside Hungary's borders'. However, this suggestion was not well received, as the diaspora elite insisted that the term '*emigráció*' referred to commitments for which unfortunately they alone were still responsible. Reinvented exilic voices called for non-communication with, and segregation from, the 'seemingly democratic' governments, and promoted independent action. A striking example is the emergence of a widely distributed pamphlet prior the visit of the then State President Árpád Göncz. The 1999 anonymous pamphlet tried to convince people to not attend the visit of the president to the Hungarian Community Centre in Melbourne. The pamphlet emphasised the president's shadowy past, and claimed that he had arrived with hidden intentions. It stated:

> Let's not go to his welcome, let's be absent from his celebration, let's not accept awards from him. If in any case we get around him, let's not celebrate him, let's not clap, let's not approach him. He and his sycophants should be followed by cool silence and reticence. That's what they deserve!

Other community members, however, considered the visit of the president an important milestone in the diaspora's inclusion into the homeland. A community member who attended the president's speech said the following:

> When Göncz started talking a couple of Hungarians who still did not realise that Communism has collapsed in Hungary long time ago started whistling. They wanted to humiliate him. They did not understand that we will lose by such actions. We have to keep connections to our homeland in order to be appreciated. We have to work on it hard. So when they started whistling, we in the front lines started clapping as a response. The room was filled with whistles and clapping, competing with each other.

Another example is the declaration of the *Ausztráliai és Új Zélandi Magyar Szövetség* (AUZMSZ or the Federal Council of Hungarian Associations in Australia and New Zealand) in October 2003. The declaration became both the accumulator of, and the springboard for, exilic voices and fear. After ex-communist parties were re-elected in Hungary in 2002 a decision was made by the representatives from all over Australia at

the federal meeting of the AUZMSZ, that Hungarian diaspora associations would cease all communication with the current Hungarian government. This decision created passionate debates within the community, as several organisations and individuals opposed the decision, depicting it as old-fashioned, irrational and contrary to the common good.

Even after 18 years, the *emigráció* still lives with disillusionment, anxiety and aspiration as defining tensions, depending on the actual political situation in Hungary. A prominent community member, Béla Kardos, who has been working on the building of the transnational bridge since 1989, bitterly concluded in a speech which was presented on the *Magyarország 2000* (Hungary 2000) meeting in 1997, where representatives of the Hungarian external and internal diasporas discussed the future of the Hungarian nation:

> The financial remittances of the Hungarian diasporas have always been welcomed in the homeland. However, our suggestions with regards to the democratic transformation were entirely disregarded. We have been completely excluded.

Three years later the same person wrote:

> Now, that Hungary is at the threshold of entering the European Union, the hundreds of Hungarian professionals who live in the West could be enormously useful in the negotiation processes. However, first we need to bind the ties together.

Similarly, ambivalence and confusion have been the hallmarks of individual return narratives. Despite all the experienced disillusionments, visiting Australian-Hungarians nevertheless struggle to carve their place in contemporary Hungary. I have witnessed several strategies by which returnees aim to enhance their feelings of inclusion and reconnection. Some migrants attempt to create an atmosphere in Hungary that echoes their memories and, thus, helps them reconnect to the 'desired' past and ignore the remaining 'undesired' past during their visits. Others try to engage with, and embrace, everyday reality in Hungary in order to revive their feelings of belonging. Similarly, returnees try to refute the *'Amerikás Magyar'* stereotype in different ways with more or less success. These attempts for reintegration are always characterised by the ambivalence of desire, disappointment and futility.

Conclusion

Hungary's newly won freedom and the expanded possibilities for transnational connections after 1989 raised new questions in the diaspora about what it meant to be a Hungarian in Australia (Satzewich 2002: 190). In considering the effects of the political transformations in Eastern Europe after 1989, we can see the Hungarian community in Australia as both a winner and a loser. Winner, because their status as émigrés officially moved from the non-accepted and neglected to an accepted but neglected status; and they were free to return and settle in Hungary, or be engaged in frequent border-crossing. At the same time, several community members feel that their

'self-sacrificing' work of decades in exile has been forgotten, their potential role as active participants in the life of the new democracy dismissed and their Hungarianness questioned after the *rendszerváltás* in Hungary. Although the emigrant community claimed the ability—material resources, ideological basis, connections, and the moral stance—to intervene effectively in Hungary's political, economic and cultural life, the desired bridge between the two communities did not materialise. The change of political regime resulted—contrary to the émigrés' expectations—neither in the development of a productive dialogue between the diaspora and the homeland institutions, nor in the formation of constructive and cooperative fora based on this dialogue. On the one hand, the new Hungarian 'discourse of the national' was characterised by inclusion; exemplified by the act of granting citizenship to émigrés and their descendants. On the other hand, it was exclusionary, as Hungarian governments and other institutions have not perceived it to be sufficiently in their interest to further build on and embody the potential for relationships and interactions theoretically enabled by moves such as inclusive citizenship. Access to and influence on powers in the homeland remained almost as remote for Hungarians in Australia as they had been formerly. In this sense, the infrastructure remains gestural only. It has offered a promise which, for Hungarians in Australia, has mostly delivered bitter disappointment. The article has demonstrated that the ambivalent experiences at the community level concur with those of individual Australian-Hungarians.

The focus on the emotional ambivalences and tensions within the diaspora enabled me to highlight and preserve the complexity of Australian-Hungarians' experiences after 1989 (Uhling 2004: 404). In turn, it is by examining this dualism and ambivalence—the simultaneous prevalence of desire, disdain and anxiety around connectedness—that this study can provide particularly fertile interpretive ground for considering ideas about migrants' sense of self and belonging (Uhling 2004: 391).

This article has demonstrated the dynamics between identification, emotions and political actions. It has shown how the initial positive emotions, such as hope and desire for connectedness, have provided a moral framework in which relations with the homeland were discussed and played out (see, for example, White 1990). Later on the political negotiations with Hungary have shaped the emotional discourses within the diaspora. The feelings of ambivalence, that is the 'double-voiced' discourses of desire, disappointment and distrust towards a relationship with Hungary continue to inform community members' thoughts and actions and impact on the processes of negotiating the *emigráció*'s relationship with Hungary, and its identity and sense of agency.

Acknowledgements

Special thanks to the many Australian-Hungarians who took time to share their opinions and assisted in my research. Thanks also go to Maruška Svašek (Queen's University), Denise Cuthbert (Monash University), Guy Doron (Inter Disciplinary Center—Herziliya), Philip Martin (University of Melbourne), Bruce Missingham (Monash University) and the anonymous *JEMS* reviewer for their extensive

comments on a previous version of this paper. This research was made possible by the Postgraduate Publication Grant from the Arts Faculty at Monash University.

References

Andits, P. (2007) The Bridges of Ambivalence: Australian-Hungarian Discourses after 1989. Melbourne: Monash University, unpublished PhD thesis.

Andits, P. (2008) 'Possible homecomings: Australian-Hungarians' attempts of reintegration in Hungary', in Nowicka, E. and Firouzbakhch, H. (eds) *Homecoming. The Study of Return Migrations.* Cracow: Zaklad Wydawniczy Nomos, 235–50.

Bakhtin, M.M. (1981) *The Dialogic Imagination: Four Essays.* Austin: University of Texas Press.

Berdahl, D. (2000) 'Introduction', in Berdahl, D., Bunzl, M. and Lampland, M. (eds) *Altering States: Ethnographies of Transition in Eastern Europe and the Former Soviet Union.* Ann Arbor: University of Michigan Press, 1–13.

Breytenbach, B. (1991) 'The long march from hearth to heart', *Social Research, 58*(1): 64–83.

Borbandi, G. (2006) *A Magyar Emigracio Eletrajza 1945–1985 (Portrait of the Hungarian Diaspora 1945–1985).* Online at: http://mek.oszk.hu/03400/03472/html/.

Bourdieu, P. (1985) 'The forms of capital', in Richardson, J.G. (ed.) *Handbook for Theory and Research for the Sociology of Education.* New York: Greenwood Press, 241–58.

Cohen, R. (1997) *Global Diasporas.* London: UCL Press.

Conradson, D. and McKey, D. (2007) 'Translocal subjectivities: mobility, connection, emotion', *Mobilities, 2*(2): 167–74.

Csapó, E. (1990) Az Ausztráliai Magyar Szövetség Javaslata Dr Jeszenszky Géza Külügyminiszter Úrhoz Az Ausztráliai Nemzeti Emigráció Szervezeteinek és a Magyar Külügyminisztériumnak Együttműködésére. Unpublished document.

Csapó, E. (1991) Letter to Pordány László, Hungarian Ambassador in Australia. Unpublished document.

Elster, J. (1996) 'Rationality and emotions', *The Economic Journal, 106*(438): 1386–97.

Emirbayer, M. and Goldberg, C.A. (2005) 'Pragmatism, Bourdieu, and collective emotions in contentious politics', *Theory and Society, 34*(5/6): 469–518.

Géfin, L. (1997) 'Still beyond the pale: Hungarian emigré writing after the collapse of communism', Special Issue: Refiguring Europe, *Symploke, 5*(1–2): 206–20.

Golanska-Ryan, J. (2006) 'Strategies of resistance in the Polish campaign against EU membership', in Svašek, M. (ed.) *Postsocialism: Politics and Emotions in Central and Eastern Europe.* Oxford: Berghahn, 159–77.

Hein, R. (2004) Humanitarian Responses in Australia to the Hungarian Revolution of 1956. Melbourne: Monash University, School of Historical Studies, unpublished PhD thesis.

Höhmann, H.-H. (2001) *Kultur als Bestimmungsfaktor der Transfromation im Osten Europas.* Bremen: Edition Temmen.

Huseby-Darvas, E. (2004) 'Extra Hungariam non est vita? The relationships between Hungarian immigrants and their homeland', in Markovitz, F. and Stefansson, A. (eds) *Homecomings; Unsettling Paths of Return.* Lanham, MD: Lexington Books, 76–90.

Kalb, D. and Tak, H. (1999) 'Out of control: a hidden history of power and water in a Polish city', *Focaal, 33*: 87–96.

Kalb, D., Svašek, M. and Tak, H. (1999) 'Approaching the new past in East-Central Europe', *Focaal: European Journal of Anthropology, 33*: 9–24.

Kivisto, P. (2001) 'Theorizing transnational immigration: a critical review of current efforts', *Ethnic and Racial Studies, 24*(4): 549–77.

Kunz, E. (1985) *The Hungarians in Australia.* Melbourne: AE Press.

Lemon, A. (2000) 'Talking transit and spectating transition: the Moscow metro', in Berdahl, D., Bunzl, M. and Lampland, M. (eds) *Altering States. Ethnographies of Transition in Eastern Europe and the Former Soviet Union*. Ann Arbor: University of Michigan Press, 14–39.

Leutloff-Grandits, C. (2006) 'Claiming ownership in postwar Croatia: the emotional dynamics of possession and repossession in Knin', in Svašek, M. (ed.) *Postsocialism: Politics and Emotions in Central and Eastern Europe*. Oxford: Berghahn, 115–34.

Lomsky-Feder, E. and Rapoport, T. (2001) 'Homecoming, immigration and the national ethos: Russian–Jewish homecomers reading Zionism', *Anthropological Quarterly*, *74*(1): 1–14.

Long, L.D. and Oxfeld, E. (2004) *Coming Home? Refugees, Migrants, and Those Who Stayed Behind*. Philadelphia: University of Pennsylvania Press.

Lutz, C.A. and White, G.M. (1986) 'The anthropology of emotions', *Annual Review of Anthropology*, *15*: 405–36.

Lutz, C.A. and Abu-Lughod, L. (1990) 'Introduction', in Lutz, C.A. and Abu-Lughod, L. (eds) *Language and the Politics of Emotion*. Cambridge: Cambridge University Press, 1–23.

Lyons, W. (1980) *Emotion*. Cambridge: Cambridge University Press.

Magocsi, P. (2005) 'In step or out of step with the times? Central Europe's diasporas and their homelands in 1918 and 1989', *Austrian History Yearbook*, *36*: 175.

Mihaylova, D. (2006) 'Social suffering and political protest: mapping emotions and power among Pomaks in postsocialist Bulgaria', in Svašek, M. (ed.) *Postsocialism: Politics and Emotions in Central and Eastern Europe*. Oxford: Berghahn, 53–73.

Misztal, B. (1996) *Trust in Modern Societies: The Search for the Bases of Social Order*. Cambridge: Polity.

Muller, B. (2006) 'The misgivings of democracy: personal resentment and alternating power in a Czech village', in Svašek, M. (ed.) *Postsocialism: Politics and Emotions in Central and Eastern Europe*. Oxford: Berghahn, 178–95.

Niedermüller, P. (1999) 'Rethinking history: time, past and nation in post-socialism', *Focaal: European Journal of Anthropology*, *33*: 25–36.

Panossian, R. (1998) *Between Ambivalence and Intrusion: Politics and Identity: Peoples in the Age of Nation-States*. London: Pluto.

Panossian, R. (2003) 'Courting a diaspora: Armenia–diaspora relations since 1998', in Østergaard-Nielsen, E. (ed.) *International Migration and Sending Countries: Perceptions, Policies and Transnational Relations*. Basingstoke: Palgrave Macmillan, 140–70.

Pomogats, B. (1994) *Nyugati Egbolt: Tanulmanyok a Nyugati Magyar irodalomrol*. Budapest: Magyar Iroszovetseg.

Reddy, W.M. (1997) 'Against constructionism: the historical ethnography of emotions', *Current Anthropology*, *38*(3): 327–51.

Ries, N. (1997) *Russian Talk: Culture and Conversation During Perestroika*. Ithaca, NY: Cornell University Press.

Rosaldo, I.R. (1984) 'Grief and a headhunter's rage: on the cultural force of emotions', in Bruner, E.M. (ed.) *Text, Play, and Story. The Construction and Reconstruction of Self and Society*. Illinois: Waveland Press, 178–95.

Rupnik, J. (1995) 'The post-totalitarian blues', *Journal of Democracy*, *6*(2): 61–73.

Rushdie, S. (1992) *Imaginary Homelands: Essays and Criticism, 1981–91*. London: Granta.

Said, E. (1983) *The World, the Text, and the Critic*. London: Vintage.

Said, E. (1992) 'Reflections on exile', in Ferguson, R. (ed.) *Out There: Marginalization and Contemporary Culture*. London: MIT Press, 357–66.

Satzewich, V. (2002) *The Ukrainian Diaspora*. London: Routledge.

Shain, Y. (1995) 'Ethnic diasporas and US foreign policy', *Political Science Quarterly*, *109*(5): 811–42.

Sevenhuijsen, S. and Brinkgreve, C. (2002) 'Trust, familiarity and otherness: how to think about trust using the work of Norbert Elias', *Focaal*, *39*: 149–60.

Skrbis, Z. (2002) 'The emotional historiography of ventologists: Slovene diaspora, memory and nationalism', *Focaal: European Journal of Anthropology, 39*: 41–56.

Skrbiš, Z. (2006) 'The first Europeans: fantasy of Slovenian venetologists: emotions and nationalist imaginings', in Svašek, M. (ed.) *Postsocialism: Politics and Emotions.* Oxford and New York: Berghahn, 138–58.

Slobin, G. (2001) 'The "homecoming" of the first wave diaspora and its cultural legacy', *Slavic Review, 60*(3): 513–29.

Stefansson, A. (2004) 'Sarajevo suffering: homecoming and the hierarchy of homeland hardship', in Markowitz, F. and Stefansson, A. (eds) *Homecomings: Unsettling Path of Return.* Lanham MD: Lexington Books, 54–75.

Svašek, M. (2002) 'Narratives of "home" and "homeland": the symbolic construction and appropriation of the Sudeten German heimat', *Identities: Global Studies in Culture and Power, 9*(4): 495–518.

Svašek, M. (2006) 'Introduction', in Svašek, M. (ed.) *Postsocialism: Politics and Emotions in Central and Eastern Europe.* Oxford: Berghahn, 1–33.

Sztompka, P. (1999) *Trust: A Sociological Theory.* Cambridge: Cambridge University Press.

Tsuda, T. (2004) 'When home is not the homeland: the case of Japanese Brazilian ethnic return migration', in Markowitz, F. and Stefansson, A. (eds) *Homecomings: Unsettling Path of Return.* Lanham, MD: Lexington Books, 125–45.

Uhling, G. (2004) 'Sitting on suitcases: ambivalence and ambiguity in the migration intentions of Crimean Tatar women', *Journal of Refugee Studies, 15*(4): 388–408.

Vasta, E. (1993) 'Multiculturalism and ethnic identity: the relationship between racism and resistance', *The Australian and New Zealand Journal of Sociology, 29*(2): 209–25.

Veenis, M. (1999) 'Consumption in East Germany: the seduction and betrayal of things', *Journal of Material Culture, 4*(1): 79–112.

Verdery, K. and Burawoy, M. (1999) 'Introduction', in Burawoy, M. and Verdery, K. (eds) *Uncertain Transition: Ethnographies of Change in the Postsocialist World.* Lanham, MD: Rowman & Littlefield, 1–18.

Wanner, C. (1998) *Burden of Dreams: History and Identity in Post-Soviet Ukraine.* Philadelphia: Pennsylvania State University Press.

White, G.M. (1990) 'Moral discourse and the rhetoric of emotions', in Lutz, C.A. and Abu-Lughod, L. (eds) *Language and the Politics of Emotion.* Cambridge: Cambridge University Press/Paris: Maison des Sciences de l'Homme, 46–68.

Emotions, Emotives and Political Negotiations: Transforming Relationships in the Bohemian–Bavarian Border Area[1]

Maruška Svašek

Since the turn of the century an increasing number of scholars working in the fields of anthropology, sociology, cultural studies, geography and political science have argued it necessary to include a focus on emotions when analysing identity formation and mobility in specific socio-political and spatial settings. Joyce Davidson, Liz Bondi and Mick Smith (2005: 3), for example, presented the perspective of 'emotional geography', defining it as a perspective that attempts to understand emotion – experientially and conceptually – in terms of its 'socio-spatial mediation and articulation, rather than as entirely interiorised subjective mental states'. Twenty years earlier, anthropologists such as Lutz and White (1986: 420) had also sought to counter the notion that emotions were nothing more than personal inner feelings. They argued that 'emotions are, in many societies, a critical link in cultural interpretations of action', and defined emotions as culturally specific discourses that inform perceptions of self and society, and shape relations of power.

While the role of emotions in many situations is subtle and elusive, in many others it is dominant and obvious. Consider, for instance the role played by emotions in state acts of mourning, and their emotional impact on the individuals participating. Can an anthropology of emotions help us better define the similarities and differences between the emotionally charged displays of heartbroken generals in North Korea, weeping with despair at the death of the Dear Leader Kim Jong-Il, and the mournful appearance and cathartic words of Tony Blair at the funeral of Princess Diana? While different cultural expectations attached to displays of emotions can vary wildly from one cultural context to the next, comparable factors often surface when analysing their impact on identity formation, and on power relations between groups. It is equally important to consider how the identities of political actors themselves might be influenced by their own emotional role play, in addition to more cynically adjudging their deftness at using emotions to their own objective political advantage.

Emotions as Bodily Experience in Spatial Settings

Margot Lyon (1995: 258) has noted that while 'social relations themselves may generate emotions', felt emotions can also have 'social consequences'. John Laevitt has similarly argued that emotions are felt and played out through embodied social action, as 'emotions are felt in bodily experience, not just known or thought or appraised' (Laevitt 1996: 526;). Inspired by the writings of Spinoza and the Russian psychologist

L.S. Vygotsky, he suggested that emotions should be regarded as 'experiences learned and expressed in the body in social interactions through the mediation of systems of signs, verbal and non-verbal' (Laevitt 1996: 526; see also Lyon and Barbalet 1994).

But how does this perspective link up to an interest in emotional geographies and mobility, in the affective dimensions of people's identifications as they create and move through multi-sensorial settings? In previous work, I have argued that mobile people and things are mutually constitutive through relationships of transformation and transition, 'transition' referring to the changing value, meanings, and emotional efficacy of objects, and 'transformation' alluding to the dynamic ways in which subjects experience and relate to the changing social and material environments they find themselves in (Svašek 2010: 65, 2012). I followed Alfred Gell in his theory of object agency, acknowledging the influence that non-human agents may have on people's subjectivity and actions. Unlike Latour's generalising network theory that, as Yael Navaro-Yashin (2009: 8–9) has pointed out, assumes that 'subjects and objects are always already engaged with and entangled in one another', Gell's approach lends itself for a historically sensitive and ethnographically detailed analysis of the emergence of concrete forms of embodied emotional engagement.

This chapter explores emotional dimensions of subjectivity and identity formation through time and space in the very specific geographical area of the Czech–German borderland, at a point when for the first time in some four decades the physical barrier between these two groups was, quite literally, lifted overnight. The analysis incorporates the view that frontiers are 'domains of contested power, in which local, national, and international groups negotiate relations of subordination and control' (Wilson and Donnan 1998: 10). Numerous studies have convincingly shown that border peoples in different parts of the world demonstrate ambiguous identities because they are pulled in different directions by political, economic, cultural, and linguistic factors (see, for example, Cheater 1998; Douglass 1998; Kearney 1998).[2] A focus on emotions helps to unravel the complexity of these processes, enriching the study of transit and transformation in border areas. Issues of mobility, translocal subjectivity and object agency are a central theoretical concern. The main question is how, after the ending of the Cold War, emotional discourses, practices and embodied experiences shaped socio-spatial life in the Bohemian–Bavaria border region, and vice versa. As we shall see, an evocative history of occupation, forced migration and marginality had left its marks, not only on the landscape but also in people's memories.

Before turning our attention to this particular border region and its complex history, two propositions about the relationship between politics and emotions need to be presented (see also Svašek 2006). First, emotions are intrinsic to politics, a proposition that runs counters to Plato's theory of rational action forming the basis of the political process, but which finds support in the work of his student, Aristotle, who convincingly argued in his work on rhetorics, that political negotiations are interpersonal processes in which people actively manipulate one another's feelings (1941: 1380). Emotional discourses, practices and embodied experiences may arise from and influence local, national and transnational power dynamics, for example in contexts of post-socialist transformation (Borneman 1998; Jansen 1998; Svašek 2006). The case discussed in this chapter will demonstrate the significance of the emotional dimensions of post-Cold War political negotiations at personal, communal, interregional and international levels.

The second proposition is that, while politics are inherently emotional, emotional processes do not always have a political meaning or impact. Privately felt nostalgia, for example, may simply express a psychological longing for a sense of safety associated with childhood. Such feelings can, however, be politicised, for instance when one ethnic group is framed as a security threat to another (Leutloff-Grandits 2006), or when public displays of frustration and anger, such as during televised street protests, function as political demands (Mihaylova 2006). But why is it that emotional expressions can become instrumental acts with a potentially political impact? Building on speech act theory, Reddy (1999: 270) suggested that emotion claims, 'emotives' in his terminology, constitute 'a special class of utterance (...) similar to performatives in that emotives do things to the world'. The practice of claiming an emotion through verbal expression ('I am angry; we are delighted') has a performative dimension that can be both self-exploring and transformative, while also being effective as a strategic act intended to shape attitudes and relationships of power. Emotives, in other words, 'are themselves instruments for directly changing, building, hiding, and intensifying emotions' (Reddy 1999: 270). Emotives negotiate subjectivity, allowing speakers to change or maintain consistency around the pursuit of certain aims ('I am angry' – But am I, I just said I was? Should I be? Yes I am truly angry, I no longer want to be accommodating).

This chapter seeks to understand how, during and after the disappearance of the Iron Curtain, Czech and German citizens, politicians, priests and Sudeten German postwar expellees used emotives within specific socio-spatial and material contexts to actively pursue personal and political aims.

The Cold War at an End: Initial Euphoria

On 23 December 1989, the West German Minister of Foreign Affairs, Hans-Dietrich Genscher, and his Czech counterpart, Jiří Dienstbier, symbolically ended Cold War relations between their countries. Just outside the village of Nové Domky, not far from the border crossing Waidhaus-Rozvadov, they ritually cut through a barbed-wire fence that for over 40 years had formed part of the heavily defended eastern bloc. To increase the festive mood, the German Musikverein Waidhaus played brass band music, and the cheering public waved flags and shouted 'Freedom, freedom!'. Responding to their enthusiasm, the ministers handed out pieces of the 'Iron Curtain', an act reminiscent of the transformation of the Berlin Wall into souvenirs of history (cf. Sporrer 1990). Their symbolic performance was intended to intensify the sense of public euphoria. The pieces of wire and chunks of concrete symbolised four decades of mutual enmity and fear, and its destruction became an expression of hope for a better future in which socio-spatial and political relations could be redefined. The Czechoslovak and German governments needed to actively reimagine and physically change the Bohemian–Bavarian border as 356 kilometres of potential contact, especially as Czechoslovakia had expressed its intention to apply for NATO and EU membership. Numerous legal and practical hurdles had to be overcome. It took another six months before the compulsory visa requirements were abolished and the heavily defended Cold War border was transformed into a less forbidding borderline.

The shift in geopolitical perception did not take place only at the level of governmental policy but also at local level, where the spatial reality of living close to a state boundary was experienced on a daily basis. For a period of over 40 years, the border populations had lived on the peripheries of two hostile ideological blocs, namely the capitalist west and the communist east. Inevitably, this had influenced and coloured perceptions of one another. While official discourses had constructed them as mutually antagonistic 'capitalist' and 'communist ' entities, curiosity to know more about one another had persisted. In the post-Cold War era, the fact that the line of separation from those on the other side was often just a few kilometres wide, created conditions of potential identification.

The Cold War had not only divided the two border populations, but had also helped maintain economic underdevelopment and political marginalisation that often characterises frontier zones. Between 1948 and 1989, the governments in Prague and Bonn had largely regarded the regions as zones of defence, investing little in their civic development. It must be noted that the inhabitants of eastern Bavaria were nevertheless much wealthier than those of western Bohemia, given the postwar boom that characterised life in much of postwar West Germany, and the government's decentralising federal policies. On the Czech side of the border, the dramatic results of economic mismanagement, overcentralisation, and strict military control were clearly visible. People lived in poor or often dilapidated housing, and to deter Czechoslovak citizens from fleeing the country, a wide strip of land beside the border was accessible only with a special military pass. With the disappearance of the Iron Curtain, many inhabitants of the Bavarian–Bohemian frontier zone hoped their economic woes would improve, and that the changing socio-spatial and political conditions would offer better prospects for them and their children. As we shall see in the next section, those living in communities close to the border particularly welcomed the changes.

Joyful Emotives and Countermemories of Fear

The sense of euphoria at the fall of the Iron Curtain had direct social and political consequences for large numbers of border communities that began to forge cross-border ties (cf. Svašek 1999). In the spring of 1990, Czechs and Germans from the Bohemian village of Broumov and the small Bavarian town of Mähring launched a series of regular meetings at the Broumov–Mähring border crossing. Co-presence in shared space was essential to building trust between old foes. People who had been expected by their governments to view each other as ideological opponents for 41 years, now chatted and drank beer while hanging over the crossing barrier. They reviewed their previous feelings toward one another that had been fuelled by Cold War stereotypes, and after several friendly exchanges during which they had to overcome their own language barriers with a combination of sign language and broken German, they agreed the best next step to deepening their new ties was to organise a communal party to celebrate the ending of the Cold War (cf. Der Neue Tag 1989; Zrenner 1990).

On the first of May 1990, two months *before* the official abolition of the compulsory visa requirement, the local border crossing threw caution to the wind and raised its barriers for one day so that the festivities could begin. On the Czech side, a banner welcomed the Germans, saying: *Broumov vítá Mähring* ('Broumov welcomes Mähring'), countered by a banner on the German side declaring: *Herzlich Willkommen* ('Our Heartfelt Welcome!'). The transformation of the physical border into an open door

invitation proved highly significant with more than 15,000 Czechs seizing the opportunity to pour across the border into Mähring, with similar numbers crossing in the opposite direction. The German newspapers described the event as a historic restoration of friendship. *Der Neue Tag* reported that Czech and German priests 'fell into each other's arms and prayed', and suggested the event marked 'the beginning of reconciliation and friendship'. The speeches by Czech and German representatives were highly optimistic about future cooperation, with the Czech Mayor reportedly declaring: 'We will build a new house without weapons, so that we can live in peace' (Sporrer 1990). The local powerholders clearly used emotional rhetoric to create an atmosphere of mutual trust and goodwill to stimulate future collaboration at both a communal and political level.

The local media claimed the optimistic mood was universally shared by all inhabitants. Subsequently, when compulsory visa requirements were officially abolished on 1 July 1990 six new border crossings were ceremonially opened, and local German newspapers declared *ein riesiges Volksfest*, *ein Festival der Lebensfreude*, expressing happiness and content about this regional transformation (Der Neue Tag 1990). The optimistic reports, however, ignored the complexity of feelings and antipathy many border inhabitants still harboured about these changes. Czechs and Germans, especially those of the wartime generation, warned their compatriots against their over exuberance, recounting their wartime and Cold War stories. Germany and Czechoslovakia had been enemies throughout significant parts of their shared history, culminating in the twentieth century with the extreme events of the Second World War and the subsequent Sudeten German expulsions. That feelings of mutual fear and loathing had not been erased highlights an important area of research in the study of emotions: the impact of past experiences on people's present perceptions. As Ilona Irwin-Zarecka noted:

> [A]s people first articulate and share the sense they make of their past, it is their experience, in all its emotional complexity, that serves as a key reference point. If their interpretive strategies are indeed products of culture, the plausibility of resulting accounts depends on the fit with the individual's emotional reality. (Irwin-Zarecka 1994: 17)

To understand people's use of emotive terms when talking about the past, a conceptual distinction between *remembered* and *re-experienced* emotions is helpful. 'Remembered emotions' refer to memories of past emotions that do not cause a (similar) emotional reaction in the person recalling them. 'Remember how angry I was?', somebody might say with a smile, while being emotionally detached from the earlier experience of anger. By contrast, 're-experienced emotions' are past feelings that are remembered *and* have the power to re-evoke the same emotions once again, possibly prompting people (individuals and their audiences) to take a particular stance on an issue. As we shall see in the course of the chapter, emotives referring to past experiences ('I was afraid', 'we were happy') might also open up space for momentary reflection on past and present subjectivity, in this case influenced by new possibilities offered by a border region in transformation.

A Troubled History

After the fall of the Iron Curtain, when the Broumov–Mähring border crossing was officially opened, thousands of people participated in the celebrations and took the opportunity to view life across the border. People living in the Bavarian districts of Tirschenreuth and Weiden, as well as the Bohemian district of Tachov could now travel relatively easily in the cross-border area. Mathilde was one of the many Germans who attended the celebrations. The event meant far more to her than to the indigenous Bavarians.

Mathilde was born in 1940 in the Bohemian village of Brand (today mainly known by the Czech name of Milíře). When I interviewed her in 1997 at her Bavarian home, she informed me that at the impressionable young age of six, her family been forcibly expelled from Czechoslovakia along with over 3 million other Sudeten Germans.[3] The Sudeten German expulsions immediately followed the liberation of Czechoslovakia from Nazi rule, two months before the signing of the Potsdam agreements. Between May and October 1945 the Sudeten Germans, whose families had lived for centuries in the Czech Lands that later became Czechoslovakia, lost their rights of domicile overnight. The confiscation of their property was given legal basis by a number of presidential decrees.

In the aftermath of the war anti-German feeling was understandably rife. There were many instances of Czechs taking revenge on the German population. From May to November 1945, a period known as the 'wild expulsion' (*wilde Austreibung*), thousands of Sudeten Germans, in particular those living in ethnically mixed areas, were terrorised, maltreated, and brutally murdered.[4] In 1946, during the 'organised expulsion' (*geregelte Vertreibung*), the Germans were generally treated in a more humane manner (cf. Hamperl 1996; Staněk 1991). The village where Mathilde came from was situated in the almost purely German district of Tachau, where the 'terror' had been less severe than in mixed Czech–German districts. Nevertheless, their sudden expulsion and loss of *Heimat* traumatised many (cf. Hamperl 1996) who often chose to settle in Bavaria in areas not far from the Czech border.

After the expulsion, Mathilde and her family had moved to Tirschenreuth, a small Bavarian town situated only 12 kilometres from the Broumov–Mähring border. Her former home of Brand had been renamed 'Milíře', and had been repopulated by Orthodox Ruthenians from Romania and Czechs and Slovaks from the Czechoslovak interior. Tachau had been renamed Tachov. Ironically, even though her birthplace was just 20 kilometres away she had never dared visit it during the Cold War. With the fall of the Iron Curtain and the opening of the borders a complete new socio-spatial context was created, which despite her painful memories of the expulsion, could now be revisited and given a more hopeful, future-oriented place in her unfolding life story.

Emotions through Space: Nostalgia, Fear and Hope

Expellees visiting the Broumov–Mähring border-opening celebrations shared feelings of nostalgia and curiosity: how had their *Heimat* changed over four decades? It was this mix of emotions that prompted Mathilde to venture into her past by cycling across the border to her *Heimatsdorf* (home village). As she recalled:

> In 1990 the border crossing Mähring–Promenhof [Promenhof is the old German name for Broumov] was opened (. . .). And when my husband and I read about it we said: 'We should really go, and have a look at the Czech side' [. . .] So we loaded our bicycles on the roof rack and drove to Mähring, from where we cycled to the border. There were so many people! Thousands! [. . .] It was a lovely, warm day.

Cycling between the two border towns, surrounded by large crowds of Germans and Czechs, Mathilde felt light hearted and experienced the event as a form of celebration. Judging from her tone of voice, cycling the first few kilometres into Bohemia, she had still felt carefree and excited about the fact that she was back in her old *Heimat*:

> We had our bicycles and it was nice weather, so we cycled, and cycled, and just kept on cycling further and further. The sun was shining brightly and we were already far inside the Czech Republic, and we saw a sign to Tachau. So we said, let's cycle just a bit further, a bit further in the direction of Tachau.

The tone in her voice changed, however, when she remarked: 'We no longer saw any Germans, because they did not venture that far as they were all on foot.' Back in a region in which the expulsions had taken place, moving away from the safety of the German border, she was increasingly haunted by memories and stories of the expulsion. Nevertheless, her desire to get closer to her home village overwhelmed feelings of anxiety, so she cycled on:

> When we saw Tachau in the distance, [we said]: 'We have to go.' When we arrived it was half past three in the afternoon ... It was not that far anymore to our home village of Brand. We did not speak a word of Czech and nobody understood us, because, until 1990, nobody went to Czechoslovakia. In Tachau, there were no Germans, and there was nothing. Today it is different, today they understand a bit of German. [But then] we asked everybody: 'Brand, Brand, Brand, where is Brand, how do we get to Brand?' [Finally] a woman understood us and directed us so we cycled on and on.

The experience of people not understanding any German, not even the German name of their home village of Brand made Mathilde suddenly feel like a stranger in her *Heimat*. She recognised only the landscape. The disjuncture between the nostalgically remembered homeland and her alienating experience of a foreign community now living in it painfully re-evoked her forced expulsion. She said it suddenly felt like a 'nightmare':

> We suddenly saw our church [of Brand] there all the time [on the hill] in front of us, but there was a new road leading around a reservoir that had not been there before [. . .] so it was much further than I remembered. It was late, almost evening, and we were alone in the Czech Republic, my husband and I. I began to cry and we were so tired as well. My husband said 'It cannot be much further any more, it cannot be far.' So finally we cycled up the Church Hill (Kirchenberg).

Mathilde was physically and emotionally exhausted. The sight of the familiar church, the landscape changed to make way for a huge reservoir where once houses had stood,

and the sudden understanding that the whole neighbouring village had been erased without a trace was an acute emotional shock. She repeated again the emotion of feeling vulnerable, of being entirely alone as a German on Czech territory. When I asked whether she had felt fear (obvious from the tone of her voice), she almost screamed and alluded to the physical dimensions of emotional experience: 'I was so afraid my heart was pounding in my chest!' As Karen Lysaght (2005: 137) noted in a study of fear and uses of space in Belfast, such bodily factors should be examined in tandem with cognitive processes, as cultural factors play an important role in the embodiment of feelings: '[I]t is only through awareness that a particular thing represents a threat, that individuals actually experience fear.' In Mathilde's case, her changed perception of the environment as a place inhabited by potentially dangerous people was also partially shaped by post-expulsion Sudeten German discourses of collective victimhood (Svašek 2005: 202; see also the introduction to the book).

When Mathilde used first-person emotives of fear to speak about her past anxiety, ('I was so scared'), her body language clearly suggested that old fears had resurfaced during the trip. Evidently, as she cycled in her former homeland, her re-experienced anxiety differed from the fear she had felt as a 6-year-old girl. As she had grown into an adult, and heard and read stories about the *wilde Austreibung*, she had reframed her past feeling as embodied proof of 'collective Sudeten German suffering'. In the light of the recent political changes in Czechoslovakia, however, her old fears were also countered by new hopes and expectations.

In the context of the interview, the claim to past anxieties arose directly out of the interview situation and functioned as an appraisal of that past. The emotive ('I was so scared') was directed at me, and she expected empathy.[5] Reddy (ibid.) has called this function of emotives their 'relational intent', arguing that 'statements about emotions in social life occur most frequently as part of (or appear to designate) specific scenarios or relationships'. This social feature of emotional claims unveils their power as tools of political negotiation, both within and outside borderlands.

When they finally reached the village, and Mathilde entered the church, she was overwhelmed by emotions. She recounted:

> We stopped near the church to have a look. My husband said 'There's a pub down there that'll have lemonade and beer. Sit down in the church, and I'll go and get us something.' So I sat down in the church, and my husband gave the sexton 20 Deutschmarks. 'For the church, it's a donation', he said. The sexton lit a few candles, and he went up and rang the bells. I was alone in the church, and I just cried!

When I suggested that she had remembered her childhood, she replied:

> Yes, I remembered, I remembered a lot of things. The church, and how I used to sit in the church, and the candles, and how they used to take photographs there, and the annual festival that used to be held on the Festplatz in front of it. It was all very moving.

Her pre-expulsion memories, that in Sudeten German texts are often referred to as a timeless, mythical paradise, temporarily pushed away her anxiety caused by the trauma of the expulsion itself. For a brief moment, her spatially mediated feelings of belonging to this place dominated her sense of self. Once outside the safe walls of the church,

however, her fears returned. 'By now it was already evening, and we were all alone in the Czech Republic! That was seriously bad!' [*Es war ganz schlimm.*] Her comment demonstrates that, when analysing socio-spatial experiences, space must not be regarded as a static location on the map, but must rather be understood in the context of physical and natural changes in the given environment. While in Mathilde's case, her personal history of forced displacement was a major influence on how she perceived her movement through the Czech borderland, other factors included the sunset, the cooling temperature, and impending darkness.

Being so close to her home village, however, her sense of longing had been greater than her sense of fear, and she had cycled on to see the spot on which her old family house had once stood. Her father who had visited the village on one occasion during the Cold War had already told her that it had been knocked down, so she was mentally prepared for that, but she explained that she had instead approached the neighbour's house expecting to experience a similar feeling of recognition and estrangement as she had felt in the church. On seeing the house she felt some relief at seeing American flags on display behind all the windows rather than any emblems of the communist east: '"Look!", I said, "thank God, everything [i.e. Western civilisation] is not so far away!" [*Es ist doch nicht so weit weg, alles.*] To me they were like rays of hope.'

As in a fairy tale, the story had a happy ending. The Czech owner of the house, Jirka, came out and invited Mathilde and her husband in. Even though the memory of fear remained, her actual fear disappeared. The owner's wife spoke a few words of German, and offered them schnitzel with bread and a glass of beer. When the German couple decided to leave because it was getting late, and they still needed to cycle all the way back to Mähring, their Czech host protested and offered to take them and their bicycles by car and trailer. The hospitality offered by Jirka and his wife, and the gratitude of Mathilde and her husband functioned as emotives that negotiated their relationship in a changing political landscape. For Mathilde, the interview provided an opportunity not only to recall, relive and share some of her feelings, but also to reflect on new affective possibilities in the redefined post-Cold War environment, as she pointed out that she and her husband had become friends with Jirka and his wife, making regular visits to each other's houses.[6]

Tackling *Mutual* Distrust: Cross-border Interaction and Cooperation

Not all Czechs, however, were as welcoming as Jirka. During fieldwork conducted between 1991 and 1993, several people told me that on the night before the official opening of the Bohemian–Bavarian border, inhabitants from the Czech village of Lesná, also known by the German name of Schönwald, had been terrified of an imminent invasion by Sudeten Germans. Arming themselves with guns, sticks and pitchforks, they had defended the forest roads leading to the border. The story, described by some of Lesná's inhabitant as sheer nonsense, illustrated that the renegotiation of Czech–German relations in the border area was not without its complexities.

The dramatic political change, however, did allow Czechs to travel back and forth to Germany, and to challenge their stereotypical views of the old enemy. Many Czechs, especially those living close to the border even began to learn German, and a considerable number found jobs in the Oberpfalz district. Temporarily living in Bavaria as migrant workers, or commuting to Germany for jobs, meant they profited from the much higher wages. They also met Germans who now travelled without restrictions to

west Bohemia to go shopping, and visit tourist attractions such as Karlovy Vary and Mariánské Lázně. Local politicians, mayors, and teachers on both sides began looking for ways to cooperate. Cities and schools formalised their contacts through community links and partnerships (cf. Giegold and Otto 1994), and in the Czech border city of Cheb, a number of intellectuals sought ways to cooperate on a larger, regional scale. Gradually, more local politicians became interested in the formation of a larger framework of euregional cooperation. The Czechs especially, regarded it as a way to increase their regional autonomy from Prague. An idea to join together four Czech and two German districts, and call it *Euregion Egrensis*, was proposed in 1992 (cf. Houžvička 1993, 1994; Svašek 1999).[7] The spatial reclassification reflected the plans to include the Czech Republic in the EU, and can be regarded as a sign of Brussels' policy of decentralisation, expressed by the slogan 'Europe of the Regions' (cf. Cooke, Christiansen and Schienstock 1997; Preston 1997: 195–209).

The propagation of euregional cooperation rested heavily on standard discourses, common in other European frontier zones. Transnational problems such as environmental pollution and illegal cross-border movements of people, goods, and money were central issues. To find support for the new cross-border policy, the adherents defined these problems as major causes of concern, and argued that they could not be tackled by individual state governments or local authorities alone. Another issue was the problem of social, political and economic marginality. As noted before, border peoples often have a peripheral existence within their own countries, and receive less financial support for the development than communities closer to state centres. The strengthening of cross-border cooperation, loyalties and identities, was presented as one solution. New symbols of shared space and identity meant to change spatial and territorial perceptions. A colourful symbol was designed as a visual emblem for the euregion, and a new map was printed outlining its territory. In the new geographic scheme, the Iron Curtain was transformed into a much less important, intra-regional boundary. The tourist guide *Museums in Euregion Egrensis: A Journey through Time and History* even printed a map of Egrensis in which the Czech–German state border had totally disappeared.

Memory and the Politicisation of Anti-German Feelings

Czechs who had experienced the Second World War, and who still distrusted their former foe, did not welcome such developments. 'You can't trust Germans', I was told frequently by Czech border inhabitants. Communists and republicans especially were sceptical of policies for closer cross-border cooperation, and found the high number of expelled Sudeten Germans who actively supported euregional cooperation disturbing. Continuously reminding people of the Nazi terror, they attempted to stir up anti-German feeling. Newspaper articles warned readers that Germany was still a nation to be feared. The communist newspaper *Halo noviny* reported that:

> [T]ransferred Germans do not hide their aim of taking back land, because without their own land, the Sudeten Germans are threatened with extinction as a national group, in as much as they are threatened by integration with the population among whom they live. They do not want to return to a Czech national state, they do not even want minority rights at a European level. They want land. It is of

> secondary importance to them whether that land will be 'Freistaat Sudetenland', or another federal land of Germany. (Čtvrtek 1992)

Halo noviny interpreted the creation of a new Czech–German geographical unit as an act of anti-Czech territoriality, an act that strongly reminded them of the assimilation of the Sudetenland by the Third Reich in 1938. Jiří Frajdl, who worked for the same newspaper, stated that *Euregion Egrensis* was 'an old Nazi plan', a conspiracy between pro-German Czechs and anti-Czech Germans, intended to undermine the independence of the Czech Republic Frajdl 1994.

The idea of a conspiracy was unintentionally reinforced by Cheb's Mayor, František Linda, when he attempted to prohibit a planned demonstration by the Club of the Czech Border Area (*Klub českého pohraničí*), an association established by Czechs who were afraid that the Germans would attempt to increase their power in the Bohemian border area. According to Linda, an adherent of Czech–German euregional cooperation, the demonstrators' (mainly communists and republicans) true goal was to increase Czech–German tension, and to 'inflame national hatred'. The Club appealed against Linda's decision to prohibit the commemoration. The High Court in Prague ruled in their favour, and the ban on the protest was repealed. On 24 September 1994 a few hundred people gathered on Cheb's main square, carrying banners with the slogan 'No Repeat of Munich', 'Cheb must stay Czech', and 'People beware of the Sudeten Germans' (ibid).

This demonstrates that the painful memories of German terror and oppression were easily evoked in the post-Cold War political arena. Through powerful rhetoric, people were reminded of past fears, and this hampered euregional and European identification. The following section will show how priests and local politicians attempted to allay such fears by creating emotional contexts in which Czechs and Germans could willingly cooperate and reconcile.

Managing Emotions through Divine Power

Czech and German representatives of different churches who regarded it as their Christian duty to stimulate reconciliation made strenuous efforts to establish cross-border contacts. Father Götz, a young German priest who headed a Catholic parish in the border town of Bärnau, told me in 1996 that: 'It is our task to retain peace. I mean, Christ says "(....) the peace given by Christ comes from the heart through the reconciliation with God [and] the forgiving of sins".'

In the same year, the Orthodox Father Hausar from the Czech village of Lesna noted:

> Up to the present day, the hatred against the Germans, against the [German] nation, is deeply rooted in some people. I always take the Christian viewpoint, [and there is] a fundamental difference between the approach taken by such people and the Christian approach. I now talk from a Christian viewpoint: there is a proverb saying that 'Christians must hate sins but love sinners.' If a German commits an offence against somebody I will condemn his deed but [at the same time] I will love that person because through love and forgiveness, the relations can be restored.

Both priests conceptualised negative emotions such as jealousy and hatred as powerful forces that should be countered by divine power and faith; feelings of hate and fear should be transformed into love and trust through personal reconciliation with God.

Priest and ministers used the performative context of the sermon to convince their congregations. To get their message across, some were quite inventive performers. 'Where is Hitler? ... where is Stalin? ... and where is Jesus?!!', shouted a German Protestant minister in Milířе's Orthodox Church during the Easter ceremonies in 1998. He had been invited to this Czech village (Mathilde's place of birth) by the local priest, Father Hausar, who had asked him to deliver a short sermon on Easter Sunday to the Orthodox congregation.[8] His powerful performance showed that:

> [T]he dramatic quality of ritual does more than define roles (...), it also provokes emotional response. Just as emotions are manipulated in the theatre through the varied stimuli of light, colour, gesture, movement, voice, so too these elements and others give rituals a means of generating powerful feelings. (Kertzer 1988: 11)

The reference to Hitler, Stalin, and Jesus undermined the image of Germans as 'the fearful archenemy' and emphasised that the Germans had not been the only enemy of the Czechs. The classification of Hitler as an evil German *individual* deconstructed the totalising image of the German Danger, and created a semantic space for more positive images of Germans. The sermon stressed that human force was limited, and God would help them find the strength to restore damaged relationships. In Reddy's (1999: 272) terminology, they would find 'emotional liberty', 'the freedom (...) to undergo conversion experiences and life-course changes involving numerous contrasting incommensurable factors'.

After 1990, an increasing number of local Catholic, Protestant and Orthodox priests established contacts with colleagues from across the border, and actively propagated political reconciliation.[9] By May 1997 35 of the 49 cross-border links between Bavaria and Bohemia were between religious parishes. The religious connections were also advocated on a higher, euregional level as, from 1993 onwards, *Euregion Egrensis* subsidized *Euregional Church Day*. This ecumenical annual event combined political and religious discourses of reconciliation. In 1996, the slogan was 'Under one heaven, we will find ways to each other.' A Czech–German booklet, published for the occasion, referred to the feelings of fear and mistrust still evident in the region (Beyhl and Libal: 1996). It included fragments from an open letter written by Wilfried Beyhl, a member of the Church Assembly in Bayreuth, in which the author tried to dispel Czech fear about a German invasion:

> As Germans we did not come with property claims, but as messengers of reconciliation, and we ask forgiveness for the crimes and damages that have been done in the name of the German nation. Let us live as reconciled sisters and brothers and as good neighbors.

The chapter also included an announcement by the Synod of the Protestant Bohemian Brothers which denounced the post-war Czechoslovak policy of collective expulsion, and stated that:

> We realize that the way to the future cannot be opened by never-ending accusations, but instead by sincere repentance, mutual efforts and understanding, and a longing for reconciliation.

It is hard to judge to what extent positive emotives and discourses of reconciliation have generated an actual change in individual cases. I realised this when I accompanied a group of expelled Sudeten Germans who had peacefully attended a religious service in Bohemia. Returning to Germany, we stopped at a *Biergarten*. After a few pints, one of the men suddenly shouted: 'The Czech nation is an evil nation!'

Love for the Old *Heimat*: Political Potentials

In the light of the geopolitical changes, many expellees enjoyed spending time in the villages or towns of their youth. Restoring the graves of close kin, commemorating the deceased in churches, they symbolically appropriated time and space, an act that strengthened their rootedness in former Sudeten German soil. Expellees from Mathilde's village also began organising annual visits, which gave them the opportunity to collectively perform their emotional attachment. She explained:

> I also have cousins, they are from Augsburg. They contact us every year, and stay with us [in Tirschenreuth] the night before. They always have tears in their eyes. They were older than me, they were 14 and 15 years old, and I was only six [at the time of the expulsion], so I did not experience it like them ... although ... it is somehow ... where one is born, that is simply one's homeland.

An expellee from the village of Labant who was 29 years old at the time of the expulsion similarly referred to his embodied feelings of belonging:

> Of course, we have a strong emotional connection with our homeland. Labant was a village in the Bohemian Forest, nicely situated, a terrific environment. The life of the farmers was tough, but somehow, communal life in the village was harmonious, and it still lives inside us, that connection with our homeland.

Evidently, the image of 'harmonious life in a beautiful world' was highly selective. It avoided accounts of Sudeten German involvement with the Nazi regime, and ignored questions about responsibility for Nazi crimes. It created a conceptual space in which the expellees could engage with their pre-expulsion past without having to deal with the darker side of their history. The discourse of 'love for our homeland' also assumed a *natural* relation between identity and place, and, as such, had compelling political connotations (cf. Malkki 1992).[10] The *Sudetendeutsche Landsmannschaft*, the biggest organisation of expelled Sudeten Germans with its seat in Munich used emotives of collective, natural love for the homeland in the representation and negotiation of political reality. Representatives of the organisation politicised feelings of embodied attachment, demanding *Heimatrecht*, the return of Sudeten property to its former owners.

At the time of my fieldwork, the organisation had approximately 100,000 members. While many were not really interested in the property claims, their leaders' calls were

loud enough to worry Czech inhabitants of the border area. The latter read frightening reports in right-wing Czech newspapers about the annual *Sudetendeutscher Tag*, a three-day ritual event which enjoyed the mass participation of many thousands of expellees. The annual event, a mixture of celebratory reunion, heritage performance and collective reliving of memories of expulsion, formed a focal point for the claims to compensation from the Czech government. Commemorations for the victims of the expulsion, and political speeches by the likes of Franz Neubauer, leader of the *Sudetendeutsch Landsmannshaft*, and the Bavarian Prime Minister Edmund Stoiber, created powerful political contexts during which remembered and re-evoked feelings of grief, loss, and anger were politicised. In 1995, the Sudeten German calls for justice were supported by influential Bavarian politicians, such as Stoiber and Finance Minister, Theo Waigel, who put pressure on the German government to accept the Czech Republic EU membership only *after* cancelling the Beneš decrees. The German government, however, had no truck with the Sudeten German demands. Instead, it signed the Czech–German Declaration in 1996, in which both governments apologized for the harm done during and after the Second World War and stressed the need to create a shared, European identity (cf. Svašek 1999).

Understandably, Czech border inhabitants followed the news with mixed feelings and some felt uncomfortable with the increasing Sudeten German presence on Czech territory. Various people I spoke with also conjured up an image of the large territory of post-2000 reunified Germany, contrasting it with their own shrunken state, after Czechoslovakia had been divided into two countries in 2003. In general, however, Czechs seemed to trust the reassurances given by the Declaration, and many younger people assured me that they saw no reason why they should fear the neighbouring German state. In an essay assignment on the theme of ethnicity and nationalism, given to students at Tachov Gymnasium in 1997, a 14-year-old female student stated:

> 'Germans.' When I pronounce the word I associate it with the Second World War and the concentration camps. I suppose I am not the only Czech with such thoughts. I also think that 50 years since the end of the war, as the older generation is replaced by a younger generation, they must distance themselves from those crimes. They are not responsible, even though they may feel ashamed. We have to try to forget the past and create a new environment.

Like many of her generation, this youngster believed in a new socio-spatial reality in which the Bohemian–Bavarian border was a space of peaceful mutual interaction.

Conclusion

This chapter focused on the spatially and materially engendered feelings that were experienced, expressed and played out in a rapidly changing frontier zone. It showed that past-, present- and future-oriented emotions and emotives were central to the renegotiation of power and identity in the region. The process was influenced by complex histories of forced expulsion, resettlement and cross-border movement and related changes in the social and material make-up of the region.

At a more general level, the distinct geopolitical situation in border areas, marked by physical reminders of state security, often has a specific influence on border peoples' outlook and experiences. On the one hand, border inhabitants live relatively close to

people who are politically linked to potentially hostile neighbouring states, which may cause feelings of vulnerability. On the other hand, the proximity of the border may be an incentive for the establishment of cross-border contacts, which can generate mutual feelings of trust and friendship. Long histories of cross-border kinship tend to increase cross-border loyalties and weaken emotional identification with the national state.

The Bohemian–Bavarian case demonstrated that geopolitical aspects alone cannot explain why specific emotional discourses and practices may strengthen or weaken identification processes in border zones. It showed that it is necessary to take a historical perspective, examining how border people remember, re-experience and reconsider the past as they live their mobile lives in changing geographical, material and social environments. Physical traces of past and present lives, such as (disappeared) buildings, roads and border crossings, partially shaped people's feelings. Both personal and collective memories of past aggression influenced Czech and German perceptions of 'those on the other side'. In numerous cases, especially in the case of traumatisation, this limited emotional liberty, the potential to change one's embodied judgements of past people and places. Re-experienced emotions in particular, evoked by memories of traumatic war and postwar experiences, influenced Czech, German and Sudeten German perceptions and hindered attempts to develop a new sense of a shared interregional, European identity.

At the same time, images of centuries of mutual cooperation were used by adherents of euregional cooperation to trigger feelings of trust, and to stimulate interregional identification. State officials and local political and religious leaders performed emotives, intending to stimulate the border inhabitants to reconsider feelings of fear and mistrust. Priests and ministers warned their congregations about the dangers caused by national hatred, while presenting ecumenic transnationalism as a way to control the situation and to encourage reconciliation. Images of fearful political personalities and traumatic historical events, such as Hitler, Nazi oppression, and the expulsion, were transformed into emotionally compelling religious metaphors. In contrast, euregional discourse focused on other major causes of fear, such as political and economic marginalisation, and environmental and social pollution. The adherents of *Euregion Egrensis* presented cross-border, euregional policy, and European identification as a political solution, and as a strong source of hope.

While the conscious politics of emotions must be welcomed as an attempt to create conditions for peaceful co-existence, it would of course be naive to analyse the dynamics of emotional liberty outside a larger context of unfolding geopolitical realities. The transformative potential offered by reflective emotional practices is always partially conditioned by the impact of newly emerging affective regimes. So while in principle the dynamics of emotional liberty may offer the possibility of cross-border reconciliation in specific spatial settings, new feelings of distrust and hatred, directed at alternative groups and individuals, may also arise. As this chapter has shown, the wider politics of emotional negotiation and identification must therefore be critically examined, both within and beyond border settings.

Notes

1 An earlier version of this paper, entitled 'Borders and emotions. Hope and fear in the Bohemian–Bavarian frontier zone', was published in 2000 in *Ethnologia Europaea. Journal of European Ethnology*, in

the theme issue on Borders (eds Hastings Donnan and Dieter Haller): 111–26. I would like to thank the journal for allowing me to publish a new version of the article in this book. The research referred to in this paper was funded by the University of Utrecht under the aegis of the Grotius Grant. Additional funding was awarded by the Catharina van Tussenbroek Fonds. Different versions of this paper were presented in July 1998 at the EASA conference in Frankfurt, and in May 2000 at the Department of Social Anthropology, University of St Andrews. I would particularly like to thank Hastings Donnan, Kay Milton and Justin I'Anson-Sparks for their critical remarks.

2 Other scholars have examined the ways in which processes such as cross-border migration, the creation of new state boundaries, and the end of the Cold War have influenced border inhabitants' perceptions both of themselves and others (see, for example, Borneman 1998; Driessen 1992, 1998; Green 1998).

3 After the liberation of Czechoslovakia in 1945, the government, headed by President Edvard Beneš, declared *all* Germans 'collectively guilty' of German territoriality and the Nazi crimes, and decided that the Sudeten Germans would be expelled to Germany. The population transfer was legally backed up by the signing of the Potsdam agreements in August 1945, which regarded the presence of ethnic Germans in states outside Germany as a danger to the political stability of Europe (cf. Svašek 1999).

4 Czech and German historians do not agree on the number of people who died during the expulsion. According to Sudeten German sources, around 250,000 people lost their lives. Czechs have argued that the number is much lower, between 20,000 and 40,000.

5 The ability to show empathy in reaction to emotives uttered by interviewees is crucial to productive fieldwork (Spencer and Davies 2010; Svašek 2010).

6 For a discussion of interviewing as potential arena of emotional remembering, performance and reflection, see Svašek and Domecka 2012.

7 Euregional policy was introduced in the 1970s by the European Union member states to encourage European integration, and to stimulate economic development in border areas. Tensions and conflicts in the post-Communist countries caused concern among the European Union member states. In particular, Germany pressed for measures to secure stability in the East and cooperation and integration with the Czechs was supported by the German government as part of European Union politics. A special subsidiary programme called Phare was established to support the reform process in most post-communist countries, and plans were made to enlarge further the European Union to the East (cf. Preston 1997: 197). *Euregion Egrensis* integrated parts of western Bohemia, eastern Bavaria, Thuringen, and Saxony (cf. Svašek 1999).

8 The latter were mainly Ruthenians from Romania who had moved to the village in 1950. The German minister was a Sudeten German from Silesia, who had been expelled with his family to Germany after the Second World War.

9 Some priests took up important positions in growing cross-border networks. The Protestant Dean Father Lubomír Libal, for example, who lived and worked in the Bohemian border city of Cheb, had connections in Bayreuth, Selb, Schönwald, Regnitzlosau, Wunsiedel, Marktredwitz, and Lautertal–Neukirchen.

10 The claim to a 'natural' connection should be examined in the light of persistent German political ideology that up until very recently still required certification of German 'blood' (normally traceable at least to one's grandparents) in acquiring German citizenship, and the *blood and soil* political discourses that predated the third Reich. See also Smith (1998: 83) on the emotional sources of national sentiment.

References

Ahmed, S. (2004a) *The Cultural Politics of Emotion*. Edinburgh: Edinburgh University Press.

Anderson, K. and Smith, S.J. (2001) Editorial: emotional geographies, *Transactions of the Institute of British Geographers*.

Bailey, F.G. (1983) *The Tactical Uses of Passion. An Essay on Power, Reason, and Reality*. Ithaca and London: Cornell University Press.

Beyhl, W. and Libal, L. (1996) *Unter einem Himmel Wege zu Einander zu Finden*. Cheb and Bayreuth: Euregion Egrensis.

Borneman, J. (1998) Grenzregime (border regime). The wall and its aftermath, in Wilson, T. and Donnan, H. (eds) *Border Identities. Nation and State at International Frontiers*. Cambridge: Cambridge University Press, 162–90.

Cheater, A.P. (1998) Transcending the state? Gender and borderline constructions of citizenship in Zimbabwe, in Wilson, T. and Donnan, H. (eds) *Border Identities. Nation and State at International Frontiers*. Cambridge: Cambridge University Press, 191–214.

Cooke, P., Christiansen, T. and Schienstock, G. (1997) Regional economic policy and a Europe of the regions, in Rhodes, M. et al. (eds) *Developments in West European Politics*. Hampshire and London: Macmillan, 190–206.

Čtvrtek, K. (1992) Štanou se z Ceskoslovenska Euroregiony? *Halo noviny*, 23 May.

Davidson, J., Bondi, L. and Smith, M. (eds) (2005) *Emotional Geographies*. Aldershot: Ashgate.

Der Neue Tag (1989) Eine Karawane in die Freiheit, *Der Neue Tag*, 27 December.

Der Neue Tag (1990) Europa blickt nach Böhmen und Ostbayern, *Der Neue Tag*, 30 June/1 July.

Donnan, H. and Wilson, T.M. (1999) *Borders: Frontiers of Identity, Nation, and State*. Oxford: Berg.

Douglas, M. (1966) *Purity and Danger. An Analysis of the Concept of Pollution and Taboo*. London: Routledge.

Douglass, W.A. (1998) A western perspective on an eastern interpretation of where north meets south. Pyrenean borderland cultures, in Wilson, T. and Donnan, H. (eds) *Border Identities. Nation and State at International Frontiers*. Cambridge: Cambridge University Press, 62–95.

Driessen, H. (1992) *On the Spanish-Moroccan Frontier. A Study in Ritual, Power and Ethnicity*. Oxford: Berg.

Driessen, H. (1998) The 'new immigration' and the transformation of the European–African frontier, in Wilson, T. and Donnan, H. (eds) *Border Identities. Nation and State at International Frontiers*. Cambridge: Cambridge University Press. 96–116.

Giegold, H. and Otto, G. (1994) *Nachbarn im Gespräch. Tschechen und Bayern*. Regensburg: Buchverlag der Mittelbayerischen Zeitung.

Green, S. (1998) Post-communist neighbours. Relocating gender in a Greek–Albanian border community, in Bridger, S. and Pine, F., *Surviving Post-Socialism*. London: Routledge, 80–105.

Hamperl, W.-D. (1996) *Vertreibung und Flucht aus dem Kreis Tachau im Egerland, 1945–1948. Schicksale in Berichten, Dokumenten und Bildern* (I and II). Trostberg: Private publication.

Houžvička, V. (1993) *Česko-Německé Vztahy Všedního Dne. Sociologická Sonda Obyvatelstva Euroregionu Egrensis*. Usti nad Labem: Sociologicky Ustav. Research Report.

Houžvička, V. (1994) *Euroregions as Factors of Increasing Cooperation within the Czech-German Relations*. Usti nad Labem: Sociologicky Ustav. Unpublished paper.

Irwin-Zarecka, I. (1994) *Frames of Remembrance. The Dynamics of Collective Memory*. New Brunswick and London: Transaction Publishers.

Jansen, S. (1998) Homeless at home. Narrations of post-Yugoslav identities, in Rapport, N. and Dawson, A. (eds) *Migrant Identity*. Oxford: Berg, 85–111.

Kearney, M. (1998) Transnationalism in California and Mexico at the End of Empire, in Wilson, T.M. and Donnan, H. (eds) *Border Identities. Nation and State at International Frontiers*. Cambridge: Cambridge University Press.

Kertzer, D.I. (1988) *Ritual, Politics, and Power*. New Haven and London: Yale University Press.

Leavitt, J. (1996) Meaning and feeling in the anthropology of emotions. *American Ethnologist*, *23* (3): 514–539.

Leutloff-Grandits, C. (2008) Claiming Ownership in Postwar Croatia. The Emotional Dynamics of Possession and Repossession in Knin, in Svašek, M. (ed) *Postsocialism. Politics and Emotions in Central and Eastern Europe*. Oxford: Berghahn.

Lutz, C. and White, G.M. (1986) The anthropology of emotions. *Annual Review of Anthropology*, 15: 405–36.

Lyon, M.L. (1995) Missing emotion: the limitations of cultural constructionism in the study of emotion, *Cultural Anthropology*, *10* (2): 244–63.

Lyon, M.L. and Barbalet, J.M. (1994) Society's Body: Emotion and the 'Somatisation' of Social Theory', in Csordas, T.J. (ed) *Embodiment and Experience: The Essential Ground of Culture and Self*. Cambridge: Cambridge University Press.

Lysaght, K.D. (2005) Catholics, protestants and office workers from the town: the experience and negotiation of fear in Northern Ireland, in Milton, K. and Svašek, M. (eds) *Mixed Emotions. Anthropological Studies of Feeling*. Oxford: Berg, 127–43.

Malkki, L. (1992) National geographic: the rooting of peoples and the territorialisation of national identity among scholars and refugees, *Cultural Anthropology*, 7 (1): 24–44.

Navaro-Yashin, Y. (2009) Affective Spaces, Melancholic Objects. Ruination and the Production of Anthropological Knowledge. *Journal of the Royal Anthropological Institute (N.S.)* 15: 1-18

Preston, C. (1997) *Enlargement and Integration in the European Union*. London and New York: Routledge.

Reddy, W.M. (1999) Emotional liberty. Politics and history in the anthropology of emotions, *Cultural Anthropology*, *14* (2): 256–88.

Smith, A. (1998) *Nationalism and Modernism*. London and New York: Routledge.

Sporrer, T. (1990) Schlagbaum hebt sich für einen Tag, *Der Neue Tag*, 2 May.

Staněk, T. (1991) *Odsun Němců z Československa*. Prague: Academia naše vojensko.

Storch, R. (ed.) (1992) *Standpunkt. Magazin der CSU in der Oberpfalz*, Special Issue on 'Brückenschlag. Die Öffnung der ČSFR-Grenze'. Regensburg: CSU Bezirksverband Oberpfalz.

Svašek, M. (1994) The Soviets remembered. Liberators or aggressors? Czech history, memory, and memorial sites, *Focaal. Journal of Anthropology* (25), theme issue on War and peace: 103–24.

Svašek, M. (1998) The ritual paradox. The construction of cultural unity and diversity in a combined Orthodox (Ruthenian) Czech/Roman Catholic (Sudeten) German religious ceremony. Unpublished paper presented at the session Multi-culturalism, ISA World Congress of Sociology, Montreal.

Svašek, M. (1999) History, identity, and territoriality. Redefining Czech–German relations in the post-Cold War era, *Focaal. Journal of Anthropology* (32), theme issue on Ten years after: hidden histories and new mythologies in post-communist east–central Europe: 37–58.

Svašek, M. (2000) Borders and emotions. Hope and fear in the Bohemian–Bavarian frontier zone, *Ethnologia Europaea. Journal of European Ethnology*, theme issue on Borders (eds Hastings D. and Haller, D.): 111–26.

Svašek, M. (2005) The politics of chosen trauma: expellee memories, emotions and identities, in Milton, K. and Svašek, M. (eds) *Mixed Emotions. Anthropological Studies of Feeling*. Oxford: Berg, 195–214.

Svašek, M. (2006) *Postsocialism. Politics and Emotions in Central and Eastern Europe*. Oxford: Berghahn.

Svašek, M. (2010) In the field. Intersubjectivity, empathy and the workings of internalised presence, in Spencer, D. and Davies, J. (eds) *Anthropological Fieldwork: A Relational Process*. Cambridge: Cambridge Scholars Press, 75– 99.

Svašek, M. (ed.) (2012) *Moving Subjects, Moving Objects. Transnationalism, Cultural Production and Emotions*. Oxford: Berghahn.

Svašek, M. and Domecka, M.D. (2012) The autobiographical narrative interview. A potential arena of emotional remembering, performance and reflection, in Skinner, J. (ed.) *The Interview: Ethnographic Approaches*. Oxford: Berghahn (forthcoming).

Veenis, M. (1995) Only because of the bananas … western consumer goods in East Germany, *Focaal*, 24: 55–69.

Wikan, U. (1990) *Managing Turbulent Hearts. A Balinese Formula for Living*. Chicago: University of Chicago Press.

Wilson, T. and Donnan, H. (eds) (1998) *Border Identities. Nation and State at International Frontiers*. Cambridge: Cambridge University Press.

Zrenner, P. (1990) Die Adressen sind schon getauscht. *Standpunkt*, special issue on Brückenschlag. Regensburg: CSU Bezirksverband Oberpfalz.

Index

Page numbers in Bold represent figures.